D0161219

Deselected Library Materia
DO NOT RETURN
TO LIBRARY
Not for Resale

Management of Hospitals and Health Services

Health Services

Strategic Issues and Performance

Management of Hospitals and Health Services

Strategic Issues and Performance

ROCKWELL SCHULZ, Ph.D.

Professor, Department of Preventive Medicine and
Programs in Health Management;
Director of University of Wisconsin
International Center of Health Services Studies,
University of Wisconsin, Madison, Wisconsin

ALTON C. JOHNSON, Ph.D.

Professor, School of Business and
Programs in Health Management;
Director, Health Services Administration Program;
Associate Director, Health Services
Fiscal Management Program,
University of Wisconsin, Madison, Wisconsin

THIRD EDITION

with 23 illustrations

The C. V. Mosby Company

ST. LOUIS • BALTIMORE • PHILADELPHIA • TORONTO   1990

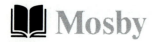 Mosby

Editor: Darlene Como
Developmental Editor: Laurie Sparks
Project Manager: Teri Merchant
Production Editor: Betty Hazelwood
Book and Cover Design: Gail Morey Hudson

THIRD EDITION

Copyright © 1990 by The C.V. Mosby Company

All rights reserved. No part of this publication may be reproduced, stored in a retrieval system, or transmitted, in any form or by any means, electronic, mechanical, photocopying, recording, or otherwise, without prior written permission from the publisher.

Previous editions copyrighted 1976, 1983

Printed in the United States of America

The C. V. Mosby Company
11830 Westline Industrial Drive, St. Louis, Missouri 63146

Library of Congress Cataloging in Publication Data

Schulz, Rockwell.
    Management of hospitals and health services: strategic issues and
performance/Rockwell Schulz, Alton C. Johnson. — 3rd ed.
      p.   cm.
    Rev. ed. of: Management of hospitals. 2nd ed. c1983.
    Includes bibliographical references.
    ISBN 0-8016-6060-2
    1. Hospitals—Administration. 2. Health services administration.
I. Johnson, Alton C. (Alton Cornelius). II. Schulz, Rockwell.
Management of hospitals. III. Title.
    [DNLM: 1. Health Services—organization & administration.
  2. Hospital Administration.   WX 150 S389m]
RA971.S36 1990
362.1'1'068—dc20
DNLM/DLC   89-13513

GW/D/D 9 8 7 6 5 4 3

Foreword

Good health is a condition of life that most people enjoy—and everyone is concerned about. We have a tendency to take good health for granted, until something adverse happens to us or to our families or friends. And, when that occurs, we assume that the system of health care service that we know and trust will respond to our needs effectively, efficiently, and compassionately.

That system, of health care delivery, has grown and changed a great deal in the past several decades. Not all of that growth and change has been for the good, and, as a result, the system and a number of its component parts are under increasing stress. Unfortunately, the response to need is not always effective, efficient, or compassionate. This is caused by a number of factors that are very complex—and that are receiving attention by an ever increasing number of people and institutions.

It is out of a recognition of these changes and the challenge involved in addressing the problems of fixing our stressed health care system that Rockwell Schulz and Alton Johnson have revised their textbook, *Management of Hospitals and Health Services*. The result is a well-conceived and well-organized book that is aimed at students in health care management and delivery programs and health care professionals, managers, and governing board members at all levels of experience.

This text differs from traditional management texts and references in its application of organization and management theory to contemporary issues in the strategic management of health services. It should be a valuable resource to those in health care management positions who want to position themselves to provide leadership at the decision-making level within health care organizations. It is a provocative and useful compendium of ideas and historic perspectives that are current and applicable. It is a worthy contribution to the health care management literature.

Good health care doesn't just happen. It is a result of a combination of dedicated and informed people and institutions functioning together, with a common purpose, within a system that really works and is responsive to human need. This book will have a positive impact on helping that take place.

David L. Everhart
President Emeritus
Northwestern Memorial Hospital, Chicago

Preface

This third edition represents major revisions reflecting the changes occurring in the health care industry. We know of no industry that is more dynamic and challenging for managers. In this book we have tried to capture this dynamism and the associated challenges.

Our combined experience represents more than 50 years of association with the health care industry as managers, teachers, and researchers. As a result of these experiences we have concluded that although the hospital still occupies a major position in the system, hospital managers must have a more sophisticated understanding of the more specialized organizations that have increased significantly in number and importance during the past decade. These organizations include such facilities as health maintenance organizations, clinics, long-term care institutions, home care services, laboratories, and outpatient units, such as surgicenters. By the same token, managers of these organizations must relate not only to the environment of their own particular facility but to others that have both direct and indirect relationships. Of course, the past 10 years have seen a tremendous increase in competition among similar providers of care. Today, to an increasing extent, hospitals compete with other hospitals in the area for patients, as well as physicians and employees. In addition, various groups, including physicians, employees, unions, patients, community leaders, and trustees, are illustrative types of stakeholders who have an interest in the operation of the health care organization. Changes in governmental regulations and societal changes have had increasingly significant impacts on the manager. We will refer to these environmental factors as the *macro* aspects of the health care industry. These will be discussed in the first section of the book.

External environmental factors have impacted on the chief executive officer and his or her staff. The position of CEO increasingly becomes one best described as that of chief strategist. This is the subject of the second section of the book. The tasks of the general manager as chief strategist include creating the culture or general ambiance of the organization, negotiating and resolving conflicts with major stakeholder groups, and developing the forward or strategic plan. There has been increasing interest in strategic management, especially in business firms. This interest has extended to the health care industry.

The third section of the book discusses the internal organization issues. It is the clinical/operating activities that are unique to a specific health care organization. For example, the clinical activities in a hospital are different from those of a health maintenance organization or a long-term care facility. However, despite the contingency or situational aspects, there are certain universal operational functions, including governance, physicians and issues, nursing, and other professionals inputs into the system (patients, supplies, equipment).

Part IV concerns managerial functions and issues. The support/business activities include accounting/finance, human resources management, marketing, supplies and equipment arrangements, and risk, cost, and quality issues. Although there are many specific objectives of a given health organization, we assume that the overriding mission is that of providing access to care and providing high quality care while containing costs of care. Management of human resources, including mitigation of conflict and labor/management relations, are also major managerial responsibilities. In the final section we conclude with an outlook to the future and with a consideration of managerial ethics in the management of health services.

This book is designed not only for hospital administrators, but also for the many people occupying managerial roles in a variety of health-related organizations and levels. It provides an overview for students who will be in managerial roles in health care organizations. Students in related disciplines, such as nursing, health economics, sociology, pharmacy, physical therapy, and social work, will find the book useful for understanding systems and issues with which they will be dealing. Also, we hope that practitioners, trustees, physicians, planners, governmental administrators, and department heads will obtain information from another perspective that they will find useful. To more properly reflect our objectives, we have changed the title of our book from *Management of Hospitals* to *Management of Hospitals and Health Services: Strategic Issues and Performance*.

Research in the administration of health services has expanded rapidly in recent years. Whenever appropriate, we have attempted to relate these findings to the many issues facing managers, trustees, chiefs of staff and medical departments, patient care departments, department heads, and planners. We have also included research from other industries where appropriate. However, the scope of this book constrains us from describing extensive theoretical approaches to management from disciplines such as sociology, economics, psychology, and computer science. Moreover, there are many conflicting theories and approaches to management. Rather than reviewing these various approaches and then applying them to health services, we somewhat boldly select those we think might be most helpful to managers in improving their performance. This is not a management text, but a text to help managers improve their understanding of issues and their performance in meeting their responsibilities through a better understanding of the broad scope of factors that affect their potential performance in a highly dynamic and challenging industry.

We acknowledge the help provided to us by Mitzi Duxbury, Gordon Johnsen, David Zilz, and Bell Oswald-Heberling.

Rockwell Schulz
Alton C. Johnson

Contents

PART V

FUTURE CHALLENGES, STRATEGIES, AND ETHICS

18 Managerial Performance and Ethics for Hospitals and Health Services into the Twenty-first Century, 305

HOSPITAL AND HEALTH SERVICES MANAGEMENT OBJECTIVES IN A RAPIDLY CHANGING ENVIRONMENT

1

The Growing Importance of Management to Institutional, Patient, and Community Health

The effective organization is that which satisfies the demands of those in its environment from whom it requires support for its continued existence.

JEFFREY PFEFFER AND GERALD SALANCIK: *THE EXTERNAL CONTROL OF ORGANIZATIONS*

The importance of health services management is a relatively recent development. Indeed, the impact of health services itself is also a relatively recent development.

Health care is now one of the largest and most complex industries in the United States in both cost and employment. In many states and communities, health care is the largest industry. Health care expends more than 11% of gross national product, and cost increases have consistently exceeded rates of inflation for the total economy. In other words, the health system has a major impact on the rest of society, just as society has a major influence over health services. As the health system continues to grow in importance, society is forced to exercise increasing influence over health services. Indeed, some theorists of organization ecology suggest that organizational success or failure is determined by historical and environmental forces and that management can do little about it but adapt to a rapidly changing environment.[1] We, however, argue that health services management can influence its environment to help achieve patient, community, and organizational health.

To appreciate the role of health services management and how roles change rather quickly, it is important to understand how the system evolved and to consider what is expected of health services, by whom, and management's* role in meeting those expectations.

STAGES IN HEALTH SERVICES MANAGEMENT

Broadly defined, the purpose of a health service is to apply appropriate technologies and provide for the delivery of care services to meet the health needs of the populations served. In the past, health services were limited primarily to physicians and to hospital inpatient services, but health services must be considered in much broader terms today. Intervening between the health service and the community it serves is an economic and political environment that is having an increasing impact. The social environment, such as community attitudes, is also important. Management, therefore, is responsible for the effective and efficient delivery of health services in keeping with the constraints and opportunities of the economic and political environment. We suggest that as health care technology has changed over the years and as the economic and political environment changes, the objectives of health services change, and, consequently, so does their management.

PUBLIC HEALTH PERIOD: Into the 1920s

We call the first period of health services management *the public health period,* recognizing that public and environmental health services were most important to improving health before and into the twentieth century. McDermott[2] described four evolutionary periods in the development of medicine, each one grafted on the other.

In stage I, the initial steps consist of environmental health advances, such as eating from a table instead of from a dirt floor. Next, more healthful practices were instituted, such as individualized clean utensils. Along with this came footpaths, roads, bridges, and then other transportation and communication devices that not only facilitated health and health services, but presented new health hazards. Stage II relates more directly to public health. It consists of purposeful attempts to affect disease by introducing a change in the nonpersonal environment. Examples of this are the provision of a safe water supply and the spraying of residual insecticides for the control of malaria. Stage III involves public health, but on a more personal although noncontinuing basis. An example of a public health intervention at this stage would include immunizations. Stage IV is personal health care services delivered on a continuing basis, that is, the doctor/patient relationship. According to McDermott, it was not until the years 1910 to 1935 that a doctor could really intervene on the course of an illness. Until then, only environmental and public health could impact on health. However, Starr[3] describes how organized medicine successfully blocked public health services from entering the

---

*We use the terms *management* and *manager* in their broadest sense to include the management team of the chief executive officer (CEO) through department heads unless positions are designated. Although the board of directors governs, its policy-making role and accountability for organizational performance make it an integral part of this broad definition of management.

private personal health care system. Management of public health services was in the hands of physicians and public health school–trained public health officers. With the exception of the Mayo Clinic, founded around the turn of the century, most physicians were in solo practice responsible for managing their own affairs. Most hospitals during this period were dominated by the trustees who donated (or invested in if they were proprietary) the hospital. Hospital owners were frequently religious orders. Indeed, very early hospitals were more an outgrowth of religion than of medicine (for example, early Roman hospitals, and the Hotel Dieu of Lyons in 542 AD and the hotel Dieu in Paris in 660 AD, which still exist today). Physicians, too, started hospitals, usually on a proprietary basis to provide needed bed services for their practices when other sources of hospital services were lacking. These physician groups controlled the resources to operate the hospitals and therefore dominated their management.

The Flexner Report (1910) signaled reforms in medical education leading toward scientific medicine. Modern surgery began to develop with advances in supporting services, such as anesthesia.

The economic and political environment had little influence on personal health care services in the public health period. Donations from philanthropists, religious orders, and free care by physicians provided most of the resources for hospitals. In addition to public health services, there were government hospitals, such as the Public Health Service for merchant seaman and Veterans Hospitals at the federal level, state custodial or teaching hospitals, and local government charity hospitals in the larger cities. Nonprofessional employees were commonly political appointees, and physician services were provided by medical schools, which in turn used the charity patients primarily for teaching purposes. Social attitudes toward hospitals reflected reverence for the humanitarian work and personal sacrifice of the medical, nursing, and other staff. Hospitals were perceived as symbols of goodness.

During the period, hospital objectives were to comfort the poor and dying who could not be cared for at home. The implications of the technological, economic, and political environment on hospital management in the period were limited to obtaining and conserving resources by soliciting donations and pinching pennies. Hospital superintendents, as they were usually called, could be seen touring the hospital, turning off the lights, counting postage stamps, and trying to collect patient's bills to meet the payroll.

PHYSICIAN PERIOD: 1930s into 1960s

The change from the public health period to the physician period was not abrupt, as the dates might imply. Indeed, one can see a resurgence today of importance of public health services to combat AIDS; drug, alcohol, and tobacco abuse; and environmental hazards to health. Advancing medical technology had a great impact on health services. With advancing knowledge and with techniques to apply the knowledge, medical specialization developed. In the 1930s, therapy progressed with the introduction of antimicrobial drugs. Laboratory medicine also developed in the 1940s and 1950s and beyond, greatly extending diagnostic capabilities and services. Physician practices were therefore moving away from the patient's home and away from physicians' offices to hospitals where the latest services could be provided. These advances in medical technology, which centered increasingly in the hospital, changed the hospital from a custodial institution to a diagnostic and curative center. Ancillary hospital services expanded in scope, size, and specialization into allied health fields, such as medical technology; physical and other therapies proliferated. These changes resulted in increases in outpatient services and the expansion and conversion of "bedrooms" into diagnostic, therapeutic, and office facilities. Since the 1930s, multispecialty physician group practices also have developed and expanded to provide a broad scope of integrated medical technologies to ambulatory patients.

The economic and political environment also began to affect health services. In the late 1930s and 1940s, Blue Cross and Blue Shield insurance were started by hospital and physician associations as a way for patients to prepay the costs of hospital and physician services. As labor unions gained power, they successfully bargained for health insurance coverage. Thus more patients now had funds for medical services, and believing medical care was a benefit they earned, they demanded more services. It also meant that hospitals and group practices had rapidly expanding income sources for additional services and facilities. The federal government also entered the scene after World War II with the Hill-Burton Act in 1946, which provided private hospitals, and especially rural hospitals, with funds to build and expand. A provision of the Act was that hospitals that received funds must provide free care to indigents. Issues over the interpretation and impact of the Act still affect hospital management.

The end of World War II saw the explosion of the discovery of new drugs, new research through the National Institutes of Health (NIH), and the birth of hospital administration as a formal university discipline. Social attitudes during this period also changed. No longer was medical care viewed as a charity service; rather, people expected diagnostic and treatment services to cure almost any malady.

Changes in hospital management mirrored the expansion of medical technology and financial resources. The mystique and glamour of medical care enhanced the prestige and status of physicians, overshadowing public health services and the dominance of hospital trustees. Physicians not only controlled knowledge about health care, but they influenced and sometimes controlled hospital financial resources as well, primarily by retaining control over patient admissions. Hospitals survived and succeeded not through cost control but through increased incomes. Patients' fees paid through insurance carriers provided the income and volume for new ancillary services, beds, and more elegant hospital facilities. Because physicians admitted the patients, they could demand a new service or more beds by showing the hospital how it would enhance its role in the community—or alternatively suggest that if these requests were not fulfilled, another hospital might attract their patients. Although physicians were frequently not on hospital boards in those days, they could wield their influence over trustees on the golf course and over the administrator in the administrator's office, doctors' lounge, or medical staff meetings.

HOSPITAL PERIOD: 1960s into 1990s

Whereas vestiges of the physician period are evident today through physician control of patient admissions, we suggest that further and accelerating changes in health care technology and in the economic and political environment created a dominant role for hospital administration after 1960. During the 1960s and 1970s, technology accelerated with an explosion in medical research. Nuclear and immunological advances, for example, resulted in radiological and transplant applications. These advances also had a dramatic effect on the role of the physician. During the previous two periods, the physician practiced as an individual in the hospital and nursing and other professional staff were oriented to the individual physician. With the advent of more intensive hospital services requiring the joint efforts of radiologists, pathologists, anesthesiologists, and all the other nonphysician professionals, hospital service has become a team effort. The physician not only relies on other professionals, but in regard to quality assurance measures, he or she is subject to surveillance from peers and is held accountable. Moreover, nurses and other health professionals expect to be viewed as colleagues rather than as subordinates.

The economic and political environment changed even more rapidly after 1960. In addition to the continued expansion of private funds into the health sector through Blue Cross and commercial insurance carriers, the federal government aided hospitals, as well as the elderly and indigents, with the inauguration of Medicare and Medicaid. Medicare and Medicaid, implemented in 1966, fund patients who were previously provided no care or free care, or whose expenses were written off as bad debts. Federal funds increased the use of hospital services. On the other hand, with the infusion of public funds into the health system, which in the 1980s accounted for more than 41% of total health care expenditures, the government gained considerable power over medical care providers. With health care representing one of the largest contributors to inflation and to rising costs for state and federal governments, there has been increasing concern for containing health care costs. Employers, too, have been expressing increased concern about rising employee health benefit costs.

The political environment since 1960 has reflected economic and social changes. In the 1960s, there was political emphasis on the underprivileged, and access to high quality care for all citizens according to their need. After experiences with the costly Medicare and Medicaid programs and increasing pressures on the federal budget, the political environment reversed itself rather quickly from access to hospital care to containing rising hospital costs. With pressures on the federal budget, efforts have been directed toward reducing resources going into hospital and other health services.

Implications for health service objectives through the 1960s and 1970s, in light of these technological and environmental changes, were an expanding scope of hospital services—increasing sophistication, volume, income, and facilities. Hospitals continued a growth posture into the 1980s by expanding revenue sources, such as through new ambulatory care services, and providing more services per patient, although bed utilization leveled off and declined in the face of expanded facilities. With excess capacity, many hospitals adopted aggressive marketing strategies to meet the competition of other hospitals and federally mandated health planning and regulation systems. By 1980, hospitals were developing affiliations and merged systems to strengthen and consolidate their positions in the face of the increased competition and regulation. Patterns of hospital control and management were rapidly changing with the development of multi-institutional hospital systems through sharing and acquisition of other hospitals and health services.

Hospital management also experienced major transformations as institutional objectives went through the rapid growth of the post–World War II period. Team medicine, increasing size and complexities, and resulting needs for coordination gave rise to the importance of management. Modern hospitals became multimillion dollar enterprises and are currently among the largest employers in many communities. Hospital technology became far advanced of most industries. Coordination of highly professionalized interests also required managerial skills advanced from previous periods. Management became the source of information about the institution, and this control of information was and is an important source of managerial power.

Control over resources shifted to management during this period. Although the patient is still the primary source of income for the hospital (and admissions are controlled by physician orders), external sources for which the administration has responsibility became increasingly important. For example, managers usually control hospital negotiations for reimbursement levels with third-party payers (such as Blue Cross, commercial insurers, health maintenance organizations [HMOs] and preferred provider organizations [PPOs], and Medicaid). Managers are also the primary influence over negotiations with rate-review and other regulatory bodies including the Joint Commission on Accreditation of Healthcare Organizations (JCAHO). As the chief spokesperson for hospital relations with these key external groups, the manager can use such forces to coerce internal groups. For example, stating (1) that unless such and such is done, accreditation will be in jeopardy or (2) that the state will take action is a source of power that was unavailable to management in the past.

In recognition of administrative dominance, most hospital administrators are considered to be CEOs. They now hold the title of president of the hospital and in many institutions are full voting members of the governing board. The hospital's management team also became more sophisticated in applying modern managerial technologies, such as accounting, finance, and systems engineering, to achieve more effective management of the complex and costly hospital organization. In addition, university graduate programs and continuing educational programs have given managers diagnostic knowledge and tools to meet the increased demands on management.

It is important to recognize the vast changes in the past 40 years and the accelerating rate of change. Assuming such changes continue, those entering careers in health services management must be prepared to cope with and take advantage of the accelerating changes in the future.

Managed Care Period: 1980s

Managed care began in the 1980s with the change from cost-based reimbursement to prospective payment and capitation systems, such as payments by diagnostic related groups (DRGs) and HMOs, described in Chapter 3. Continued improvements in health care technology, increasingly complex delivery services, increasing demands from an aging population, increasing counterpressures to contain costs, potential surplus of physicians, increasing competition, and consolidation of services demand more and better management of health services. Because of the importance of these forces on management, we devote Chapter 3 to them.

FRAMEWORK FOR A STRATEGIC MANAGEMENT ROLE TO IMPROVE PATIENT OUTCOMES AND COMMUNITY HEALTH

Fig. 1-1 proposes a framework of factors that explain *organizational performance* (Box 8). We argue that organizational performance in health services is not just a goal in itself, but a means to improve *patient outcomes* (Box 9) and *community health* (Box 10). Normally one might assume that improvement of patient outcomes is left to physicians and other health professionals. Management's role in such an assumption is to get resources to these professionals, to see that such resources are used efficiently, and to ensure that professionals evaluate and improve patient care. However, we propose a more proactive management to improve patient outcomes and community health than simply managing resources. In the next chapter we examine inputs to health and in later chapters we describe opportunities for intervening on these inputs to improve patient outcomes and community health.

We suggest that there are a variety of interacting forces that predict organizational performance and effectiveness in improving patient outcomes and community health. Let us examine the variables shown in Fig. 1-1 that might determine health services performance to improve patient outcomes and community health, starting with Box 1, *environmental forces*.

1. Environmental forces help to determine institutional characteristics, characteristics of professionals in the organization, management, organizational culture, and organizational effectiveness. Environmental forces have varying degrees of support and hostility for the health service organization. Environmental forces include many variables, among them financial and personnel resources available to the organization. Organizations in poor rural and innercity areas will have substantially more difficulty obtaining both financial and professional resources than organizations in more prosperous locations. Regulation, such as that which tries to contain costs, may make for a hostile environment, preventing the organization from obtaining what it needs to achieve its goals effectively and efficiently. Competition from other organizations for resources or service provision is a major environmental force in health services operation today. There are many other environmental variables that help to determine an organization's effectiveness that are unique to the type of organization and community in which it operates. As noted, a number of theorists who study organizational ecology believe that the environment is the overwhelming determinant of organizational success, and the best that management can do is to try to adjust to it. We, on the other hand, believe that there is much that strategic management can do to manage the environment through interorganizational relationships and organizational performance that satisfies demands of the environment.

2. Institutional characteristics are at least in part determined by environmental characteristics, but they too are precursors to other variables, such as the types of clients served, professionals in the organization, management practices, organizational culture, and organizational effectiveness. Organizational size helps to predict scope of services that might be offered to patients. It is also an important determinant of management staff specialty services, such as marketing, risk management, and other managerial skills. However, management of a small organization can intervene to arrange affiliations with larger organizations to obtain such services. On the other

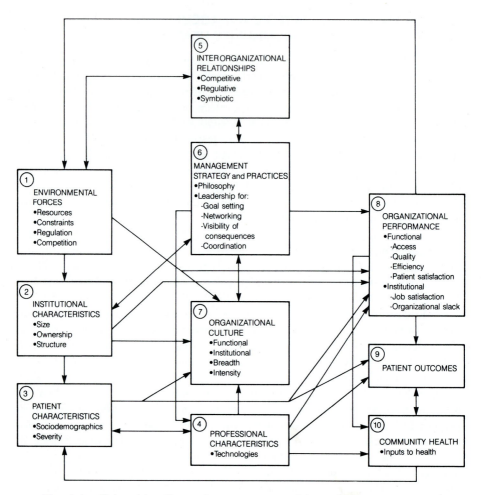

Fig. 1-1   Role of health services management in patient outcomes and community health.

hand, a large organization might be handicapped in terms of its flexibility to adjust to environmental changes. Organizational ownership and its mission influence the type of clients served, types of staff professionals, management practices, organizational culture, and its measures of organizational effectiveness. A for-profit organization will naturally differ from a governmental or church-owned institution. Organizational structure is another important institutional variable. For example, how the medical staff is organized and whether it is independent or organized into a vertical system affects other factors.

3. Patient characteristics are basic predictors of patient outcomes. The aged, poor, drug and alcohol abusers, smokers, and others in high-risk categories will have less favorable outcomes. Management information systems comparing outcomes should consider case mix. Case mix can be managed by demarketing and rationing processes to help achieve favorable performance indicators. We argue for a focus on needs, not merely outcome measures. Managers who strive to serve needs must convince evaluators of the organization to view outcomes in relation to needs and patient inputs.

Not only are patient characteristics most important to their outcomes, but the mix of patients in the organization helps to determine other organizational factors. For example, do patients come from deprived populations, how severely ill are they, and how old are they? What needs to be done to prevent the health problems facing them? How might the health service contribute to preventing such problems? Although health services seldom ask themselves such basic questions, answers consciously or unconsciously influence the professional characteristics and technologies used to care for such persons. They also influence organizational culture and measures of performance. Patient characteristics are in turn influenced by the inputs to health presented in Chapter 2.

4. Professional characteristics, such as numbers and types of specialties and the technologies they use, influence management practices, organizational culture, measures of effectiveness, and, of course, patient outcomes. The higher the technologies and the more specialties in the organization, the more complex the organization is likely to be. A university hospital naturally differs from a nursing home in types of staff and technologies used and consequently affects other variables.

Management, however, frequently abrogates its responsibilities for professional characteristics in the organization, leaving that to the doctors and nurses. A shameful example of board and administrator negligence to professional characteristics and to the purpose of a health service was presented to us a few years ago when a small rural hospital asked for help in recruiting a general surgeon. The surgeon who had recently left the community and a general practitioner had accounted for most of the admissions to the hospital. The town did not want to lose its hospital, which was its largest employer and an attraction for its tourist industry. We proposed that they affiliate with a nearby major multispecialty clinic. The hospital refused to do so because the clinic insisted that surgery be done in their hospital. Board members themselves confessed they went elsewhere for care. Moreover, the administrator admitted that the previous surgeon left because there probably wasn't a gall bladder left in the county. Nevertheless, the hospital did recruit another surgeon. Although few managers would be accomplices to such desperate practices, many practice benign neglect to improvements that may be needed in medical and other professional staff characteristics and practices.

Characteristics of incumbent professionals can facilitate or impede efforts to improve the health services products, that is, patient outcomes. Managers cannot "clean house of the bad apples" on the medical staff or board, or even very easily among employees, such as nurses, who are in scarce supply. On the other hand, working with the "good apples," exposing problems with information systems, and using criteria of the accrediting bodies, management can be a powerful force in improving the production system that leads to patient outcomes. Professional characteristics can also be influenced by managers in terms of who they recruit to serve patients. Moreover, managers are responsible for motivation of all staff, including professionals. Behaviors, attitudes, knowledge, and skills can be changed.

5. Interorganizational relationships are major determinants of organizational effectiveness. Pfeffer[4] found a relationship between environmental linkages and hospital effectiveness. Interorganizational relationships are the ways in which management influences its environment. Health services depend on many groups in their environment, including patients, employers, regulators, and volunteers. Communities also depend on health services. Interdependence exists when one actor does not entirely control all conditions necessary for achievement of an action or outcome desired from actions. Fig. 1-1 suggests that there are competitive, legal, and symbiotic interorganizational relationships. Competitive relations exist when organizations compete with each other for resources. Legal relationships include regulating agencies. Symbiotic relationships are those where organizations complement each other, such as one providing financial resources and the other medical care—both of which are needed for patient care. Comprehensive care in a continuum requires interorganizational linkages. For example, community mental health care requires strong interorganizational relations among, for example, inpatient services, community mental health centers, halfway houses, police, employers, and sheltered workshops. Such organizations are both competitive and symbiotic, requiring considerable effort for effective relationships.

Pfeffer and Salancik[5] suggest that mismanagement of an organization's environment occurs when management does the following:

Has an incorrect perception of its environments and the relative importance of each group

Misreads demands and expectations

Has conflicting demands

Does not determine interest groups

Neglects weighing of interest groups

Does not recognize priorities of groups

Neglects to relate impact of actions to group's priorities.

Ways in which health services provide linkages to their environments is through governing boards, external activities of the CEO, marketing studies, and evaluation procedures. Pfeffer and Salancik suggest a number of ways that environments are managed (some more ethical than others). They include the following:

Control demands—for example, control information or give at least an illusion of satisfying demands; Thompson[6] suggests demand for services can also be controlled by forecasting, buffering to other services, leveling demand, and rationing

Control the definition of satisfaction—for example, define quality in terms of technology that only providers can define

Control the formation of demand—for example, through marketing programs

Control discretion in behavior—for example, prevent an influencing organization from using its power by isolating it from observation

Avoid dependence—for example, broaden resource groups

Employ strategies for merger or growth that result in diversification and less dependence on single sources

Negotiate with environments through collective structures—for example, hospital associations and political action committees

Lobby for laws or social sanctions to protect the organization from demands—for example, laws to limit malpractice suits or occupational licensing

While the environment in which health services operate has become more hostile in recent years, these are ways managers have coopted their environments. Managing the organization's environment is an important managerial function, but it must be done in an ethical manner to ensure that the organization is truly a service and not a burden on society. Establishing broad and frequent communication networks through interorganizational relationships are constructive ways to link the organization with its interdependent environment. Informal social and work networks are among the most effective means for supportive interorganizational relationships.

6. Management practices can influence organizational culture, organizational effectiveness, and in turn patient outcomes and community health. Fig. 1-1 suggests that strategic management with an appropriate management philosophy, implemented with goal setting, and proactive leadership are important predictors of organization culture and effectiveness. Leadership should be proactive in networking with the external environment, making consequences of operation visible and coordinating efforts to achieve goals. Management philosophy is discussed in Chapter 18 in relation to managerial ethics.

There is overwhelming evidence that goal setting and management to achieve goals contribute to organizational performance.[7] We have described ways that networking with other organizations can help to achieve a more supportive environment for the health service. Shortell et al.[8] found that organizations' practice of making the consequences of their operations visible to key individuals in the organization (providing information on how well the organization was doing to achieve goals) was important to explaining hospital performance for quality and efficiency. There is also evidence that coordination practices that include physician and staff participation in management information and decisions relates to job satisfaction.[9] Preliminary evidence suggests that participation may also relate to performance in health services.[10,11] Our own research finds that a combination of goal setting, making consequences visible, and certain coordination practices relates to performance in health services.[12,13] They are essential components of strategic management and are elaborated on later in this book.

7. Organizational culture has been of increasing interest to organization theorists, stemming from studies of factors contributing to the success of Japanese companies[14] and "excellence" in certain U.S. corporations.[15] "Culture is to the organization what personality is to the individual—a hidden, yet unifying theme that provides meaning, direction, and mobilization"[16] (p. 9). Organizational culture might be defined as "shared values" in the organization. Weick[17] asserted that strategy and culture are essentially synonymous. Whether culture is related to organizational performance is debated.[18] Although cultures are hard to describe, let alone measure, they do exist.

Cultures are established by leadership, and they can evolve into a tradition of culture. Organizational cultures tend to be self-perpetuating. For example, the selection of managers are influenced by culture. However, by the same token, managers can influence culture, as described in Chapter 6. In most medical services, physician and/ or board leadership was instrumental in establishing organizational culture historically. More recently, administration has had increasing influence over health services organizational cultures. External political forces, such as changes in values, influence organizational culture as, of course, does ownership of the organization. There are several dimensions to organizational culture. The *breadth,* that is, the number of members in the organization who hold central values, and *intensity* of values vary among organizations. Cultures also vary according to priorities for *functional values,* that is, products of the organization (for example, who is served and how they are served) and *institutional* or *elitist values,* for example, being the biggest or the best.[19]

We argue that organizational culture is important to the management of health services, and we speculate that it is important to staff satisfaction, quality, and at least indirectly to access and cost performance dimensions proposed in our model. We hypothesize that organizations with strong central functional values would tend to be more successful than organizations with weak and disparate functional values. Conversely, those with higher priorities for institutional values would be expected to have more difficulty over the long run. Functional values for better patient outcomes and improved health of citizens of the population served address needs of the community that must support the health service and should facilitate obtaining resources for organizational success to do just that. On the other hand, organizations without common and strong value systems and those that focus on their own health as much or more than the community's are not likely to gain lasting resource support.

One can criticize an organizational culture as (1) promoting "group think," that is, blindly following the group, (2) limiting individuality, and (3) developing rigidity.[20] On the other hand, one of the advantages of a strong organizational culture is that it gives a framework for unifying an organization with less reliance on rules, regulations, procedure manuals, and exhortations from management. It should provide autonomy for individuals to manage their own responsibilities and to manage them with peer support to help implement common goals.

8. Organizational performance (which we use synonymously with organizational effectiveness) is very difficult to measure in health services. Little agreement exists among organization theorists as to what organizational effectiveness means, let alone how to assess it. Different stakeholders have various priorities for what they expect of a health service. For example, payers favor efficiency, whereas physicians and other professionals favor technology and quality. Definitions vary over time, measures differ, time frames for achieving performance differ, as do referants for performance.[21] There are multiple preferences for organizations, such as "doing good deeds" versus "doing deeds well," attaining desirable results versus desired results, and doing things right (efficiency) versus doing the right things (effectiveness). Nevertheless, effective management is at least implicitly based on attaining a certain measure of performance. Defining what this is is an essential element of strategic management, as described in Chapter 5.

In Fig. 1-1 we propose two levels of organizational performance: one at the functional (societal) level and the other at the elitist (institutional) level. Functional performance (at the societal level) might include providing programs and technologies that will improve patient outcomes and community health, providing access to such programs for persons most in need and who can benefit most from them, providing such programs and technologies with appropriate quality and cost (that is, appropriate to meeting goals and not in excess of those needs), with equity, and to the client's satisfaction. Each organization has to define what this means as a part of its strategic plan. Institutional (or elitist performance) might include capturing resources from the environment (that is, financial, staff, and patient resources), job satisfaction among workers, organizational slack (that is, operating margins to expand or undertake new programs to meet changing needs), and ultrastability (as defined in Chapter 4). Institutional performance also needs to be defined in the strategic planning process.

CONCLUSIONS

Health services organizations are complex, multifaceted operations. Whereas their overriding mission is to improve health of the people they serve, their operating objectives reflect pressures and incentives from their environment. These pressures and incentives have been changing and will continue to change. Organizational objectives are reflections of the people in the organization—especially of management, which has the power to influence directions. In this text, we propose that management rededicate itself to the purposes for which health services were originally created, that is, to improve health of the individuals and community served. To do this, it is necessary to understand the factors that determine a person's health, that is, the inputs to health. Inputs to health are presented in the next chapter.

REFERENCES

1. Medical Care Review 44:2, 1987: a series of articles on organizational ecology and its relevance to health services.
2. McDermott, Walsh: Demography, culture, and economics and the evolutionary stages of medicine. In Kilbourne ED and Smillie WG, editors: Human ecology and public health, ed 4, London, 1969, Macmillan Publishing Co.
3. Starr P: The social transformation of American medicine, New York, 1982, Basic Books Inc, Publishers.
4. Pfeffer J: Size, composition and function of hospital boards of directors: a study of organization-environment linkage, Admin Sci Q 18:349, 1973.
5. Pfeffer J and Salancik G: The external control of organizations, New York, 1978, Harper & Row Publishers, Inc.
6. Thompson JD: Organizations in action, New York, 1967, McGraw-Hill, Inc.
7. Locke EA and Latham SP: Goal setting: a motivation technique that works, Englewood Cliffs, NJ, 1984, Prentice-Hall.
8. Shortell S, Becker S, and Neuhauser D: The effects of management practices on hospital efficiency and quality of care. In Shortell S and Brown M, editors: Organization research on hospitals, Chicago, 1976, Blue Cross Association.
9. Schulz R and Schulz C: Management practices, physician autonomy and satisfaction in mental health services in the Federal Republic of Germany, Med Care 28(8):750, 1988.
10. Linn SL et al: Physician and patient satisfaction as factors related to the organization of internal medicine group practice, Med Care 23(10):1179, 1985.
11. Weisman CS and Nathanson CA: Professional satisfaction and client outcomes: a comparative organizational analysis, Med Care: 23(9):1179, 1985.
12. Schulz R, Greenley J, and Peterson R: Management, cost and quality of acute inpatient psychiatric services, Med Care 21(9):911, 1983.
13. Schulz R, Girard C, and Harrison S: Management practices and priorities for mental health system performance: evidence from England and West Germany, University of Wisconsin, 1989, (submitted for publication).
14. Ouchi WG: Theory Z: how American business can meet the Japanese challenge, Reading, Ma, 1981, Addison-Wesley Publishing Co, Inc.
15. Peters TJ and Waterman RH, Jr: In search of excellence, New York, 1982, Harper & Row, Publishers, Inc.

16. Kilmann RH et al: Gaining control over the corporate culture, San Francisco, 1985, Jossey-Bass, Inc, Publishers.
17. Weick K: The significance of corporate culture. In Frost P et al, editors: Organization culture, Beverly Hills, 1985, Sage Publications, Inc.
18. Ott JS: The organizational culture perspective, Chicago, 1989, The Dorsey Press.
19. Wiener Y: Forms of value systems: a focus on organizational effectiveness and cultural change and maintenance, Acad Manage Rev 13(4):534, 1988.
20. Saffold GS: Culture traits, strength, and organizational performance: moving beyond "Strong" Culture, Acad Manage Rev 13(4):546, 1988.
21. Cameron KS and Whetten DA: Organizational effectiveness: a comparison of multiple models, Press, San Diego, 1983, Academic Press, Inc.

2
Health and the Health System

A common mission for a health service is to improve health of individuals. But what determines health, and can health services do much about it? What is the health system to which management must relate in both a competitive and symbiotic way? Inputs to health and the system that delivers health services are presented in this chapter.

INPUTS TO HEALTH

The World Health Organization (WHO) defines health as a state of "complete physical, mental, and social well-being and not merely the absence of disease."[1] Although there is some disagreement as to whether this is a useful definition because it presents an unattainable and unmeasurable ideal, it is unquestionably a desirable objective for the health industry. It is clear that health is indeed a comprehensive concept and that hospital care is but a small component in the provision of complete physical, mental, and social well-being.

An alternative approach to defining health is the ecological one, which considers health to be a state of optimal physical, mental, and social adaptation to one's environment. For example, an individual with a chronic disease condition, such as arthritis or chronic mental illness, can never return to complete well-being but can adjust and adapt quite adequately. A more direct example is a patient with a terminal illness. Facilitating adaptation in this case would mean helping to prepare for and adjust to the realities of death.

Blum[2] suggests that the ultimate needs and goals for the health system are the following:

Prolongation of life through prevention of premature death

Minimization of departures from physiologic or functional norms for optimal health (such norms have yet to be defined)

Minimization of discomfort (illness)

Minimization of disability (incapacity)

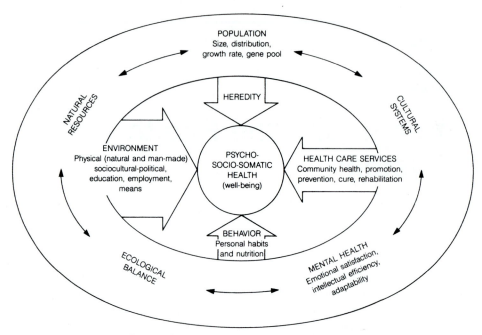

The width of the four huge input-to-health arrows indicates assumptions about the relative importance of the inputs to health. The four inputs are shown as relating to and affecting one another by means of an encompassing matrix, which could be called the "environment" of the health system.

Fig. 2-1 Inputs to health. (Adapted from Blum HL: Planning for health: development and application of social change theory, ed 2, New York, 1981, Human Sciences Press, Inc.)

Promotion of high-level "wellness" or self-fulfillment (internal satisfaction)
Promotion of high-level satisfaction with the environment (external satisfaction)
Extension of resistance to ill health and creation of reserve capacity (positive health)
Increasing capacity for the underprivileged to participate in health matters

Fig. 2-1, adapted from Blum,[2] presents the health spectrum showing environment, behavior, heredity, and health care services as inputs to psychosocial (emotional and mental) and somatic (physical) health or well-being. These four inputs relate and affect one another through ecological balance, natural resources, population characteristics, cultural systems, and mental health.

Environment

Natural physical characteristics of the environment, such as climate, soil conditions, and topography, relate to health directly, as well as interacting to affect the economy, the culture, and other forces that contribute to a state of healthfulness. Moreover, manmade aspects of the environment have an increasing influence on health. Inadequate housing, for example, contributes to disease. The (Wisconsin) Governor's Health Policy and Planning Task Force identified inadequacies in transportation and communication as major barriers to the adequate delivery of health services.[3] Because accidents are the fourth leading cause of death in the United States, safety in work and leisure is another major factor. Sanitation in its broadest sense, that is, the control of air, water, and noise and aesthetic pollution, obviously contributes to good health. Although advances in technology have had a major impact on improving health, they sometimes lead to new hazards, for example, the noise pollution associated with airplanes.

Sociocultural factors are inputs to health. Cultural patterns affect nutrition, exercise, personal habits, and other factors related to health. Social stress and the responses of cardiovascular, respiratory, gastrointestinal, and other systems have been widely researched and relationships detected.[4] Most authorities now agree that life-style contributes in a major way to health status more so than income or medical care. Fuchs, for example, suggests that life-style may account for otherwise unexplained differences in health between males and females, races, middle-aged adults in Sweden and the United States, those with differing marital status, people with varied occupations, and the populations of Nevada and Utah.[5] Politics as reflected in laws on alcohol and safety, for example, contribute to health. The reduction in deaths on the road as a result of the reduction in speed limits is a recent example.

There is substantial evidence that after age and heredity, individuals' educational levels are correlated with their health.[6-8] Although a number of researchers have found that family income is not directly correlated with health, the capacity of an individual to obtain an education, live in a healthful area, and purchase other services contributes to a high quality of life and health. Occupations have an important relationship to health. For example, 33% of farmers over 44 years of age have work-limiting chronic conditions as compared with only 7% of professional workers.[9]

Behavior

Personal behavior and habits, such as smoking, drinking, dangerous driving, over-eating, abuse of drugs, neglect of personal hygiene, and delay in seeking medical care, are major influences on health and well-being. The physiological responses to personal emotions, such as a face flushed with anger or loss of energy and desire caused by sadness, have been observed by all of us. The effect of personal behavior on an individual's health reflects the way in which he or she reacts to environmental, hereditary, and health care services influences.

Nutrition is one of the more important inputs to health. In the United States, where inadequate food is not the primary barrier to good health (as it is in much of the rest of the world), personal behavior is the primary influence on nutrition. Overeating and eating the wrong kinds of foods relate to the dietary problems that contribute to ill health. Higher educational levels are again linked to personal behaviors of beneficial nutritional practices.

Heredity

Heredity or genetic endowment, that is, the intrinsic nature of the individual, is increasingly recognized as having a primary influence on susceptibility to disease and inheritance of disease. Genetic endowment interacts with both environmental and behavioral factors. Cultural considerations, such as ethnic or racial proclivities, limit the choice of marital partners and so influence the genetic potential of offspring and their susceptibility to certain diseases. An example would be sickle cell anemia, which occurs almost exclusively among blacks. However, this disease can be diagnosed and treated through personal behavior and health care services. Problems arising from genetic factors can be controlled through screening, increasingly through genetic counseling, and potentially through genetic engineering.

Health Care Services

Among the four major inputs to health, health care services have the least influence on health and are portrayed as such by the narrowest arrow in Fig. 2-1. Health care services include the community health services delivered by environmental and public care agencies. These services can intervene, for example, on environmental problems of pollution, occupational safety, and housing conditions. Health promotion delivered by public and personal health services is another major input to health. Health promotion activities are directed at behaviors such as exercise, rest, attitudes, and good nutrition. Current interests in jogging, *vita* courses, and other physical fitness programs, emphasis on good nutritional practices, and increasing emphasis on attitudinal influences on health have all contributed to improving health in the United States. Community health campaigns, employee health programs, and efforts of individual physicians all help to deliver health promotion services. Scrimshaw[10] and others have reported on the importance of nutrition on health and on the outcomes of contracted disease.

The prevention of disease includes health screening and early diagnosis, and good personal habits. For example, smoking has been shown to increase the risk of death from cancer, bronchitis, and chronic heart disease. The cancer of the lung death rate for persons smoking 21 to 30 cigarettes a day was found to be about 17 times greater than for those who never smoked.

However, though health promotion and disease prevention probably have the greatest impact on health, cure or diagnosis and treatment factors, that is, physician and hospital services, receive primary attention when health is studied. Of the billions of dollars expended for health care, most is expended for personal health services and supplies, primarily for hospital and physicians' services. Of the balance, less than 5% is spent on public health services and research. A large part is spent to correct the problems caused by demographic, behavioral, physical, and genetic factors, and health promotion and prevention deficiencies. Medical and hospital services are usually crisis care, sometimes referred to as "heroic medicine" or "too late medicine;" they are concerned with illness, not health. This is partly a result of health insurance that encourages crisis care, and the lack of promotion and prevention services; it is also caused by personal attitudes—people respond only when they must. Moreover, as Scrimshaw[10] notes, "No matter what is done most patients get well most of the time. Therefore, anything done in the name of health [cure] will be successful most of the time. This includes prayer, incantations, copper bracelets, manipulations of joints, special foods, prescription drugs, anything at all!"

Rehabilitation or restorative services designed to return patients to their maximum state of health are provided through hospitals, extended care facilities, and rehabilitation centers. Custodial care delivered by institutions and home health services also provide inputs to health.

To complete the picture of health inputs it is important to note that individuals' health is also affected by environmental factors, such as their employment and housing. It is also important to point out that we are not suggesting there is always a cause and effect relationship between inputs and health. Although there is good evidence of correlation, because the inputs are intricately interwoven, it is difficult in most cases to determine the relative influence of each factor.

Questions are frequently raised regarding the emphasis on treatment services in the United States. Winkelstein et al.[11] suggested that ". . . medical care is largely unrelated to health status of the populations . . . that ecology is the primary determinant of the health status . . ." McKeown[12,13] suggested that neither personal nor public health care services have had much influence on reducing deaths. He attributed the great strides made since the 1700s in reducing premature deaths to improvements in food supply, birth controls, and hygiene. The late F.J. Inglefinger, M.D., former editor of *The New England Journal of Medicine,* put the role of medical care into perspective with this excerpt from a 1977 editorial[14]:

> Let us assume that 80% of patients have either self-limited disorders or conditions not improvable, even by modern medicine. The physician's actions, unless harmful, will therefore not affect the basic course of such conditions. In slightly over 10% of cases, however, medical intervention is dramatically successful, whether the surgeon repairs bones or removes stones, the internist uses antibiotics or palliative measures (e.g. insulin, vitamin B_{12}) appropriately, or the pediatrician eliminates a food that an enzyme-deficient infant cannot absorb or metabolize. But alas in the final 9%, give or take a point or two, the doctor may diagnose or treat inadequately, or he may just have bad luck. Whatever the reason, the patient ends up with iatrogenic problems (adverse affects induced by medical care), so the balance of accounts ends up marginally on the positive side of zero.

One might ask that if the conclusion is that health is related for the most part to heredity, environment, and behavior, does the health service have a role in health? Or, is its role only to minimize discomfort and attempt to repair disease? Repair and help in coping with illness is, of course, an important and primary function of most health services and as such contributes to individual and community health. Quality assurance efforts described in Chapter 15 contribute to this goal. Opportunities for broader roles to improve community health are proposed also in later chapters.

THE HEALTH SYSTEM

In Fig. 1-1 we noted that external relations and interorganizational relationships were essential to the management of health services. It is important therefore to understand the system that contains both the competitive constraints and symbiotic opportunities for the management of health services. In the balance of this chapter we begin with an overview of the system, followed by a description of the public and

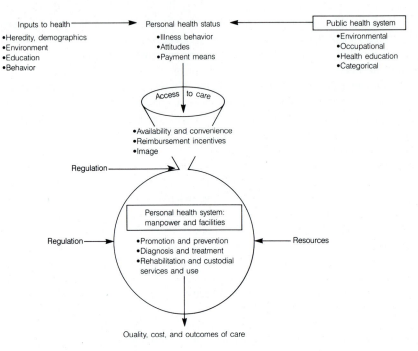

Fig. 2-2   The health system.

personal health systems, including different physician delivery models, hospitals, and other services.

It is difficult to portray the health system, which touches so many facets of society. However, a simplified presentation is shown in Fig. 2-2. It shows the health system from a patient flow perspective. What systems affect a person's health? How do they get into the system if they need personal health care services? What affects the system and the system's ability to serve patients?

An individual's health status is the primary determinant of whether he or she gets into the system. The top of Fig. 2-2 shows two primary forces affecting personal health status. On the left side are the heredity, demographic, environmental, behavioral, and educational inputs to health status described in the previous section. On the right is the public health system, which provides services to improve the health status of its population. Public health services are described on pp. 23-25. Although an individual may need care, whether it is sought relates to personal socioeconomic variables, such as illness behavior, attitudes, and ability to pay for service. Access to care is portrayed in Fig. 2-2 as a funnel. Access to care includes the five A's: availability, accessibility, accommodation, affordability, and acceptability. Availability reflects the supply of services available in the area to obtain care. There is a widely recognized maldistribution of health services in the United States—many metropolitan areas have a surplus of physicians while some rural and urban inner-city locations have a severe shortage. Accessibility concerns location and ease of transportation to the service.

Accommodation includes, for example, convenience of hours the service is available, ease of obtaining appointments, and presence or absence of bureaucratic barriers. Affordability concerns cost to the patient as a barrier, and acceptability is how the patient views the provider and the provider views the patient. For example—are there cultural, ethnic, or medical (such as AIDS) barriers to obtaining service? A health service has financial incentives to serve paying patients on a fee-for-service basis, but it has disincentives to serve the uninsured and prepaid patients and it may restrict such persons from obtaining service. The image the service presents is a way to restrict or market access to service.

The personal health care system shown in the bell of the jar in Fig. 2-2 consists of health workers and facilities for promotion, prevention, diagnosis and treatment, rehabilitation, and custodial services. The external environment is crucial to the performance of the health system and its abilities to meet needs of the sick and injured. The size of the system and its quality and cost outcomes are determined by the resources available to it and regulatory constraints, as shown by the arrows in Fig. 2-2. For example, the National Health Service (NHS) in Great Britain controls resources into the system, and with fewer resources, it is a smaller system relative to its population, with a smaller neck to get into the system. The United States by contrast used regulation to control the size of the system and access into it. In the United States a primary rationing mechanism is ability to pay for care. In the United Kingdom it is a queue at the funnel manned by general practitioners who determine who needs and can benefit most from specialist and hospital service.

Health Services in the United States: Direct and Indirect Competition

The United States has a private competitive (or fragmented) system. A hospital, for example, may view another hospital as direct competition and may view an HMO as indirect competition but increasingly direct, as both compete for the growing ambulatory market. The hospital may view public health services as indirect competition, for example, competition over legislation, regulation, or for resources.

Within the health system there are two main delivery subsystems. One of these is the *public and environmental health systems,* which are concerned with populations. A public health service is a designated government agency concerned with health of the general population in its jurisdiction. The environmental health system is related to public health services but includes a number of other agencies that contribute to a healthy environment for the population. The second subsystem is the *personal health care system,* which is concerned with health of individuals.

Public Health Services

The primary objective of a public health service is to improve the health of the population for which it is responsible, such as a state or local community. Performance is measured by vital statistics, such as incidence and prevalence of disease, mortality and morbidity, and longevity. A second objective is to protect public interests. An example is licensing to protect the public from incompetent practitioners and organizations. A relatively new objective is to protect the public from exorbitant costs of health care. Regulation of rates and capital expenditures of health services are examples of implementing this objective. A third objective of public health services is to implement expectations of elected officials, especially the executive branch. For example, a conservative government may give priority to cost containment, whereas a liberal government may focus on access to care.

Environmental health is a responsibility of public health departments, but such services are also provided by a number of different and fragmented agencies. The objective for environmental health is to reduce pollutants and hazards from the environment. A variety of agencies are responsible for ridding the environment of air, water, and ground pollutants. Different agencies are also responsible for reducing hazards to the health of a population, such as road and occupational dangers.

Public health services have traditionally included the following:

Communicable (infectious) disease control

Sanitation

Maternal and child health

Public health nursing

Public health education

Vital statistics

Administration of funds for local public health services

These programs have been administered through state, county, and local health districts.

Increasingly, public health services provided by government go beyond the basic services listed above. They now include programs and activities for the following:

Health planning and policy determination

Health maintenance

Continuous assessment of community ecology and resources

Reduction of health hazards

Research

Environmental health programs relate to public health and are carried out through a number of governmental and private organizations. They include more than public health services, and frequently there is overlap and conflict among public health agencies, industry, labor, conservation, and other governmental and private agencies. This has handicapped the development of effective and efficient programs. Environmental health programs include the following:

Water supply and pollution control

Solid waste disposal

Insect and rodent control

Milk and food sanitation

Air pollution control

Noise pollution control

Control of radiological hazards

Housing and land use

Occupational health

Public health made substantial contributions toward the great improvement in the health of populations in the ninteenth and early twentieth centuries. Although less has been spent for public health services than for personal health care, public health measures, such as sanitation, have probably had a greater impact on improving health in the past hundred years than have personal health care services.

However, today "the nation has lost sight of its public health goals and has allowed the system of public health activities to fall into disarray," according to a 1988 report by the Institute of Medicine of the National Academy of Sciences in Washington, D.C.[15] They reported that the public health system is fraught with problems as a result of shrinking funds, inadequate program administration, and inconsistent health goals. Consequently, the system has not been able to respond adequately to problems such as AIDS. The report recommends organizational changes at the state level to give a more organized prominence to public health. The report also recommends greater federal support. The root of many of our health problems, as described in Chapter 1, regarding inputs to health are public concerns. It is hoped that in the future more effort will be placed on solving and preventing the conditions that lead to personal health problems and to the high cost of treating them.

PERSONAL HEALTH CARE SYSTEM

Personal health care is usually provided, for example, by private physicians, hospitals, and nursing homes. As suggested in Fig. 2-2, it can be classified as: (1) promotion of health, (2) prevention of accidents and disease (both of which overlap with public health), (3) cure or diagnostic and treatment services, and (4) rehabilitation or restorative care and custodial care. Personal health care systems will be considered in some depth in the rest of this chapter and in the next, for it is in this area of responsibility that most health services function.

Promotion of Health

Promotion of health is usually considered the responsibility of the individual. It includes such factors as diet, exercise, and rest. In most cases, information and prescriptions regarding these important aspects of health are provided by the individual's cultural environment, family, and schools, and through the mass media. Management is usually by the individual. Pediatricians, concerned with well-baby care, and dentists are among the few providers of personal health service that appear actively concerned with the promotion of health. Others who are concerned with the promotion of health are usually outside the health system; they include physical and mental health educators. Recognizing relationships between employee health and productivity, increasing numbers of employers are offering health promotion and disease prevention programs related to such matters as physical and mental fitness, diet, drug abuse, alcohol and tobacco prevention, and rehabilitation services.

Evidence to the benefit of health promotion activities is overwhelming. It is interesting and at the same time disappointing to note role reversals between the higher-educated and the less-educated population groups. Whereas obesity and tobacco, drug, and alcohol abuse, for example, were problems of the affluent, they are now mostly problems of lower socioeconomic groups.

Prevention

Cooperation between professional health services and the individual for the prevention and early detection of disease is more common than for promotional health purposes. All diagnostic and therapeutic activity has a preventive component in that it seeks to forestall or prevent further deterioration of an individual's health. Here again, the individual has a responsibility to be alert to hazards and to emotional and physiological changes and to seek professional assistance.

Early detection of disease through mass screening services among higher-risk populations is another component of preventive medicine. It is favored by some and may have potential for greater application. However, others question this approach from an economic standpoint, noting that the cost of detecting pathology through multiphasic health screening units is high, particularly when it is considered that most individuals with pathology detect changes in themselves.[16,17] However, other studies have shown that selective screening could save both lives and dollars.[18]

Prevention of disease and accidents by controlling personal habits, for example, refraining from smoking and wearing seatbelts, is usually an individual and political matter. However, certain preventive programs can be delivered, such as physicians' recommendations for life-style changes and various employee health programs.

Primary prevention is a direct and specific service designed to protect against a specific disease, and its prototype is immunization, for example, against polio or tetanus. Leavell and Clark[19] also include health promotion as a part of primary prevention. Early disease detection is considered to be secondary prevention. Health screening by multiphasic clinics or an annual physical examination, and surveillance of individuals with a suspected proclivity toward certain diseases all fall into this category. Rehabilitation is considered tertiary prevention by Leavell and Clark.[19]

Cure Services

Cure, that is, diagnoses and treatment services, can be categorized as ambulatory outpatient care or inpatient hospital care. Outpatients services are usually provided in physicians' offices or clinics, although hospitals increasingly provide them as they compete for rising ambulatory services in a declining inpatient market. Specialized diagnostic and treatment services have also attracted such ambulatory patients as alcoholics and drug abusers to hospitals. Inpatient services are usually provided by hospitals. Home care services offer an alternative that has a potential for more development among hospitals.

Treatment services are also categorized as primary, secondary, and tertiary care.[20,21] Primary care can be defined as the site of entry into the health system and coordination through it. It is usually obtained through the family physician, who may be a family or general practitioner, internist, pediatrician, or general surgeon. Primary care services are usually provided on an ambulatory or office visit basis. The WHO takes a broader view of primary care, defining it as ". . . essential health care based on practical, scientifically sound and socially acceptable methods and technology made universally accessible to individuals and families. It is the first level of contact of individuals, the family and the community . . . and constitutes the first element of a continuing health process."[22] The National Academy of Sciences, Institute of Medicine examined 38 different definitions of primary care and developed its own definition in terms of attributes of primary care: "The five attributes essential to the practice of good primary care are accessibility, comprehensiveness, coordination, continuity and accountability."[23] Secondary care services are consultant services that are intermediate in generality. The services of a classically educated internist or general surgeon would fit in this category.* Tertiary care refers to subspecialty or categorical referral services provided in a regional medical center, such as a university hospital.

Dental health is another important curative service. Though many hospitals have dental surgery services and some group practices offer dental service, dental care is usually isolated from other health care services.

PHYSICIAN SERVICES

A growing surplus of physicians, especially in nonprimary care specialties, suggests there will be increasing direct competition among physicians. For example, there will be increasing competition for patients; turf conflicts, such as medical versus surgical treatment of heart problems, will grow; and competition with nonmedical practitioners, such as chiropractors and other practitioners and healers, will continue. Moreover, physician organizations compete directly with hospitals and public health services for preventive, diagnostic, treatment, and rehabilitation services.

There are many different models for delivering physician services. We summarize them within four basic models: (1) solo practice, (2) single-specialty group, (3) multispecialty group, and (4) community health center (CHC) practice. Fig. 2-3 lists these four models, relating them to components of comprehensive services in a continuum, that is, promotion of health, prevention of disease, treatment, and restorative and custodial services. The provider component in the square suggests the unifying core organization for vertical integration of health services (note: this is distinguished from horizontal system integration, such as an association of hospitals).

There are, of course, variations on each of these models, as well as other models not shown, such as hospital-based physician delivery models of the Veterans Administration system, university hospitals that employ faculty-member physicians, the large, public, city hospitals, and the community hospitals that employ hospital-based specialists as pathologists, radiologists, and emergency room physicians. However, the majority of citizens in the United States receive their personal health services through one of these general models or some combination of them. Although only the HMO and CHC models tend to be formally integrated on a vertical basis, other models have informal integration and a potential for more formalization.

---

*This is but one of the many examples of the difficulty in classifying the health services delivery systems. In this case a single physician could fit into all three categories at various times.

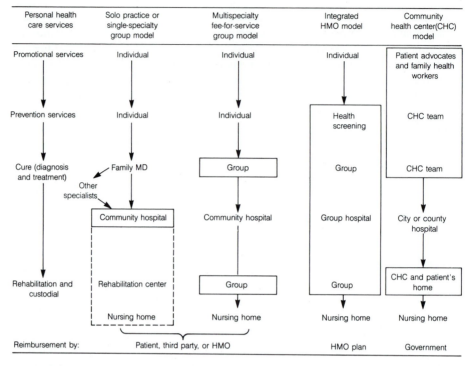

Fig. 2-3 Basic models for delivering personal health care services under different physician organization models and reimbursement practices.

Solo Practice

Although increasing numbers of physicians enter group practice, solo practice (the physician who practices alone or with others but does not pool income or expenses) still dominates in many communities. In many respects, solo practice is a misnomer. Much of a physician's practice centers around the hospital where he or she practices in association with other health professionals. Moreover, increasing numbers of solo practitioners provide care to HMO and PPO patients in a managed care setting.

Solo practice has certain advantages for both the physician and patient. Though autonomy is diminished, the physician has more than in other models of care. The solo practitioner also has more referral freedoms for fee-for-service patients. This may be an advantage to the patient to ensure referrals are to the most competent physician rather than limited to the physician's group if the group is small. Patients also report closer doctor/patient relationships in solo practice settings. Some of the disadvantages of solo practice may be less coverage for both the doctor and patient, and less professional interaction and quality review. With the growing surplus of doctors in a managed care environment, it is increasingly difficult for physicians to enter solo practice. Other solo practitioners are joining groups (1) because of the increasing administrative hassles of managing complicated insurance, fiscal, and regulatory matters and (2) to be in a more price-competitive HMO.

Single-Specialty Group

In a single-specialty group practice, physicians in the same specialty, for example, pediatrics or orthopedic surgery, pool their expenses, income, and offices. The average size of the single-specialty group is about four physicians, which is sufficiently large to employ a business manager. The single-specialty group model resembles the solo practice model more than the multispecialty group model in its impact on the physician and patient except for better coverage and at least informal quality reviews and interaction.

Multispecialty Group Practice

The Mayo Clinic in Rochester, Minnesota, was a pioneer in the development of multispecialty group practice. This model provides for more professional interaction for quality assurance and the potential for skilled management. On the other hand, there is less autonomy for physicians, perhaps more limited referrals in smaller groups, and frequently higher costs as a result of greater use of ancillary services. Methods for dividing incomes between procedural-based specialties, such as surgeons, and time-based specialties, such as pediatrics, is a frequent source of conflict in multispecialty groups.

Many of the larger multispecialty group practices have added a group model HMO to their fee-for-service practice. Having an organization that has pooled income and expenses and having experience of practicing together have facilitated adoption of a managed care HMO practice. Some group practices have also vertically integrated their group with hospital services, such as the Cleveland Clinic and Hospital, and more recently where the Mayo organization acquired the Methodist and St. Mary's Hospitals in Rochester, Minnesota.

Integrated HMO Model

HMOs are primarily a financing scheme and are discussed further in the next chapter. However, they also provide for different organizational arrangements. The integrated HMO model or prepaid multispecialty group is a health care financing plan tied to physician (and in this example also hospital) services. Group Health Associates of Puget Sound, Washington, is a "staff model HMO" example (physicians are employed and salaried by, in this case, consumer owners). Another example is the Kaiser Health Plan, which began in California and is currently the largest HMO in the United States. In the Kaiser Permanente HMO, physicians are organized as a prepaid group practice that contracts with the Kaiser Health Plan and limits its patients to the HMO members. This model comes close to providing vertically integrated comprehensive care in a continuum from screening through treatment services. A single patient record for all health services is an important advantage of this system (although an impersonal one as far as the patient is concerned), along with primary care coordination from family and other practitioners. Control is by the group, which may be provider-dominated, as in the Kaiser Plan, or consumer-dominated, as in Group Health Associates. The Group Health and Kaiser plans have saved from 10% to 40% of traditional "unmanaged" fee-for-service (FFS) systems;[24] there is no evidence that quality of care is lower in these organizations, but care tends to be less personal and both the doctor and patient have less autonomy than in the solo models.

Community Health Center Practice

Community Health Centers (CHCs) were developed with federal funding in the early 1960s (originally named Neighborhood Health Centers). The CHC model comes closest to addressing environmental inputs to health. These centers have addressed themselves to environmental health care issues, such as education, housing, jobs, and behavior. They were targeted by the Reagan Administration in the early 1980s for extinction because they were viewed as costly public programs. However, whereas there were only 112 such centers in the United States in 1978, the number actually grew to 642 centers with 6 million clients by 1988. Each center is unique, some with physicians, others referring clients to physicians when appropriate. The centers serve as a safety net for the disenfranchised, such as the poor; those with "new morbidities," such as AIDS; the homeless; and the addicted.

It is important to note that most of the different delivery systems could be provided in an HMO or PPO setting. However, because the primary objectives of HMOs and PPOs are cost containment, they are discussed in the next chapter.

Mental Health Services

Mental Health Services are provided by both public and private organizations. There is a broad scope of mental health services from health promotion to rehabilitation and custodial care provided by different organizations and agencies. A study sponsored by the National Institutes of Mental Health reported in 1988 that almost one third of all Americans suffer from acute mental illness during their lifetime. Many patients suffering somatic illnesses also have serious mental illnesses. In 1986 Torre and Wolfe[25] reported there were about 2 million seriously mentally ill persons (sometimes referred to as chronically mentally ill) with diagnoses such as schizophrenia, bipolar disorders, and other psychoses. About half of the severely mentally ill are on their own or live with their families, 300,000 are in nursing homes, 300,000 are in group or foster homes, 200,000 are in hospitals, and nearly 200,000 are in public shelters, on the streets, or in jail. Schizophrenia alone has been estimated as costing the United States $18 billion annually, including lost wages but excluding costs to the afflicted "who must endure incompetent professionals, uncaring support staff, inadequate hospitals and housing, and unsafe streets."[25] (p. 2).

There are a number of professions devoted to treatment of the mentally ill, such as psychiatrists, psychologists, social workers, psychiatric nurses, and occupational, recreational, and music therapists. Within the professions there are a variety of optional interventions among practitioners who have different preferences for treatment. Nevertheless, the evidence is overwhelming that deinstitutionalization with strong community support systems is not only better for patients, but it is more efficient.[26] Torre and Wolfe[25] surveyed all states for mental health service effectiveness. They found, for example, that Wisconsin, which was ranked the best system, had lower expenditures per patient than many other states. Through policy and management improvements, mental health services in all states could be more effective and efficient with community psychiatry and support systems. However, current public and private reimbursement practices still favor inpatient care. As a result, inpatient psychiatric services have been profitable for hospitals, and at the time of this writing many hospitals are expanding inpatient psychiatry beds to improve their competitive positions. Meanwhile, other patients without third-party funding are being forced from public inpatient facilities into the streets. Providing for coordinated services to the mentally ill presents an important goal and challenge to health services managers.

HOSPITAL SERVICES

Of the 6841 hospitals registered with the American Hospital Association in 1986 in the United States, 342 are federally owned (for example, Veterans' Administration [VA] and Public Health Service [PHS]), 634 are psychiatric hospitals, and 5728 are short-term, general hospitals of which 3338 are not-for-profit, 834 for-profit, and 1556 state and local government.[27] As noted in chapter 1, hospitals have been at the center of the health system, consuming more than 40% of personal health care expenditures,[28] providing the highest medical technologies, and employing more than 5.7 million full-time equivalent (FTE) persons, in 1985.[29] Hospitals were originally established by religious orders, doctors, and governments at considerable sacrifices to those involved to serve unmet needs of the sick and injured. After World War II and with assistance from Hill-Burton federal funds, hospitals expanded rapidly to meet increasing demands. In spite of facilities planning and regulation, hospitals overexpanded. This, coupled with inpatient need reductions from cost-containment activities and new alternatives to inpatient services, has resulted in increasing hospital competition, mergers, and closures. Many hospitals are in a fragile position. However, the hospital remains as one of the more important and complex organizations in our society. Although we are concerned with health services broadly, hospitals will be a major focus in the balance of this book.

Restorative and Long-Term or Custodial Care Services

Restorative services are organized in a variety of institutions, such as hospitals, convalescent centers, group practice clinics, separate rehabilitation centers, and public agencies. Long-term care facilities have been categorized according to reimbursement definitions used by Medicare and Medicaid. A "skilled nursing facility" as the name implies must provide registered nursing services around the clock. An "extended care facility" is a skilled nursing facility that provides posthospital services to be reimbursible by Medicare. An "intermediate care facility" provides mainly maintenance services; these facilities include homes for the aged and rest homes. With an aging population, the number of nursing home residents is expected to about double in the next 25 years, making this the fastest growing sector of the health care system. Because the aged are the source of patients for most hospitals and long-term care services add to the comprehensiveness (also size and income) of hospital services, there is increasing hospital interest in long-term care. Management of long-term care facilities is different from management of acute facilities. In long-term care, the emphasis is on living and the quality of life; it is not limited to emphasis on sickness or wellness. The whole person and particularly his or her psychosocial environment are especially important in the long-term care facility. Administration of a long-term care facility has important benefits and obligations for the manager in that he or she must be in contact with the persons being served. Managers of hospitals seldom receive the rewards of seeing the fruits of their efforts, that is, care to individual patients.

Each of the above components of personal health services involves a variety of independent individuals and governmental, proprietary, voluntary, and church institutions. The financing of such services is just as diverse. Because of the diversity in health service delivery in the United States, some refer to it as a nonsystem. Certainly it is a pluralistic one.

There are many other competitive and supportive forces in the health care environment. Many of the readers of this text may now or in the future be managers or policymakers in one of the health services support or regulatory agencies. Such organizations include "third-party payers," for example, Blue Cross/Blue Shield plans, commercial indemnity carriers, HMOs, PPOs, and Medicare and Medicaid agencies. They also include local, state, and federal agencies that regulate health services, and employer health benefit plan managers who are concerned with cost and quality of care to employees are a growing force. Such organizations are discussed in the next two chapters.

CONCLUSIONS

Health services feel threatened. A study released by Touche Ross & Co., New York, in 1988 reported that nearly half of hospital executives surveyed feared their institutions would fail in the next 5 years.[30] It is no wonder that many health service managers view their environment as hostile. Nevertheless, one would hope that such managers can look beyond this to how environmental resources can be related symbiotically to meet common goals of more effective and efficient health services.

Health services compete for limited resources. They compete for paying patients to increase revenue and they compete for capital to expand and improve facilities and for programs and staff to enhance quality and prestige. However, unlike other industries, health services to date have limited incentives to compete on the basis of price or cost. Rather, the primary method of competition is based on images of quality.

There are a number of arguments against competition in health services. Health care is more like education and other essential public services than competitive market good industries. The health system is cited as an example of market failure. For example, there is not freedom of entry of suppliers, consumers are not knowledgeable buyers, there is little opportunity for substitution, and there is the belief that health services should be delivered on need, not effective demand. Competition exacerbates inequities in the system. Competition for paying patients means that the uninsured and underinsured have difficulties gaining access to care. Some hospitals use demarketing strategies to minimize services to the uninsured and underinsured, who contribute to bad debts. Competition forces health services to focus on their own institutional needs above those of the community it was originally designed to serve. The hospital industry is now market driven rather than service driven.

On the other hand, some argue that competition is a way of achieving community goals that have not been attained by regulation. For example, inefficient hospitals are no longer as protected as they were under regulations such as rate review. The least efficient hospitals are now forced into mergers or closure. Competition for patients is a powerful incentive for physicians to join HMOs and PPOs, which appear to be more efficient than traditional models. Competition is very consistent with the basic foundation of the United States' economic system. By competing on the basis of quality and cost, an organization must continually improve or die. Substantial improvements have been made in our system, and many more are needed. Competition may or may not help achieve improvements in quality and efficiency.

Although competition is currently in vogue, it is by no means the final answer. Indeed, as system policy evolves, we seem to retain some of the old and never go as far as planned in policy changes. For example, we never had a totally regulated system; regulation may have failed because there was not enough of it. By the same token, the current system is not totally competitive. Indeed, Altman and Rodwin[31] suggest that the United States has both halfway competition and ineffective regulation. Nevertheless, there has always been some competition in the United States' health system, and there always will be. Even in nationalized systems there is competition for resources. Strategy is an important managerial skill to obtaining resources for meeting community service needs.

REFERENCES

1. World Health Organization: Primary Health Care, Geneva, 1978.
2. Blum HL: Planning for health: development and application of social change theory, New York, 1974, Human Sciences Press, Inc.
3. Wisconsin Governor's Health Planning and Policy Task Force: Final Report, Madison, Wis, Nov 1972, Wisconsin Department of Administration.
4. Graham S and Reeder L: Social factors in chronic diseases. In Freeman H, Levine S, and Reeder L, editors: Handbook of medical sociology, ed 2, Englewoods Cliffs, NJ, 1972, Prentice Hall.
5. Fuchs V: Who shall live? New York, 1974, Basic Books Inc, Publishers.
6. Fuchs V: Economics, health and post-industrial society, Milbank Mem Fund Q Health Soc 57(2):153, 1979.
7. Lefcowitz ML: Poverty and health: a re-examination, Inquiry 10(1):3, 1973.
8. Survey: confirming health connections to income, education, etc, The Nations Health, ISSN:0028-1496, pp 1, 10, 1988.
9. Limitation of activity and mobility due to chronic conditions, Vital and Health Statistics, Pub No 1000, Series 10, No 45, pp 48-49, Public Health Service, Washington, DC, 1968.
10. Scrimshaw N: Myths and realities in international health planning, Am J Public Health 64(8):792, 1974.
11. Winklestein W and French F: The role of ecology in the design of a health care system, California Med 113(5):7, 1970.
12. McKeown T: The role of medicine: dream, mirage or nemesis, Oxford, 1976, Basil Blackwell.
13. Mckeown T: Seminar, University of Wisconsin, Madison, April 14, 1980.
14. Inglefinger FJ: Health: a matter of statistics or feeling? N Engl J Med 296:448, 1977.
15. Institute of Medicine: National Academy of Sciences: The future of public health, Washington, DC, 1988, National Academy Press.

16. Felch W: Does preventive medicine really work? Prism, Oct 1973, p 26.
17. Forst BE: An economic analysis of periodic health examination programs, Arlington, Va, AD-735-949, Institute of Naval Studies.
18. Collen M et al: Dollar cost per positive test for automated multiphasic screening, N Engl J Med 283(9):459, 1970.
19. Leavell HR and Clark EG: Preventive medicine for the doctor in his community, ed 3, New York, 1965, McGraw-Hill, Inc.
20. White L: Life and death and medicine, Sci Am 229(3):23, 1973.
21. Hansen M: An educational program for primary care, J Med Educ 45:1001, 1970.
22. World Health Organization: Primary health care, Geneva, 1978.
23. National Academy of Sciences, Institute of Medicine, A manpower policy for primary care, Washington, DC, 1978.
24. Luft H: Trends in medical care costs: do HMOs lower the rate of growth? Med Care 18(1):1, 1980.
25. Torre E and Wolfe SM: Care of the seriously mentally ill: a rating of state programs, Washington, DC, 1986, Public Citizen Health Research Group.
26. Kiesler CA: Mental hospitals and alternative care: non-institutionalization as potential public policy for mental patients, Am Psychol 37(4):349, 1982.
27. Hospital statistics: 1987 edition, Chicago, 1987, American Hospital Association.
28. Letsch S, Levit K, and Waldo D: National health expenditures, 1987, Health Care Financ Rev 10(2):1988.
29. US Bureau of Census: Statistical abstract of the United States: 1985, Washington, DC, 1987, Table 156, US Government Printing Office.
30. Touche Ross' survey, AHA News 24(26) June 27, 1988.
31. Altman S and Rodwin M: Halfway competitive markets and ineffective regulation: the American health care system, J Health Polit Policy Law 13(2):1988.

3

Environmental Pressures from Cost Controls and Consolidation

The rising cost of health care is probably the strongest environmental force affecting health services. Payers find rising health care costs intolerable. They are forcing many organization, management, and procedural changes on the system. Are health care costs too high? Why are costs rising rapidly? Who pays for health care, and where does it go? And, what are ways to control costs? Managers need an understanding of these basic questions to develop and implement strategies to cope with external forces.

ARE HEALTH CARE COSTS TOO HIGH?

When one is ill, health care is a priceless commodity. There have been dramatic advances in medical science, but high technology is costly. Nevertheless, we have come to expect the application of these advances to curing any illness we may have, regardless of cost. We are prepared to pay any price when seriously ill. However, few individuals are aware what health care really costs because funding is channeled through third-party payers, such as private insurance, employer benefit programs, or the government.

Health care expenditures in the United States are 11% of gross national product (GNP), or about $2000 per person per year.[1] In other words, this is an average of $2000 a year that an individual cannot spend on other goods and services. Health care represents a large portion of the taxes an individual pays, and it is also a part of the cost of everything he or she purchases. Only what a person has to expend from his or her own pocket is exposed, and that seldom represents total costs.

Whether health care costs are too high depends on the perspective of the beholder, for example, that of a patient with full insurance coverage versus that of a patient with little or no insurance, or that of a hospital social worker with a relatively low wage trying to find resources to help an uninsured or underinsured person obtain needed care. When comparing health care costs with those of other advanced societies, the United States is often criticized as spending more but getting less. For example, Macrae[2] noted that the United States expended $1500 per person in 1984—considerably more than West Germany, which spent $900; France, $800; Japan, $500; and Britain, $400. Yet health status in the United States did not compare favorably with many of these countries. It did not compare favorably for life expectancy, infant mortality, or deaths from heart disease. Japan, which at that time expended one third of that of the United States for health care, had the best record on these indices. On the other hand, if one judged health status by the occurrence of cancer of the colon, Japan has the worst record. However, as noted in Chapter 2, medical care has little bearing on health status indicators compared with the impact from genetic, environmental, educational, and behavioral variables.

Whatever one's viewpoint, it is clear that payers are finding rising costs unbearable and they are forcing changes on the health system.

WHY ARE COSTS RISING?

An aging population requiring more services is an increasing contributor to rising costs. Advancing technology is also an important force to an increasing intensity of medical care services. For example, coronary artery bypass graft surgery today extends productive lives of persons who 20 years ago had prognoses for debilitation and early death. However, such surgery is likely to cost more than $50,000. On the other hand, there is uncertainty and controversy surrounding the effectiveness and efficiency of surgical versus more conservative medical interventions for certain cases.[3]

WHO PAYS AND HOW DO THEY TRY TO CONTROL COSTS AND QUALITY?

Fig. 3-1 lists who pays health system costs in the United States, how they pay them, and how they attempt to control costs and quality of the care for which they pay.

Who Pays?

Defenders of health services in the United States point to the fact that about 92% of all citizens have some form of third-party payment by the government, employers, or private insurance and only 8% are uninsured. However, the uninsured group represented nearly 40 million people in the late 1980s. In addition, there was another large group of underinsured persons.

Fig. 3-1 shows that about 29% of total system costs are supported through the federal government. This includes public health, research, construction, and other system costs, but about two thirds of total federal health care expenditures are for Medicare and Medicaid. Medicare was inaugurated in 1966 as part of the Social Security system to provide health insurance for persons over age 65. Benefits have since been extended to the disabled and their dependents and those suffering from

Who pays?			How pay?		How to control?			
			DOCTORS	HOSPITALS	SUPPLY	PERFORMANCE	PRICE	DEMANDS
Federal government 29%	Tax payers	Direct & Medicare &	FFS	PPS/DRG	Planning and facility regulation	UR/PRO	Wage and price controls (1971-1973) (RVS*1990)	PPS/DRG
State's local government 13%		Medicaid	FFS HMO	FFS,HMO, or PPS	Planning and facility regulation	UR/PRO	Rate review	PPS/DRG and HMO
Private insurance 32%	Employers		FFS,HMO, or PPO	FFS,HMO, or PPO		UR/PRO, protocols, case management	PPO	Deductibles and copay, HMO
Out of pocket 26%	Individuals		FFS	FFS		Litigation		
(Uninsured) 8%								

*Relative value scale

Fig. 3-1   Health care costs.

chronic kidney disease. Part A of the program, financed by payroll taxes collected under the Social Security system, provides a portion of hospitalization expenses and, to a very limited degree, some nursing and home care costs. Part B is a voluntary supplemental program that pays certain costs of physicians' services and other medical expenses. It is supported in part by general tax revenues and in an increasing part by contributions paid by the elderly.

Medicaid was inaugurated in 1967 also as part of the Social Security Amendments. However, unlike Medicare, Medicaid is a program run jointly by federal and state governments; the name is more or less a blanket label for 50 different state programs. It is designed to provide funding for the poor and medically indigent. Initially it was designed to bring them into the mainstream of medical care—in other words, to provide a one-class health service for all citizens. Medicaid covers hospital, physician, and skilled nursing home services. However, the program varies widely by states with the ratio of Medicaid recipients to individuals living below the poverty level ranging from 115% in Massachusetts to 24% in several states.[4]

State and local governments account for about 31% of public expenditures for health care. States, in addition to their portion of Medicaid, and localities fund public health services, public hospitals, and health services to the poor not covered by Medicaid.

The private sector covers approximately 58% of health care costs. Philanthropy, which funded most hospital costs in the nineteenth century, is now negligible in relation to total costs. Private health insurance, such as the not-for-profit Blue Cross and Blue Shield and for-profit commercial carriers and self-insured employers, provide about 32%, with premiums paid by employers and individual subscribers. The balance, about 26%, is not covered by third-party payers and therefore is paid either by individuals at the time of service or provided without reimbursement to those giving care. Uncompensated care is a serious financial burden on many providers, although providers attempt to shift such costs to private payers. The uninsured and underinsured represent an increasing problem. It is, of course, a problem for the individuals without means who are hesitant to seek care. It is a problem for financially stressed providers to give care regardless of ability to pay. Furthermore, it is an increasing problem for private payers who have such costs shifted to them. Neither Medicare nor Medicaid will support uncompensated care costs, and few health services have endowments for free care. The public/private partnership soured in the 1980s. Initially the government supported private care with Medicare and Medicaid rather than building a separate government health system. However, in the 1980s government support of care for the elderly and poor diminished, shifting increasing costs to private payers and providers.

Although payers complain that health care costs are too high, multiple funding sources have meant that no one group has had control over costs of the system. Hospitals, physicians, and other providers have been relatively free, or creative, to increase their revenues to meet rising costs. Most of the high costs are hidden from consumers through third-party payers, taxes, and in the price of goods they purchase. Health insurance carriers for the most part have been able to pass on rising costs to subscribers in the form of higher premiums or increasing deductibles and copayments. State and local governments have limited eligibility for public programs as a way to control their rising costs. The federal government has shifted rising Medicare costs to the elderly. Federal and state governments have tried a variety of means to help contain rising health care costs, but with little success. By contrast, Great Britain, with a single government source funding the National Health Service, has controlled the amount going into the system, controlled its wage scales, and delegated to regions and districts how limited monies are to be allocated. However, while Britain expends about half as much as the United States on health care, such savings take its toll in terms of long waiting lists, outdated facilities, and limited incomes of health professionals, even though there are no measurable penalties on the health status of its population.

HOW ARE PHYSICIANS PAID?

Fee-for-service (FFS) is historically and still the most prevalent payment mechanism for physicians. HMOs and PPOs are recent alternative payment mechanisms designed to help contain costs by means of competitive pricing and managed care.

Fee-for-service is, as the name implies, reimbursing the provider whatever fee he or she charges on completion of a specific service. When a patient has indemnity health insurance, he or she usually pays the doctor directly and the indemnity carrier reimburses the patient according to insurance benefits, which are usually less than medical care charges. Providers may also be paid FFS, but by the insurance carrier when the patient has a service benefit plan, such as Blue Cross and Blue Shield. Insurance carriers have more control over provider charges in a service benefit plan, but considerably more so in an HMO. Both indemnity and service benefit plans reimburse on the basis of FFS; they also allow for freedom of choice of doctors— unlike HMOs. Organized medicine has argued that FFS is important to bonding the patient/doctor relationship and that the doctor should focus only on the patient's need and not be distracted by third parties. Some doctors are concerned that third party payers with access to patient records could breach confidentiality of the patient/doctor relationship. Moreover, they argue that FFS is a control mechanism for the patient to obtain and reward provider services. The FFS financial incentive for the physician is to do as much as possible for the patient. However, more services may not necessarily be better or in the best interest of either the patient or payer. While Medicare and in some states Medicaid have changed reimbursement mechanisms to hospitals, they have to this date only threatened changes from FFS for physician reimbursement.

Prepaid health care is an alternative payment mechanism, of which HMOs are the most prevalent model. The concept of prepayment on a per capita basis can be traced back to 1721.[5] However, the term HMO was introduced by Paul Ellwood in the early 1970s based on the Kaiser Permanente model in California. The HMO concept was adopted by the federal government as a way to contain costs. HMOs have grown rapidly, representing less than 12 million members in 1982 to more than 31 million by 1988.[6] The federal government requires employers to offer an HMO alternative if they have employee health insurance benefits and if HMOs are available.

Simply stated, the HMO providers receive payment in advance for whatever care may be needed for a group of subscribers. In HMOs, patients may receive care only from those doctors who are members of the plan,* and the provider is at risk for the annual cost of care. The incentives are to maintain health of patients because providers have already collected their money. Less medical expense means higher provider income. Potential dangers for HMOs are fiscal incentives for underuse contrasted with fiscal incentives in FFS for overuse.

There are many variations and definitions of categories of HMOs, but the three categories most frequently used are (1) staff model, (2) group model, and (3) Independent Practice Association (IPA). In the *staff model,* the HMO employs physicians to provide services exclusively to HMO plan enrollees. Staff physicians are usually paid a salary. *Group model* physicians usually own the HMO or contract with it. In a prepaid group practice, such as in Kaiser Permanente, the group limits its patients to those in the HMO. Physicians in other group models may also treat a mixture of FFS and HMO patients, but all practice expenses are shared and income is distributed on a capitation or some formula basis. A variation of the group plan is the network model, where a number of groups network for purposes of the HMO. In an *IPA,*

---

*Recently many HMOs have begun to offer an indemnity option to allow patients to refer themselves to providers outside of the HMO.

physicians retain their independent practices but jointly share HMO expenditures and income while retaining their FFS practice. Income is usually distributed on the basis of physician charges, with the HMO retaining a certain percentage to cover expenses and potential losses. In fact, IPAs function much like FFS for the doctors; they bill the HMO as they would any other insurance carrier. IPAs offer a means for FFS physicians to market HMO services, but IPAs, which usually distribute income to physicians on a FFS basis, have not shown the savings found in the staff and group models.[7] Within the IPA model there are open and closed panel plans. Open panel plans are frequently sponsored by medical societies. They are open to any physician who chooses to join. Closed panel plans restrict physician membership and usually manage utilization of services more closely.

Preferred Provider Organizations (PPO) are somewhat similar to IPA HMOs in that the PPO is a corporation that receives health insurance premiums from enrolled members and contracts with independent doctors or group practices to provide care. However, it differs in that doctors are not prepaid, but they offer a discount from normal FFS charges. The advantage to the doctor in joining a PPO is access to more patients while retaining FFS. The advantage to subscribers is freedom of choice of doctors, but at higher cost if their choice is not in the PPO. PPOs, however, have few incentives to control utilization unless they adopt case management or other control procedures.

There are a number of variations and combinations of HMOs and PPOs, but objectives for such plans are to stimulate price competition and to manage care for greater efficiency. Managed care and alternative payment mechanisms to the traditional FFS and more managed care represent substantial changes in reimbursement, organization, and relationships among physicians. It has resulted in new and more influential roles for health services managers to achieve growth, cost containment, profitability, and physician satisfaction. Although HMO enrollments are increasing at a slower rate at the time of this writing, it is projected that HMOs could represent one half of the private insurance market by 1997.[8]

HOW ARE HOSPITALS PAID?

FFS has been the traditional reimbursement for hospitals, as well as physicians. While FFS remains a commonly used method of private insurance reimbursement for hospitals, other payers have imposed more cost-containment incentives on hospitals.

The prospective payment system (PPS) using diagnostic related groups (DRGs) is the current method by which hospitals are reimbursed for Medicare patients (except psychiatric patients). The 1982 and 1983 amendments to the Social Security Act established PPS, whereby hospitals are paid a preestablished amount per case treated, with payment rates varying by some 470 diagnostic groups, based on the patient's age, sex, and other clinical information. PPS and DRGs have had important implications for both hospitals and physicians. Under PPS, hospitals have incentives to attract Medicare patients who are in more profitable DRG categories, and to discharge them from the hospital as soon as possible, using fewer rather than more hospital services. Similar to HMOs, PPS fiscal incentives are to earn more by doing less for more patients. PPS has forced hospital management to improve information systems to control expenses and utilization. The medical staff organization has had to monitor utilization more closely for both quality and efficiency, and enact sanctions on physician deviants. PPS has contributed to a further decline in physician autonomy. There are conflicting arguments regarding the impact of PPS and DRGs on cost savings to the government, quality of care to patients, and solvency of hospitals. To date it appears that PPS has helped to restrain rising inpatient costs for Medicare with little empirical evidence of compromising quality of care.[9]

State reimbursement to hospitals for Medicaid patients is mixed. In some states Medicaid has adopted PPS, some require recipients to join HMOs, and in some FFS has been retained.

HOW DO PAYERS CONTROL COSTS AND QUALITY OF CARE?

The ideal way to control costs is to improve health and reduce the need for medical care. Health status of the United States' population has improved, but improvements in health status in some ways increased, not decreased, needs for medical care. For example, longevity has increased and an aging population requires more medical care. On the other hand, advances in treating heart disease have not only improved survival rates, but patients are returned to productive lives in a matter of days rather than months. Rationing medical care, that is, not meeting all needs, helps to control costs but at the expense of those who might benefit from medical care. The U.S. government has never articulated a national policy for health care, for example, that it is or is not a right of all citizens. In the United States, care has been rationed by ability to pay, whereas in the United Kingdom, it is rationed by age, delays, and need priority screened by general practitioners. In countries such as Sweden and West Germany and in the Eastern Block, medical services are essentially available to everyone, limited only by physician orders for services.

Federal and state governments have been most vulnerable to effects of cost increases on Medicare, Medicaid, and other direct care services. Since the implementation of Medicare and Medicaid, governments have attempted to control costs and quality of care by controls over (1) the supply of services, (2) performance of services, (3) price of services, and (4) most recently the demand for service (see Fig. 3-1). All of these control activities have affected the management of health services.

Controlling the Supply of Services

Until the 1980s the assumption was that demand for medical care was insatiable. Roemer's somewhat facetious law, "A built bed is a filled bed," was widely quoted. A hospital building boom after World War II was facilitated by federal construction funds from the Hill-Burton program. It was later perceived to have resulted in unnecessarily duplicated services and unnecessary costs. In 1966, along with Medicare and Medicaid, the Partnership for Health Act to accomplish comprehensive health planning was passed. Its intent was to "focus on all the people's total health needs" in planning for efficient development of facilities. In 1974 the National Health Planning and Resources Development Act was passed requiring states to institute certificate of need (CON) programs, with further requirements for limiting the development of health care facilities. The planning mechanism was costly and appeared to have little impact on costs or much even on facility development. During the Reagan Administration, most of the facility planning and regulation mechanism was dismantled.

The surplus of physicians is a more recent concern on the supply side of health care costs. It has been estimated that each physician results in medical care expenditures of at least $500,000 per year. Physicians, not patients, order services. Considerable time was required to expand the needed production of physicians after World War II. However, once needs were met, it was difficult to scale back production of physicians while trying to improve their distribution. It is possible for physicians to create their own demand within some limitations. A surplus of surgeons therefore suggests a potential increase in unnecessary surgery. However, in a free society it is difficult to prohibit qualified persons from pursuing careers of their choice.

Controlling the Performance of Health Services

Payers are concerned about efficiency of services they are purchasing, that is, that recipients obtain high quality care. The federal government legislated structures and procedures to monitor quality, as well as cost factors. In a 1972 amendment to the Social Security Act (PL 92-603), physicians were directed to establish and operate Professional Standards Review Organizations (PSROs). PSROs had three major objectives: (1) to certify that health services were necessary; (2) to ensure that quality of services met professionally recognized standards of care; and (3) to ensure that the type of facilities used were the most economical in keeping with needs of patients whose care was paid for under Medicare, Medicaid, and other federal programs. The primary operating goal was to control utilization of hospital services and thereby expenditures. It was consistent with the peer review system established by the medical profession itself and managed through the voluntary Joint Commission on Accreditation of Healthcare Organizations (JCAHO). There were mixed reviews regarding the effectiveness of PSROs. In 1982, as part of the antiregulatory program of the Reagan Administration, legislation created a successor system of Peer Review Organizations (PRO) to replace PSROs. Changes to PROs were mainly structural but in effect resulted in more regulation having a more direct, "interfering" impact on medical practice. PROs have considerable power with their ability to deny payment. Moreover, data from PRO reviews have enabled the Health Care Financing Administration (HCFA), which administers Medicare and Medicaid, to publish mortality data (controlling for severity), indicating which hospitals appear to be questionable. HCFA also has data on every physician, which is made available to hospitals for quality review purposes.

State governments' licensing role has been an ineffective monitoring mechanism. In most states, only after criminal charges are litigated can a doctor's license be removed. However, some states are becoming more active in evaluating licensed professions. Moreover, within Medicaid systems many states adopted the PRO system to monitor doctor and hospital services. Additionally, nursing home services represent a large portion of Medicaid expenditures, and states have quality reviews of such facilities and services.

Since the mid-1980s employer payers have increasingly adopted performance review as a means to help contain costs and assure quality of care. Many of the large employers have contracted with PROs or one of the proliferating private utilization review companies to monitor care received by their employees. Based on such reviews, some employers designate which providers they find effective and efficient and in some cases fully reimburse employee medical expenses only at approved services. Some employers also require authorization before a physician can perform costly treatment services. A few have even gone so far as to establish protocols that doctors must follow to be reimbursed by the insurance carrier. Although such protocols are determined by panels of doctors, it is labeled as practicing "cookbook medicine" and is an obvious restriction on physician autonomy and the exercise of professional judgment. Case management is another means employers have used to control utilization of health insurance benefits. For example, a self-insured employer might contract with a case management firm that would require a doctor to obtain approval from the case manager before specified surgical procedures, and the case management firm would then monitor the patient's progress and utilization of services while under treatment. Case management represents further intrusion on the physician's autonomy, but it can serve as an advocate for the patient. Utilization review services can cost an employer from $1.25 to $2.50 per employee per month, but savings are estimated to be $2.63 for every dollar invested.

Health care costs represent substantial expenditures for employers in the United States. For example, a few years ago the Chrysler Corporation reportedly expended nearly $6000 per auto worker for employee and retiree health and retirement benefits, whereas a Japanese competitor Mitsubishi Motors expended less than $400 per worker. American employers find they cannot afford such burdens in international markets. On the other hand, German manufacturers have even greater employee benefit costs that do not appear to overburden them.

Controlling performance is the one place that an individual patient has influence. It is very difficult for a patient to evaluate technical quality or efficiency of care. However, if they perceive they have been harmed by the provider, patients can sue for malpractice. Malpractice suits are a major threat to physicians. In addition, the high cost of malpractice insurance (more than $50,000 annually for some specialties in some cities) and defensive medicine to avoid suits add to rising costs of health care. Contingency cases, where the plaintiff pays lawyer and court costs only if he or she obtains an award, contribute to the frequency of malpractice suits in the United States. Other countries do not allow contingency cases; consequently, aggrieved parties are more cautious about bringing suit. The implications of malpractice litigation for health services managers are a further complication for management. On the other hand, protecting the organization from suits increases the importance of management and is a source of managerial power. Managers can use the threat of patient or employee litigation to obtain support for managerial requests, although ethics of such tactics may be questionable if there is no real threat.

Controlling the Price of Services

Price controls have been a primary source of cost control in countries with nationally mandated health insurance. In Japan, for example, national health insurance fee schedules do not reimburse surgical procedures and high technology at high rates, such as received by providers in the United States. There is less financial incentive to develop such services in Japan, and costs are contained by reimbursing surgical procedures at lower rates. In West Germany, the various sickness funds negotiate medical fees with doctor and hospital associations, arriving at a consensus that costs shall increase by a given amount that year. Doctors are limited not only by fee schedules, but doctor associations monitor utilization to guard against doctors doing more procedures to increase income. Hospitals are reimbursed on a per diem basis, providing incentives for long lengths of stay but disincentives to intensive care. Canada too, with its national health insurance, uses control over prices as one means to contain rising costs.

In 1971 to 1973 during the Nixon Administration, controls were imposed on wages and prices of medical care and other goods and services. Health care cost increases were contained during that period. However, after controls were lifted from other industries, the health industry claimed it was being discriminated against and quality of care was suffering. When wage and price controls were removed, health care costs shot up, wiping out any savings from 1971 to 1973. Price controls are currently being considered by HCFA. The commission that recommended a relative value scale system proposed a fee schedule that would reimburse physicians, for instance, on the basis of time and training. It is expected to have a major impact on redistribution of physician fees in which time-based practices would gain and procedure-based specialties, such as surgery, would have reductions.

At the state level, controls over hospital prices were enacted in a number of states. Rate review in New York and New Jersey were shown to have helped to contain hospital costs, whereas in others it had little impact and later was abolished under the assumption that competitive systems would obviate the need for rate review.[10]

Many employers have contracted with PPOs, which are competitive price control methods. Negotiating discounts with PPOs provides employers some influence over prices and, coupled with monitoring utilization, prior authorization, and protocols, gives larger employers considerable influence over both prices and utilization. Such controls also limit the autonomy of providers. Individuals also have some influence over the price they pay for insurance when there are choices among FFS, HMOs, and/or PPOs.

A major objective of PPOs and HMOs is to establish price competition to help contain rising costs. They have extracted discounts from hospitals and other referring agencies, but to date most hospitals and others have been able to compensate for losses by increases to fee-for-service patients and by general price increases. Moreover, preliminary evidence suggests that HMOs and PPOs do not compete on price but focus their marketing on quality of care.[11,12] There is little evidence that HMO competition has contained costs.[11] Price competition may have lowered premium costs to some employers who implemented direct provider bidding, but to date health services have apparently been able to increase income from other sources to make up for premium savings.

Controlling prices has implications for health services managers. First, the service must be efficient if it cannot freely raise prices to cover costs. Price competition means increasing attention to product line management, targeted marketing, and utilization controls. Price competition also enhances the power, as well as burdens, of management to limit wage increases and to decrease staff. Such competitive pressures have resulted in United States' health services changing from a service-driven system to a market-driven system.

Controlling Demand for Health Care

With the failure of government controls over supply of services, performance, and prices, efforts in the 1980s focused on the control of demand. Previously, individuals with full-coverage health insurance had no financial disincentives to use the benefits available to them. Certainly, providers who were reimbursed FFS had no disincentives to apply all services that could possibly help a patient. Recognizing that both providers and consumers had disincentives to containing costs, payers inaugurated incentives for cost containment.

The federal government inaugurated PPS and DRGs as incentives to hospitals to reduce the demand for long lengths of stay and use of hospital services. As noted, hospitals gain by shorter lengths of stay and less intensive care than projected by DRGs. Hospital management through utilization review processes monitor physician treatment services to help keep them within DRG limits. This represents a further intrusion on physician autonomy.

State governments reduced demand for services by reducing eligibility for Medicaid and other state services in the 1980s. This placed burdens on the poor and near poor who no longer had coverage to demand medical services. State governments have also placed incentives to reduce provider demands for intensive and lengthy service to Medicaid patients by adopting PPS or HMO payment systems. States that require Medicaid recipients to use HMOs also require HMOs to establish quality assurance systems. Quality assurance systems represent management intrusion on physician autonomy in outpatient services, an area previously exempt from control.

Most employers have put the burden for cost-containment incentives on the patient. That is, they have increased the copayment and deductible portion that must be paid by the patient. By bearing more of the cost of care, patients demand less service. They are more likely to postpone seeking care and request that doctors take a more conservative approach to treatment. A Rand Corporation study that randomly assigned patients to full-pay and copay plans found as much as 50% reduction in costs with minimal negative impact on health status of the copay patients.[13] Many employers have adopted direct provider bidding to HMOs and PPOs, placing the burden for reducing demand for care on the providers. In such cases employees are penalized financially if they select plans that provide freedom of choice of physicians and fees-for-services.

Reducing demand for service also had a major impact on management of health services because of problems with uncompensated care. The uninsured and underinsured suffer when they do not seek care when it is needed, but when they do obtain care for which they cannot pay, providers have problems shifting such costs elsewhere.

Reduced demand means that those who do receive care are sicker and require more intensive services. Reduced demand with excess medical care providers also contributes to increasing competition.

FUTURE PROSPECTS FOR COST CONTROLS

Is it possible to gain control over health care costs? So far there is little evidence that it is possible. Twenty years ago when health care costs started to rise so dramatically, many thought it was intolerable to go above 6% or 7% of GNP. Today some say 15% is the limit. In the near future, an aging population, "medicalization" of social problems such as substance abuse, and increasing numbers of AIDS patients (whose lifetime medical care costs are estimated at about $62,000 per patient in 1991)[14] suggest continued acceleration of health care costs. There is a relation between national wealth and health care.[15] If the United States continues to prosper, it can probably afford continued increases, including coverage for the uninsured and underinsured population.

However, should the United States face a serious depression, major war, or similar calamity, it is conceivable that the financing and even the delivery of health care could be nationalized. If private insurers find health care no longer to be profitable, the government will have to assume that responsibility. If physicians realize that because of their surplus, they can no longer make it in the private sector, they will accept government service to survive and practice what they have been trained to do. Hospitals too could be nationalized as have railroads, schools, and other essential services that can no longer survive as private industries in a difficult economic environment. Although such a scenario may seem remote now, it is worth remembering that the United States is unique among most developed nations in not having a governmentally organized health care system (although a few, such as Great Britain, have in recent years taken tentative steps toward privatization).

IMPLICATIONS OF COST CONTROL ON MANAGEMENT OF HEALTH SERVICES

Forces for cost containment have in the last decade or so had a major impact on the management of health services. Health services values have changed from solely a service orientation to one of a business enterprise; information systems have become as sophisticated as those of commercial industries; the number of generalist and clinical managers and management specialists has grown rapidly; and power within health services has shifted from trustees and physicians toward management. In the near future the trend toward increasing importance of management is likely to continue. However, there is nothing so certain as change. Should a national disaster, such as a depression, occur, savings could be made in the $24.5 billion administrative component of health services expended in 1986. Although reductions in administrative costs would be beneficial to the economy, the specialty of health services management could be one of the casualties with reduced job opportunities.

Perhaps the greatest effect of cost containment and competition has been the consolidation of health delivery services into large horizontal and vertical multi-institutional health systems.

CONSOLIDATION OF HEALTH SERVICES

Hospital mergers and closures have been experienced in many cities and rural areas. For example, ten hospitals in Chicago closed in just 3 years, between 1985 and 1988. Many of these were hospitals that served mainly the poor. The number of HMOs grew rapidly in the early 1980s, but this growth slowed by 1990 as many of them merged into larger organizations. Physicians are entering group practices at a rapid rate as HMO and PPO managed care systems grow. In the 1970s and early 1980s, investor-owned, for-profit hospitals became aggressive buyers of hospitals. Not-for-profit hospital corporations also acquired a number of hospitals and for-profit related organizations. Why has consolidation occurred, how have services consolidated, is consolidation into vertical, horizontal, and for-profit services beneficial, and how has consolidation affected management of health services?

Why Have Health Services Consolidated?

Historically and until the 1980s most health services were autonomous units. For decades, the United States' public demanded that hospitals be built so that travel distance and time were at a minimum. For example, Congress enacted the Hospital Survey and Construction Act (Hill-Burton) in 1954, which in policy stated that Congress would provide the means to meet the needs of citizens and increase access to medical care through financing the construction of new hospitals. However, in the 1960s and 1970s a number of health planning laws were enacted in attempt to consolidate and control health services facilities as a way to reduce unnecessary duplication and costs.

Government policies, however, failed to achieve consolidation of services. Rather, it was cost containment and market forces to which multisystem developments can be attributed.[16] Consolidation was not unique to health services in the 1980s. Air lines, newspapers, breweries, and many other industries experienced a wave of mergers and buy-outs. Some of the same reasons for consolidation in those industries apply to health services, as well as some different reasons. Indeed, in the late 1980s the federal government, fearing too much consolidation, began to apply antitrust laws to hospital mergers. For example, the U.S. Department of Justice challenged the merger of two of the three Rockford, Illinois, hospitals on the grounds that it was anticompetitive and would increase health care costs to consumers. The two hospitals, on the other hand, testified that merger would result in elimination of duplicated services and savings of more than $40 million in 5 years.[17]

There are a number of reasons why consolidation has occurred. Cost containment has been a major factor underlying the need for consolidation. Medicare and Medicaid no longer merely cover whatever the hospital finds are its costs. Many rural and innercity hospitals serve mainly the elderly and poor and have limited opportunity to

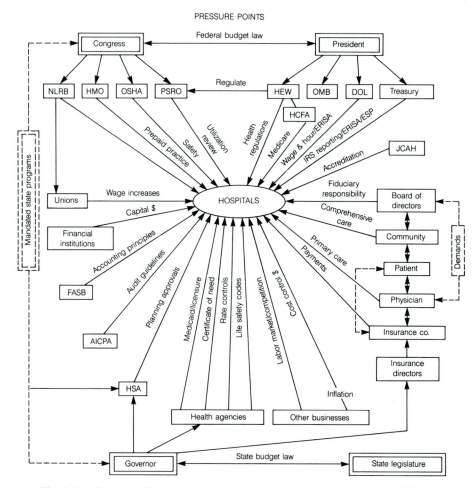

Fig. 3-2   External influences and constraints on hospital management. (From *Managerial cost accounting for hospitals*, published by the American Hospital Association: AHA, Chicago, 1980. Reprinted with permission from AHA.)

shift costs of uncompensated care to others. Such hospitals are frequently absorbed by other institutions or go out of business entirely. Smaller organizations have particular problems competing with larger facilities. Fig. 3-2 shows some of the pressure points on hospitals from a variety of sources in 1980. Since that time, even greater pressures have been added, such as business coalitions that organize business interests to intervene on hospital costs and services. Pressures from competing hospitals, physician-owned organizations, and multihealth service systems are not shown on the figure and are major factors in problems of smaller organizations. It takes a large organization to hire the management specialists needed in a competitive environment for finance and accounting, marketing, risk management, information systems, and others. Larger organizations extract more favorable prices from suppliers. High technology services require a larger volume to provide quality care. Consequently, patients requiring higher technology services are referred to subspecialists in large medical centers.

In predicting that only half of the hospitals in existence in 1988 will be needed by the year 2010, Jeffrey Goldsmith expects medical advances will concentrate on helping patients to live with their illnesses rather than on curing them.[18] As a result, he suggests, the home and other residential settings, such as retirement centers, will be the dominant places for health care delivery in the future.

How Have Health Services Consolidated?

Health services have consolidated both horizontally and vertically. Johnson[19] describes a vertically integrated system as a combination of "different kinds of health care delivery units, such as clinics, hospitals, ambulatory care institutions, long-term care, and/or mental health facilities" (p. 405). An HMO, such as the Kaiser Permanente system, is an example of a vertically integrated system. An advantage of vertical systems is that they formalize arrangements for comprehensive services in a continuum. Thus formal understandings are reached regarding referrals. However, services in a vertical system are likely to give up autonomy. In addition, patients may feel that they have given up choice of sources of care.

Horizontal integration involves the combination of similar health care units, such as a number of hospitals or long-term care facilities, in order to share administrative and medical technology. An investor-owned or Catholic hospital multihospital system is an example of horizontal integration. By 1987, 45% of community hospitals in the United States belonged to systems defined as two or more hospitals with a common form of ownership, according to the American Hospital Association.

Starkweather[20] suggests seven dimensions of facility combinations in a range from pluralism to fusion. Table 3-1 shows general models for combining and/or regionalizing hospital services on a vertical, horizontal, or regional basis. The models are based on scope and depth of services and referral patterns. There can be modifications or combinations of these models, and within each one the arrangements can vary from informal pluralism to fusion.

INVESTOR-OWNED HEALTH SYSTEMS

Another development of the corporation of United States' medicine is the growth of for-profit health services in the 1980s. Depending on an individual's feelings toward such organizations, they have been called "the medical-industrial complex"[21] or for-profits, investor-owned, and tax-paying health services. We use the more neutral term of *investor owned,* or IO. The IOs had rapid growth in the early and mid-1980s into horizontal hospital or HMO systems at first, and later into vertical systems. However, some of the large IO hospital systems that ventured into HMO insurance and physician services lost millions of dollars, and they retreated back into hospital services. Some of the largest IO HMOs also sustained huge losses in the late 1980s, some of them filing bankruptcy and/or extracting losses from participating physicians.

A lesser publicized development of IOs was the unbundling of not-for-profit (NFP)

Table 3-1 Seven dimensions of health facility combination on scale of pluralism to fusion

Dimension	Pluralism		Informal (latent)	Mergers	Fusion
	Informal (preformal)	Shared services, joint undertakings, cooperatives, affiliations	Consolidations, multiple units under single management, satellites, branches, chains		
I Organizational pattern	Informal relationships, complete formal integrity	Voluntary subscriptions, joint development of support services	Tradeoff agreements Common delegation of authority to outside agency	Absorption Fusion	
II Legal bonds	Preformal relationships, formal independence	Implied agreements Contracts Formal agreements with escape provisions	Formal agreements, permanent, which preserve self-sufficiency of prior organizations	Formal agreements, permanent, which prohibit independent operation Replacement agreements	
III Nature of combined services	Informal arrangements, no formally shared services	Support and administrative services only	Professional services	Direct patient care services ambulatory inpatient both	
IV Stages and forms of production	Natural exchanges formal separation	Affiliations	Vertical combinations	Horizontal combinations, transformations	
V Geography of population served	Natural regionalization and localization	Dispersed populations	Common geographic population, partial services	Common geographic population, all types of services Geographic expansion	
VI Facility location	Distant	Same community	Approximate, adjacent	Contiguous, integrated	
VII Organizational impact	Unofficial relationships, status quo	Minimal to changes of tasks, jobs, rules	Substantial—new function, reorganization of departments	Evolutionary—system-wide changes, deliberate restructuring Spontaneous—sudden impact, unpredictable consequences	

From Starkweather D: Health facility mergers: some conceptualizations, Med Care 9(6):473, 1971.

hospital services into for-profit (FP) services. For example, a hospital might spin off its laboratory into a FP corporation with better access to capital and, through sales to physicians and smaller hospitals, a source of contributions to the hospital. This usually meant first establishing an umbrella corporate organization of which the hospital, laboratory, and other FP and NFP facilities would be a part.

ARE HORIZONTAL, VERTICAL, AND FOR-PROFIT CONSOLIDATIONS BENEFICIAL?

Table 3-2 lists some of the advantages and disadvantages of horizontal, vertical, and for-profit consolidations. Advantages and disadvantages vary, depending on the evaluators perspective, for example, that of the institution, a physician, or the community and patient. Evaluations will also vary from organization to organization, but Table 3-2 presents some general advantages and disadvantages. Generally, consolidated services offer (1) more access to capital to improve facilities and (2) economies of scale to improve technical services. On the other hand, the institution's staff, physicians, and community lose considerable autonomy in consolidated services.

There has been considerable research into the benefits of multi-institutional systems. Shortell in a review of these studies concludes[22] (p. 183):

> Thus, there is little support for any of the alleged advantages of system hospitals relative to their nonsystem counterparts. Little, if any, economic or service "value added" appears to be present. This is consistent with the view, mentioned before, that the major reason for most system affiliation has been the search for security and protection—a defensive retreat from a highly uncertain, complex, and hostile environment.

Investor-owned organizations have been accused of "cream skimming," that is, serving only the more profitable patients; they respond that they pay taxes that equate the cost of care for such patients in other institutions. Moreover, findings suggest that in areas where the IO is the only facility, it is just as likely to provide free care as NFPs and just as likely as NFP chains in competitive environments.[23] We suggest that the difference between the FP and NFP is not great. It is our belief that the NFPs who have to focus on bottom lines and markets function as FPs. Based on our anecdotal evidence and also that of others who have surveyed a number of multihospital systems, the NFP system that has clear priorities for service over bottom line financial success is rare. As one administrator told us, "Most hospitals have floated bonds to finance our facility development. What really drives us and our counterparts at budget allocation time is our bond rating." With such motives it is not surprising that there are federal, state, and local efforts to remove tax-exempt status of hospitals.

IMPLICATIONS OF CONSOLIDATION ON MANAGEMENT OF HEALTH SERVICES

It is predicted that instead of the 300,000 or so current systems of independent doctors, hospitals, and other services, before the year 2000 there will be less than 100

Table 3-2 Advantages and disadvantages of consolidation of health service to the institution, physicians, community, and patients

Type of consolidation	Institution		Physician		Community and patients	
	Advantage	**Disadvantage**	**Advantage**	**Disadvantage**	**Advantage**	**Disadvantage**
Horizontal, e.g., multihospital system	Access to capital Economics of scale Management resources Improved recruitment More political power Hospital survival	Loss of autonomy	Higher technology Access to specialists Hospital survival	Less influence over management Easier for management to close the hospital	Higher technology Less duplication of services	Higher costs Less influence over management Easier to close the hospital
Vertical systems, e.g., HMO, clinic, and hospital	Offer full range of services More competitive Economics of scale Articulation of services More political power	Loss of autonomy	Unified support systems Marketing support to retain patients More peer review	Less autonomy Less freedom of referrals	Less costly Continuity of care Less duplication of services	Less freedom of choice Less personalized service
Investor-owned	Access to capital More freedom to serve organization goals	Stock holder and corporate control	Responsive to phys. requests that increase income	Less autonomy	Pay taxes	Profit priorities

and possibly only 20 supermedical corporations. Such predictions appear unrealistic at this time; nevertheless, the trend toward consolidation of services at least at the local level continues. Physicians are joining HMOs and joining or forming group practices to cope with cost-containment forces and increasing competition. Other health services, such as home care, long-term care, and rehabilitation services, are affiliating if not merging with hospitals and other services. Managers in larger systems have less autonomy. They must be responsive to the management strategies of the umbrella organization, they must be adept with management information and control systems, and they must have networking and negotiation skills to obtain resources required for the service.

We now move from the environment to implementation of strategic management and the internal management of hospitals and health services to cope with and utilize the forces of change for health services performance.

REFERENCES

1. Letsch SW, Levit KR, and Waldo DR: National health expenditures: 1987, Health Care Financ Rev 10(2):109, 1988.
2. Macrae N: Health Care International: better care at one-eighth the cost? Economist, April 28, p 17, 1984.
3. Sawitz E et al: The use of in-hospital physician services for acute myocardial infarction, JAMA 259(16):2419, 1988.
4. Muse DN and Sawyer D: The Medicare and Medicaid data book, HCFA Pub No 03128, Washington, DC, 1981, US Dept of Health & Human Services.
5. From a letter to Cadwallader Colden: Letters from Dr. William Douglas to Cadwallader Colden of New York, Collections of the Massachusetts Historical Society, 4th Series, 2:164, 1854.
6. Inter Study Center for Managed Care Research as reported in: Data watch: an HMO industry profile, Business & Health, p 6, June, 1989.
7. Luft HS: Health maintenance organizations: dimensions of performance, New York, 1981, John Wiley & Sons, Inc.
8. AHA News 24(28):3, 1988.
9. Davis CK and Rhodes DJ: The impact of DRGs on cost and quality of health care in the United States, Health Policy 9:117, 1988 and Hellinger FJ: Reimbursement under diagnostic-related groups: the Medicaid experience, Health Care Financ Rev 8(2), 1988.
10. Morrisey MA, Sloan FA, and Mitchell SA: State rate setting: an analysis of some unresolved issues, Health Aff 4(2):36, 1983.
11. McLaughlin CG: Market responses to HMOs: price competition or rivalry? Inquiry 25:207, 1988.
12. Feldman R et al: The competitive impact of health maintenance organizations on hospital finances: an exploratory study, J Health Polit Policy Law 10(4):675, 1986 and Luft HS, Maerki S, and Trauner JB: The competitive effects of health maintenance organizations: another look at evidence from Hawaii, Rochester, and Minneapolis/St. Paul, J Health Polit Policy Law 10(4):625, 1986.
13. Newhouse JP et al: Some interim results from a controlled trial of cost sharing in health insurance, N Engl J Med 305(25):1501, 1981.
14. Hellinger FJ: Forecasting and personal medical care costs of acquired immunodeficiency syndrome from 1988 through 1991, Public Health Rep May-June 1988.
15. Maxwell RJ: Health and wealth: an international study of health care spending, Lexington, Ma, 1981, Lexington Books.
16. American Medical News: Big firms seen dominating health care, p 2, March 1, 1985.
17. AHA News: Antitrust trial on hospital merger wrapped up, 24(29) July 18, 1988.
18. AHA News: Goldsmith: half of today's hospitals won't be needed two decades from now, 24(33), August 15, 1988.
19. Johnson AC: Management of health institutions. In Bittle R, editor: Encyclopedia of professional management, New York, 1978, McGraw-Hill, Inc.

20. Starkweather D: Health facility mergers: some conceptualizations, Med Care 9(3) Nov-Dec, 1971.
21. Relman AS: The new medical-industrial complex, N Engl J Med 38(17):963, 1980.
22. Shortell SM: The evolution of hospital systems: unfulfilled promises and self-fulfilling prophesies, Med Care Rev 45(2):177, 1988.
23. Shortell SM: The effects of hospital ownership on nontraditional services, Health Aff 5:97, 1986.

II

STRATEGIC MANAGEMENT

4

Strategic Management Defined

We deliberate not about ends but about means. For a doctor does not deliberate whether he shall heal, nor an orator whether he shall persuade, nor a statesman whether he shall produce law and order, nor does anyone else deliberate about his end. They assume the end and consider how and by what means it is to be attained; and if it seems to be produced by several means they consider which it is most easily and best produced, while if it is achieved by one only they consider how it is achieved by this and what means this will be achieved, till they come to the first cause, which in the order of discovery is last. For the person who deliberates seems to investigate and analyze in the way described as though he were analyzing a geometrical construction, all investigation appears to be deliberation—for instance, mathematical investigation—and what is last in the order of analysis seems to be first in the order of becoming. And if we come on an impossibility, we give up the search, e.g. if we need money and this cannot be got; but if a thing appears possible we try to do it.

ARISTOTLE: *NICOMACHEAN ETHICS*

Although the word strategy implies long-range change, it also has some other intriguing implications. The definition appearing in the *Random House Dictionary of the English Language* (Unabridged, 1967) is most appropriate: "a plan, method, or series of maneuvers or stratagems for obtaining a specific goal or result; a strategy for getting ahead in the world."

The word *strategy* comes from the Greek word *strategia,* which means general or generalship. This military relationship has continued through the centuries, and you will find strategy and the related word *tactics* in present-day military leadership training programs. The military has made a useful distinction between strategy and tactics. Once again using the Random House dictionary definition, we note that *strategy* is the utilization of a nation's forces, through large-scale, longrange planning and development, to ensure security or victory. *Tactics* deals with the use and deployment of troops in actual combat. We will use *strategy* to refer to the long-range plans an organization requires and *tactics* to mean the implementation through daily operations to reach those plans but, of course, drop the military connotation.

There is one additional footnote that should be added to our exploration of the word *strategy*. You have noted that the definition of strategy contained a reference to strategem. An alternative definition of strategy is the skillful use of a stratagem. A stratagem can be considered as "any artifice, ruse, or trick devised or used to attain a goal or to gain an advantage over an adversary" (Random House dictionary). Thus a skillful use of a stratagem could be for a husband or wife to *seem* always to agree with his or her spouse to gain some ulterior goal. In a business setting a stratagem could be to gain an advantage over competitors by skillful advertising.

Note that a stratagem could also utilize unethical behavior, which raises the question of social responsibilities of health care organizations. We explore this further in the last chapter.

Earlier we said that strategy had been substituted for long range in the identification of long-range planning. More recently management has been substituted for planning. Hence, long-range planning has evolved to *strategic management*. Note the shift from the noun *strategy* to the adjective *strategic*. This implies a unique approach to management as indeed it is. Furthermore, in actual practice the development of a strategy (plan of action) cannot realistically be isolated from the mission or goal of the organization or the operationalization or implementation of the strategy. The development and utilization of a strategy does not take place in a vacuum. The characteristics of *strategic management* include the environmental or situational analysis to ascertain the organization's posture, the utilization of resources to gain the goals of the organization, and the operationalization of strategic management to implement and evaluate the adequacy of the resultant actions and outcomes. The key words are *environment, goals, resources,* and *operationalization*. A modern interpretation of Aristotle!

We believe that various interpretations, the evolutionary development of concepts, and the results of research activities have produced a modern definition of strategic management. By strategic management we mean the establishment of the organization's missions or goals, the formulation of a strategy or strategies (plan[s]) congruent with the environment both internal and external to the firm, and the operationalization (implementation of tactics) of the strategy or strategies, including the evaluation of the results and the possible redeployment of resources. This strategic management approach will enable health care managers to meet the challenges embodied in the changing environment for health care delivery outlined in previous chapters.

THE CONCEPT OF ULTRASTABLE EQUILIBRIUM

An underlying assumption in our definition of strategic management is that an organization is an open system; that is, it exists in a constantly (potentially, at least), changing relationship with its environment. In a changing environment an open system either changes with the environment or perishes. The system or organization "survives" these changes in the environment through adaptation by means of the processes of learning and innovation. As the learning and innovation processes are successful, the organization achieves a state of ultrastability. Great Britain is an example of a survival organization as it met the changes entailed in medieval, mercantile, capitalistic, and

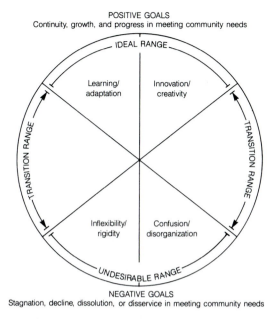

POSITIVE GOALS
Continuity, growth, and progress in meeting community needs

IDEAL RANGE

Learning/
adaptation

Innovation/
creativity

TRANSITION RANGE

TRANSITION RANGE

Inflexibility/
rigidity

Confusion/
disorganization

UNDESIRABLE RANGE

NEGATIVE GOALS
Stagnation, decline, dissolution, or disservice in meeting community needs

Fig. 4-1   Achieving ultrastability through strategic management.

socialistic periods. Companies such as General Motors, Du Pont, and General Electric have survived similar kinds of changes in the environment. The concept of ultrastability or dynamic equilibrium permits us to employ some of the concepts of the science of cybernetics with its concerns of regulation, control, and homeostasis to explain the structure and behavior of organizations using the strategies they develop and implement. The basic problem is to incorporate the opposite concepts of change and order relative to a state of stability. However, if stability in an organization is a moving state toward the achievement of ultrastability, an explanation of the necessity for strategic management is possible. The following paragraphs sketch the process. The discussion generally follows an approach versus avoidance, or positive versus negative, format.

Fig. 4-1 is a schematic conceptualization of the organization and its operations. Primary consideration must be given to the goals or mission. The positive goals are continuity, growth, and progress in meeting community needs, whereas the negative goals to be avoided are stagnation, decline, and dissolution and disservice or irrelevance in meeting community needs. Within this framework the process of strategic management is enacted. Obviously the goals or mission are affected by the values of top management of the organization, and more will be said about goals, missions, and objectives in a later chapter.

How does the strategic manager operate? Basically he or she manages by pursuing strategies ranging from innovation/creativity and learning/adaptation. Innovation and creativity involve the introduction of new strategies (plans), stratagems (courses of action), research and development (procedures and technology), and operating procedures (participatory management or computerization). Learning or adaptation is a more stabilizing activity that attempts to control the system. Some of the rationality ideas embodied in scientific management (training) and the administrative management model (management by objectives) are illustrative examples. We do not agree with some theorists studying natural systems who conclude that there isn't much that managers can do because external events control and managers react. Our premise is that there is rationality relative to open systems, and therefore management does make a difference.

It is important to our discussion that (1) both innovation/creativity and learning/adaptation be considered positive in their orientation with respect to achieving the positive goals or mission of the organization or health care system, and (2) that each is equally desirable at any one point in time. In achieving positive goals, each health care organization and unit within the organization must include elements of innovation and learning. The dynamics of the situation are such that as progress is made, there is in the actual operating situation an oscillation or shifting in emphasis between these two basically desirable concepts. An indication of progress can be suggested by reference to a person walking up an unending staircase. A step upward represents innovation or creativity and is followed by a period of learning and adaptation. The moment of pause or rest when climbing stairs can be thought of as the period of equilibrium in preparation for the next step upward. As progress up the stairs is made, the position of ultrastability is achieved without sacrifice to stability or stagnation. In other words, there is a blending of innovation/creativity and learning/adaptation to changing community needs and the utilization of resources for meeting those needs.

In the undesirable range are inflexibility/rigidity, confusion/disorganization, and disservice. These are negative goals and are to be avoided. They may be the result of inappropriate management. Note also in Fig. 4-1 that there are operating limits. The ideal range for most organizations is relatively small, but the transition period into the undesirable range is quite large. Many organizations have fallen into the transition range but have recovered. The U.S. automobile industry in the early 1980s is a case in point. Whether all organizations can successfully navigate the transitional range and achieve continuity through a combination of learning and innovation may not be evident for many years. It should also be pointed out that once the transition stage is reached, great care is required so that the downward flow of the "roller coaster" does not quickly land a health care organization in the dissolution stage. Just as a roller coaster picks up increasing speed in the downward descent, so does the organization. This has been evident in some of our major industries, such as railroads and steel. Care must be exercised so that a similar kind of development does not occur in health care to the detriment of present and prospective patients, for example, just because we have overcapacity in some hospitals and in some medical specialties. A major factor in achieving ultrastability and the positive goals of continuity, growth, and progress is through strategic management. The next section outlines the major components in the strategic management process.

THE STRATEGIC MANAGEMENT PROCESS

The act of discovery can be physical, perceptual, or intellectual. For the explorer, whether of the universe, the planet Earth, or the world of ideas, the excitement comes

Table 4-1   The strategic management process

Major components	Processes
Planning	Determining mission, goals, and objectives Surveillance External environmental analysis Internal analysis Determining capabilities Strategic choice Developing the strategic plan
Implementation	Motivation Change Structure Resource deployment Policies Culture
Evaluation/Control	Evaluation Effectiveness Strategic plan revision Redeployment

from seeing something one has not seen before, from seeing familiar things in a new and different light, or from bringing things together in a fuller conceptual framework. Strategic management is such an exploration—an exploration of the dynamic process, whereby managers interact with the everchanging environment in which the health care organization exists.

Strategic management can be thought of as three fairly distinct but interactive stages: (1) the planning stage—the estimate of the situation and formulation of guiding strategies (plans); (2) the implementation (operational) stages—basically who will do what, where, when, and how; and (3) the evaluation/control stage—supervision of the strategies to ensure that "the best laid plans of mice and men don't 'gang oft agley,'" and that gains don't lapse, that momentum is maintained, that goals and plans are adjusted with environmental changes, and that plans will benefit from the experience.

The major components of the strategic management process are outlined briefly here but will be discussed in more detail throughout the book.

THE MAJOR COMPONENTS OF THE STRATEGIC MANAGEMENT PROCESS

Table 4-1 presents a model of the strategic management process. Although the figure and our discussion suggest discrete steps and a time frame of reference in terms of orderly progression through the model, it should be remembered that the process is continuous and complementary. However, for purposes of presentation and discussion, it is necessary to analyze each unit separately. Each will be reviewed briefly here and in more detail in subsequent chapters.

The first major component of the strategic management process involves planning leading to the development of the strategic plan. Planning begins with an examination of the mission and goals of the health care organization. What does the organization seek to accomplish? Why is it in existence? Who will be the people served? In light of the mission or purpose of the organization, the external and internal environmental information is analysed to ascertain short-term, as well as long-term, goals and objectives. In this book, a goal or an objective will be used to indicate an end to be accomplished to achieve the mission of the organization. Although it is possible to distinguish between a goal and an objective, they will be used interchangeably.

An appreciation of the necessity and breadth of objectives can be ascertained by reference to Drucker's[1] conclusion that objectives are necessary in a number of areas for the firm to survive. Because Drucker was referring to business organizations, we have taken the liberty to paraphrase his set of "survival" objectives slightly for them to be pertinent to health care organizations. We also suggest they be considered "service" objectives in keeping with a mission of a health care organization.

Quality of care—efficiency and effectiveness
Innovation—avoidance of obsolescence
Professional relationships—physicians, nurses, for example
Human organization—selection and development
Social responsibility—external/internal environment
Marketing—creating patient access
Financial resources—financial management
Physical resources—adequacy and efficiency (p. 100)

An underlying activity in the strategic management process is surveillance. For the strategist to make wise decisions and plans, it is necessary to obtain information about both the external and internal environment. The CEO's staff must establish the intelligence units. This may be very informal, involving employees and reports, journals, and friends. In some large units the network is formalized to include surveys, special studies and reports, and consultants. Whatever approach is used, it is necessary that a communication network be established because no health service establishment is a unit unto itself at this time when there is such turbulence in the environment.

The second component of the strategic management process is implementation or operationalization of the strategies. The first major consideration relates to the resources that are needed—human, material, and financial. Obviously these require some type of budget commitment and also policies (courses of action) related to each area.

Operationalization of strategy (sometimes referred to as tactics) usually requires change of some sort. Managers therefore become change agents in the accomplishment of the strategies. Change must permeate the organization, and it often requires great finesse to obtain a positive response to change—especially at lower levels in the organization where communication networks have considerable static.

Another aspect of operationalization involves establishing the proper structure wherein the strategy operationalization occurs. Rigidity of structure can produce stagnation with considerable "dead-wood" and obsolete offices and departments. Matrix organization structures have sometimes produced good results by permitting a person to hold a position in his or her parent department and also participate in a new project

or program, which may be of limited duration but will, for example, meet the conditions of a government contract. This is quite usual in patient care team arrangements.

The third major segment of the strategic management process is evaluation/control. Evaluation requires the measurement of the effectiveness of the strategy. Did the strategy meet the objectives, and if not, why not? Related to the effectiveness issue is whether resources should be redeployed and/or a new strategy established. Obviously this requires constant surveillance by the intelligence unit and feedback to the interested parties. Control is needed to assure that performance is as expected. If change in the strategic plan is needed or redeployment of resources is necessary, change should be made as quickly as possible, even to reworking the entire strategic plan.

We now turn our attention to the actions or activities of the strategic manager in the system.

THE ROLE OF THE STRATEGIC MANAGER

Successful managers develop a style that suits their particular experiences and their overall situation. Management style involves being an entrepreneur—initiating and controlling change in the organization. It involves leadership and setting direction through the strategic plan and the supervision of people so that they can be innovators themselves but not at the expense of the organization failing to achieve its mission. The manager must develop a style that provides motivation for the employees of the health care organization to achieve its mission. From time to time conflicts will arise, and the manager must resolve them in a way that results in equity and fairness. Finally, the strategic manager must provide the resources so that employees can perform. This is often a problem if resources are limited or if employees believe they require what are actually excessive resources. Indeed, with the development and use of computers (information systems) and similar technical equipment, the subject of resources and their deployment may become even more important in the future.

The transformation of the organization to meet changes and challenges in the environment may indeed require new leadership skills. The impact of environmental changes results in organizations that are increasingly open systems—the relationships with stakeholders discussed in Chapter 1. This situation and the resulting development of strategic management necessitates a new look at leadership skills. To this end Byrd[2] suggests the following categories of leadership skills:

- *Anticipatory skills*—accept that the "world" is constantly changing, networking with constituencies and building coalitions, or as Robert Greenleaf[3] states in *Servant Leadership,* "The leader needs two intellectual abilities that are usually not formally assessed in an academic way: he needs to have a sense for the unknowable and to be able to foresee the unforeseeable. Leaders know some things and foresee some things which those they are presuming to lead do not know or foresee so clearly."
- *Visioning skills*—inducing a group to take action in accord with the leader's purposes involving people in shaping the vision of the future, and developing "pictures" for employees of desirable future states.
- *Value-congruence skills*—the importance of values and beliefs in motivating and giving meaning to people at work, and developing consistency in applying values.

■ *Empowerment skills*—sharing of power but not giving away a finite portion of his or her power, releasing power in others, unlocking motivation in others and developing people.

■ *Self-understanding skills*—introspective skills, developing frameworks for understanding self as well as others, and developing an inventory of self.

Legend has it that General Nathan Bedford Forrest, one of the most successful cavalry officers in the Civil War, was guided by his simple motto, "Get there firstest and the mostest." In a similar vein, Peters and Waterman's study[4] of 37 well-run organizations identified eight attributes of excellent management, and "a bias toward action" headed the list. Good planning is difficult enough, but people who are planners without this "bias toward action" are more fitted to staff positions than for major line decision–making positions. As the Peters and Waterman's report[4] says of their well-managed companies (p. 13):

. . . the excellent companies were, above all, brilliant on the basics. Tools didn't substitute for thinking. Intellect didn't overpower wisdom. Analysis didn't impede action. Rather, these companies worked hard to keep things simple in a complex world. They persisted. They insisted on top quality. They fawned on their customers. They listened to their employees and treated them like adults. They allowed their innovative product and service "champions" long tethers. They allowed some chaos in return for quick action and regular experimentation.

We believe these comments are most appropriate for health care organizations whose goals include quality, efficiency, and effective operations in the modern environment of deregulation.

Although strategic managers are people of action, this does not mean that they are not concerned with investigation, evaluation, negotiation, and communication. Decisions based solely on intuitive judgment stemming from experience will not suffice in a rapidly changing environment. Today's strategic managers in health care organizations must complement intuitive judgment with rationality based on logical study, fact finding, and consultation. This combination of rational approaches with intuitive judgment is what distinguishes today's strategic manager. Rational approaches include the following:

Investigation and fact finding

Evaluation

Negotiation

Communication

The following summarizes these basic competencies that strategic managers require in today's environment.

COMPETENCIES
Investigation and Fact Finding

Every manager must make a number of decisions each day. Some are made after much fact finding and analysis; others must be made immediately and are based on knowledge and experience. To assist them in this, managers often have staffs or perhaps departments of advisors who are specialists in certain areas or who provide them with advice and assistance when continual research and evaluation are necessary. These units, for example, budgets and finance, personnel, and marketing are usually referred to as staff or functional departments. Managers, in fact, delegate a degree of authority to obtain the facts and to be assured that certain services are provided for their staff and for the organization. In addition, managers are constantly acquiring facts through their own observations, through reading, or through studying the situation in their departments or divisions.

An important aspect of fact finding is its innovative potential. Too little attention has been given to innovation because so much time and effort is spent on problem solving. The idea seems to be that if all problems are solved, there is a viable department. In most situations this is not necessarily correct. Perhaps a better approach would be to give more attention to innovation or *opportunities*. All the problems might not disappear, but the attitude would be positive rather than negative. There is a need for effective innovation both in managing workers and organizing work; despite the progress made in this area, it may still be the most neglected subject and have the most potential for improving and increasing productivity.

Managerial style in fact finding and investigation is an important element. Situations where consensus is important call for attention to group decision-making processes, whereas situations calling for immediate decisions that cannot be delayed necessitate individual decision making usually based on managerial experiences in similar situations. In a health service where many decisions are based on judgment and implementation of decisions depends on commitment from others, group decisions are (or should be) more prevalent than those made unilaterally.

Fact finding and investigation are the most important ways of identifying community needs and expectations. Much information is available from other sources in the community, such as planning and public health agencies; however more attention must be given to this important responsibility of management.

Evaluation

Another competency needed by managers is the ability to evaluate people, programs, and the overall effectiveness of the health care organization in meeting community needs and expectations. Evaluation of people is necessary not only with regard to prospective employees, but also in terms of clientele relationships and interpersonal behavior. In addition, managers are constantly required to evaluate progress in terms of expected achievement, merit, and continuation.

Certainly managers must constantly make judgments about others. Often this is done with great reluctance, but this reluctance does not remove the responsibility. Invariably managers ask how the evaluation or appraisal process can be improved. *Motivation* is probably the most important requirement—if we are motivated to judge our subject accurately and if we feel free to be objective, we are likely to achieve our aim, provided we have the necessary experience and/or training and can use appropriate judgmental norms.

In making evaluations, the manager must first establish the general organizational structure and the jobs to be performed. Then individual employees must know what is expected from them on their jobs. This management-by-objectives approach based on objectives is essential to evaluation of institutional effectiveness.

Negotiation

There is little doubt that the manager spends much time negotiating both with agencies outside the health service and with staff members within, especially regarding their working arrangements and in conflict resolution. It is somewhat unfortunate that the term *negotiation* has become associated to such a great extent with the collective bargaining process. The term actually implies reaching a mutual agreement or consensus between the two parties involved, either individuals or groups.

There are many examples of negotiation in management. Increasingly managers must negotiate, for example, with third-party payers, regulatory agencies, and planning groups. Internally, for example, there are elements of negotiation in the hiring functions. Often certain adjustments are made in the duties assigned, depending on the interests and abilities of the person to be hired and the needs of the health care organization. If no agreement is reached, it is either because the person is not acceptable or the organization or the position is not acceptable to the person. A similar negotiation activity often exists in salary determination.

Now, what can be said in connection with developing the competency of negotiation? First, one should recognize the part that emotions play in a negotiation session. Ideally this activity is or should be as rational as possible. Unfortunately, tempers are likely to be short, and sometimes critical attitudes are present that are not conducive to objectivity.

A second consideration relates to the kind of authority exercised. If the negotiation conference is one-sided in favor of the manager, a unilateral decision will be reached. In fact, we can say this is an arbitrary decision and the manager is in the role of an arbitrator. On the other hand, the decision may be tossed to the other party, whose answer will be accepted by the manager. True negotiation should be somewhere between these extremes.

Ideally the manager will strive for a positive problem-solving situation. This implies moving away from a win/lose (I win—you lose, or vice versa) situation to a win/win (I win—you win) result. In this case the manager will turn from a "choice" to a "creative problem-solving" situation, with both parties focusing on mutually agreed-on goals.

Communication

Someone once said that if we could solve the problems inherent in communications, we would indeed solve most of the problems not only of the organization but of the world. But it is somewhat disconcerting to note that as we improve communication facilities, we seem to achieve less understanding.

A key problem in communication is the assumption that others hear and understand what we say and write. Usually we make no effort to ascertain whether our message is received. Too, if we discover that our message is not understood, we usually conclude that it is not our fault, but that the problem rests with the receiver for not listening or for being too obtuse to understand.

The manager who discovers that he or she is not communicating effectively to the staff often resorts to memoranda or policy statements. Before long, these means become standard and very little attention is given to face-to-face communications, and a means of checking for understanding is lost. For many people the written word is more difficult to understand than the spoken one. This is true because, in most cases, the reader who encounters an obscure passage does not have the opportunity to question the writer (the communicator). A high level of understanding is not achieved by using unintelligible language.

Most people can think about 5 times as rapidly as they can speak. This suggests that there is all kinds of room for static, ranging from "turning off one's hearing aid" to rewriting or restating the speaker's message. Thus we sometimes rely on visual aids to help keep the listener's attention. But often the listeners give so much attention to the visuals that they do not hear the message!

A final thought related to communication involves the art of listening. Communication is a two-way street, and managers must listen to what their employees tell them both directly and indirectly. Much of what has been said about the receiver applies to the transmitter of information, because it concerns the feedback of understanding in words and behavior.

A variety of tasks are performed by managers that naturally vary from position to position. The manager must develop the competencies to perform these tasks. The primary aim is to develop an effective organizational managerial system in which all the people components function as a team to meet the needs of the community, institution, physician, patient, employees, and government, as well as the manager.

SUMMARY

In Chapter 1 we traced the major changes in the health care system, pointing out the significance of external forces. In this chapter the concept of strategic management was introduced, a rationale was presented for the strategic management process, and a model of the process itself was developed.

The goal of the strategic management process is to recognize the significance and impact of external factors and to energize actors involved in the clinical/operating sector of the health care institution, as well as the management sector, to provide high quality, effective, and efficient health care.

REFERENCES

1. Drucker P: Management: tasks, responsibilities, practice, New York, 1973, Harper & Row, Publishers, Inc.
2. Byrd RE: Corporate leadership skills: a new synthesis, Organizational Dynamics 16(1):34, 1987.
3. Greenleaf RK: Servant leadership, New York, 1977, Paulist Press.
4. Peters TJ and Waterman RH, Jr: In search of excellence: lessons from America's best-run companies, New York, 1982, Harper & Row, Publishers, Inc.

5
Strategy Formulation

Planning is a tool that should lead to strategy formulation, but unfortunately a plan may be nothing more than a piece of paper. For example, you may have planned to read this chapter several days ago. However, that plan does not become a reality until it relates to a direction, an action, and a commitment. Cannon[1] clearly defined the nature of a strategy and described the concept as "directional action decisions which are required competitively to achieve the company's purpose" (p. 9). We urge you to substitute *health care organization* for *company,* because the definition is most appropriate to all organizations including those in health care. The key to the concept is "directional action." All of us attempt to provide direction for our lives. Some of us succeed better than others. It is safe to assume that aimless wandering will usually result in a chaotic situation evolving into failure and despair. An organization must have a basic direction and a commitment to reaching its mission, goals, and objectives. Strategies are the means for achieving the mission, goals, and objectives, and these means should be known within the organization for effective implementation of the strategy.

A reader who is familiar with the health planning history in the United States might well ask, why this emphasis on strategy formulation. Is it not only a reinterpretation of the long history of planning? Our response is that the early planning period was primarily regulatory in nature and/or concerned with expansion of service. The system reimbursed cost and guaranteed a daily payment.

It is important to reiterate that the present health care national climate for planning is no longer a cost-based reimbursement system, but a price-based system. Weintraub[2] very aptly describes the impact of the price-based system in the following components (p. 21):

> The new reimbursement schemes give incentives to hospitals to improve and enforce stricter utilization reviews. This, combined with physician peer review programs to assure the delivery of appropriate services, has had substantial impact on lowering admissions, census and lengths of stay. Expanded technology has also had a significant impact on reducing occupancies. . . . Because of the effects of the federal initiatives, private industry and other health care payers also moved to a fixed price system. In addition, these payers created incentives to foster more widespread use of outpatient

services. Recognizing that hospitals might have more beds available than patients to fill them, the payers began to negotiate special rates with hospitals in return for a guarantee of that group's patients. This further intensified the competitive environment. For hospitals operating under the DRG reimbursement program, survival became directly related to their ability to market services and compete successfully. Those hospitals able to provide the best combination of cost and quality became more successful. Competition and marketplace forces dramatically downsized the system and accomplished in a remarkably short time what regulation had attempted to achieve in a more cumbersome and costly manner.

It is within this climate of competition and marketplace forces, similar to those facing business organizations, that today's managers of health care organizations exist. The following material in this chapter outlines a strategy formulation approach relative to this situation.

DETERMINING THE MISSION, GOALS, AND OBJECTIVES

Motives, as the root of the word implies, are what move people. Motives explain the direction and intensity of activity. People are motivated. Organizations are not. Organizations are collectivities of people, and the directions that organizations take and the amount of effort expended are the result of a coming together of people in organizations, each bringing to the organization his or her own particular set of needs. How much they give to the organization in the early stages of membership and indeed whether they join in the first place depend on the needs of the individuals and the expected payoff when weighed against perceived alternatives. In later stages of membership, expectations change partly in response to the payoffs received. But expectations and motives change as the organization itself begins to impact on its members. The organization embodies and manifests the desires of its members, but the organization also shapes its members.

People interact with other members (1) through conflict and cooperation, (2) through giving and receiving rewards, recognition, and approval, and (3) through shared experiences. One manifestation of this takes the form of identification with the organization, which seems to have a personality of its own despite changes in the membership even at the top. The dichotomy between "me" and "them" gives way in even a moderately successful organization to a view of the organization as "us." Collective goals and values are internalized by individuals: "we" win the football game or get the contract even though "I" played no part except as a spectator.

Mission

The organization's mission or purpose identifies what it is about—the nature of its relationship to the whole of society. It appears that many organizations never acknowledge the subject. However, for long-run continuation of the organization, it must continually keep its mission as a guiding star and continually review whether there should be a change in the mission to better serve society.

The mission is thus, in the final analysis, shaped by the relationship between the present or potential capabilities of the organization and the present or potential needs and desires of the community. Some organizations falter or fail because they attempt to produce a service that lies outside their capabilities, others because the demand fails to materialize or declines. In the former, for example, the urge to diversify sometimes leads organizations into fields where they lack technical expertise, access to professionals, or technology. In the latter and probably more common instance, they either misread the needs or fail to reach the community.

How then do organizations arrive at a sound formulation of mission?

The organization must answer the three fundamental and practical questions that follow:

1. What services are we providing? What are we really about?
2. For what purpose are we in this activity?
3. What tasks must be carried out to meet community needs, provide services, and survive?

Goals and Objectives

Health care organizations exist to accomplish a purpose, or "to attain a goal or objective." This implies a goal formulation process. There generally are two approaches to goal formulation expounded by both practitioners and academicians. They are (1) an objectively rational approach and (2) subjectively political. Probably in most situations, there is a combination of the two. The rational approach advocated by the prescriptive theorists stresses the need for rationality, logic, and comprehensiveness. For example, Ansoff[3] prescribed an approach designed to narrow the gap between current objectives and future prospects for the organization. At the other extreme, Cyert and March[4] suggested that organizational goals are determined by bargaining among coalitions in the organization. Today many argue for a contingency approach based on where power is concentrated. The various approaches include: problem solving, when power is concentrated among policy makers; coalition formation, when power is dispersed or parties are in conflict; and bargaining, when power is balanced between policy makers and other active parties and there are conflicting goals among parties to the goal-formation process. We believe that the contingency approach is the viable alternative for health care organizations, where the environmental situation is rapidly changing.

Management is faced with the constraints imposed by the availability of funds, by the labor supply, by interest rates, and by the state of the underlying technology. Thus top management seems almost hemmed in by a set of material and social constraints. However, the goal-setting process achieves maneuvering room because of two closely related phenomena—(1) what Barnard[5] called the "zone of indifference" and (2) what March and Simon[6] called "satisficing."

The Zone of Indifference. Barnard's theory of authority[5] posits that the successful execution of an order depends on if the person or unit to which it is directed can and is willing to carry it out. Given the ability to carry out the order, the acceptance of the order is a matter of whether it falls within a certain range— a "zone of indifference," which he defines as follows (pp. 168-169):

If all the orders for actions reasonably practicable can be arranged in the order of their acceptability to the person affected, it may be conceived that there are a number which are clearly unacceptable, that is, which certainly will not be obeyed; there is another group somewhat more or less on the neutral line, that is, either barely acceptable or barely unacceptable; and a third group unquestionably acceptable. This last group lies within the "zone of indifference." The person affected will accept orders lying within this zone and is relatively indifferent as to what the order is so far as the question of authority is concerned.

Expanded beyond the area of authority, the zone of indifference defines the range of goals or objectives that will be accepted by the various parties to the organization's survival and well-being. For example, physicians in a staff model HMO may not accept protocols but would accept prospective peer review for elective surgical procedures as a way to reduce utilization of referred services. The stockholders in an invester-owned hospital may act to remove a management that promises them a 50¢ dividend but may accept a $2 instead of a $3 dividend without a murmur. In this situation the executive may argue successfully that the value of a $3 dividend has to be weighed against alternative uses of that added dollar for price reductions or wage increases. On the employee side of the ledger, in a given state of the economy, a 3% salary increase may activate a job search on the part of key employees. A majority may be satisfied with a 7% increase.

Satisficing. Closely related to the zone of indifference concept is the idea "satisficing," which played a part in earning the Nobel Prize in Economics for Herbert Simon. Classical economic theory was built on the idea of "economic man" as a rationally maximizing or optimizing creature. Economic man enumerated the alternatives, set a value on each, and selected the one that would maximize the return. In effect March and Simon[6] said that economic man was an ideal type, which at most was only approximated in the economic behavior of real people. Instead, he said, real people satisfice; that is, they settle for something less than the maximum or optimum goal, objective, or monetary level.

Thus the concepts of satisficing and the zone of indifference suggest that the appropriate reaction to social constraints to goal setting is to estimate a lower limit within the zone of indifference for each group and to allocate basic inducements accordingly. The residual resources then become the parts of the total output that remains for discretionary allocation by top management. Likewise with respect to the material inputs, the extent to which management can hold these elements to a lower cost also increases the resources available for discretionary allocation. In Barnard's terminology[5] he covers the assessment of what is possible in his "theory of opportunism" and the value-laden judgment as to what *ought* to be done in his theory of "executive responsibility." For example the executive might conclude that he or she could hold cost and quality down by substituting an aide for a registered nurse position and that this would reduce cost without affecting patient satisfaction. At the same time he or she might decide that the commitment to quality should not be compromised and that a substitution will not be made. Alternatively he or she might decide to make the saving and lower the cost of service to patients or increase employee benefits.

With respect to the zone of indifference, one important point should be remembered.

It is not immutable. External circumstances and leadership may influence the boundaries. For example, an economic recession may affect the lower limit of acceptable wages or a charismatic leader may get people to accept a work situation or hazards that would be unacceptable under different circumstances.

Barnard[5] has developed a theory of opportunism describing executive action. He describes effective action as "the control of the changeable strategic factors," that is, the exercise of control at the right time, right place, right amount, and right form, so that purpose is properly refined and accomplished. There are two types of responses to conditions in the environment—those that require no decisions and those that involve decisions related to the purposes, goals, ends, or objectives of the organization. The decision situation involves two basic classes of decisions—the moral element group and those with an opportunistic element. The moral element is indispensible because no organization, especially a health service, can operate without it. Opportunistic elements are premised on the assumption that everything takes place in the present, under conditions of the present, and with means presently available. The search then is for the strategic factor or the limiting factor. When ascertained, it will establish a new system, a new line of action, new implementing process, or, in general, a new strategic plan and management. The strategic or limiting factor is the center of the environmental decision—to act or not to act is the basic question. Strategic action and decision making become processes of successive approximations—the closer and closer discrimination of facts until a satisfying state is achieved.

Of course a key to this is the ability of executives to recognize the strategic factor (the limiting factor). Today, because of the complexities in the environment, professional planners are used in our organizations. The need remains, however, to determine and take advantage of the opportunity through ascertaining the limiting factor. If the goals are to improve quality of care, provide improved service to the community, or add additional services, long-range planning is involved, as well as sequential development of implementing strategies.

SOCIAL RESPONSIBILITY

As stated, every health care organization, business firm, government agency, and private, not-for-profit organization exists to serve a need or needs of society. If the organization serves even a small constituent group, it must still, as a minimum condition for survival, avoid doing so at a significant cost to the larger society of which it is a part. From this perspective, a social contract exists between organizations and society that embodies understandings and expectations on the part of both parties. Many elements of this social contract were written in the past and made explicit, if at all, only in the common laws. Recently, however, there is evidence that the social contract has undergone considerable change, especially in the expectations of society. The advent of consumerism has given a larger voice to the consumer relative to product and service performance. Antipollution laws have been passed, aimed at reducing the pollutants entering the atmosphere, the water, and the human body. Environmental impact studies are required in most states before large buildings can be erected. Health planning and peer quality review regulations were established to help ensure health service responsibility to the community.

More recently, attention has been directed toward social responsiveness, a concept that stresses social response processes and ethical behavior. Wartick and Cochran[7] suggest two aspects of social responsibility:

- *Constituency theory*—corporate decisions should enhance the welfare of both its economic and noneconomic constituents (patients, physicians, employees, general public, employers, payers, etc.). This tends to conflict with economic responsibility.
- *Social performance*—the organization should "manage" its approach to social pressure by (1) anticipating social issues and selecting the line of least resistance (issues management) and (2) sacrificing short-run gains, where necessary, to obtain long-run gains. This tends to conflict with economic performance expected of investor-owned, for-profit health service organizations.

There are no hard and fast principles associated with social responsibility. A key consideration, however, is the important role of managers in establishing a strong commitment to ethical behavior and providing leadership among the employees to that end. More will be said about social responsibility in subsequent chapters.

COMPETITIVE POSITION

Whether one approves or not, health services compete with each other—at least for resources. A key to strategic thinking and managing is competitive position. To be competitive it is necessary to obtain and analyze information or data.

Competitive position cannot be understood by looking at an organization as a whole. It stems from the discrete activities an organization performs in designing, marketing, delivering, and supporting its services. Each of these activities can contribute to an organization's relative cost position and create a basis for differentiation. A cost advantage, for example, may stem from such disparate sources as a low-cost purchasing system, a highly efficient record-keeping system, or superior utilization of staff. Differentiation can stem from similarly diverse factors, including the development of high quality physician staff, a responsive patient care system, or an efficient delivery system. Competitive responsiveness requires examination of both the external and internal environments of the health care organization.

The External Environment

In today's situations it is usual to be cognizant of changes in the external environment of the health care organization. To properly formulate strategic plans, the strategic manager must obtain information about the external environment.

However, there is no question that information available to the strategic manager relative to the external environment is imperfect. The reader will recall from Chapter 1 the economic, societal, and political changes. How these will affect an individual health care organization cannot be determined with 100% accuracy. A manager must identify and interpret the available information with the understanding that it may be imperfect. Although the imperfect information problem presents a dilemma for the strategic manager, a course or courses of action must be decided. The important task is to make a decision, right or wrong; avoiding a decision is a decision by default. But this does not completely resolve the problem. Managers need to identify the dominant components of the environment. These are identified as those items that, if exploited, controlled, or satisfied, will result in more autonomy or control, which in return effects an improvement in performance of the health care organization.

Michael Porter[8] and many others believe that the secret to attaining a competitive advantage stems from the generic strategies of developing and maintaining a lowcost operation, differentiating service from other competitors, or focusing on a unique niche or service area in the community. As health care organizations are increasingly involved in the competitive marketplace, the situation described by Porter becomes increasingly significant. Indeed, in some cases in light of the risk involved, it may be necessary to pursue a less ambitious goal or even settle for a lower degree of performance. The old adages "Quit when you are ahead" and "Limit your losses" say it all.

Finally, the interdependence of the actions of others is a key characteristic of the free marketplace and accounts for the unruliness and unpredictability of the market, as well as stress on constantly improving competitive performance, quality, and cost effectiveness.

It is interesting to note the change in the health care system relative to competition. Not too many years ago many health care organizations held a monopoly position in the community; there was no competition. Now with changes in physician and patient expectations, improved transportation, increased technology and treatment modes, and cost initiatives, most if not all health care organizations are in a competitive situation.

The Internal Environment

We will devote relatively little space to internal sources of data. Our rationale is that we will devote a chapter to internal functional specialists, who will supply much of the internal information. A usual approach is to establish an internal audit task force consisting of managers from different units of the health care organization. Their charge could be to develop a list of sources of information and actually obtain and then analyze the data from those sources. It is recommended that the managers identify the 10 to 20 significant strengths and weaknesses of the organization, with a short explanation of the reason for such a designation. Some organizations hire management consulting firms to conduct the internal audit. Of course, the audit and especially the analysis may be performed by the CEO and staff.

Among the areas that would ordinarily be considered in an internal audit are the following: top management (goals, values, and organization, for example); functional programs (such as patient care, central supply, laboratory, therapy, and pharmacy); medical staff (for example, their specialties and their concerns); physical facilities; the human resources of the organization; and interrelationships among the areas. Some of the data may be readily available, such as financial information. Other data may require more time to acquire, such as employee attitudes.

It is true that external and internal environmental sensing, intelligence, and surveillance are terms that conjure up negative images in the minds of many. We call the readers' attention to the concepts of social responsibility, social responsiveness, and

Strengths	•Excellent location and new hospital •Reputation for providing high quality care, coronary, oncology, and hematology •Good cash reserve and financial position •Slightly above average occupancy rates •Excellent laboratory •Excellent financial foundation
Weaknesses	•Poor relationships between administrative and medical staffs •Increasing costs •Indecisive administration •Old section of hospital disliked and underutilized •Problems with pharmacy and food service •25% of physicians account for 60% of patients •Many "old timers" on board of trustees
Opportunities	•Eliminate underutilized section of hospital •Incorporate as a profit-making HMO •Remodel old section •Acquire other institutions •Emphasize cardiac, cancer, and other specialties •Increasing population in area, younger families •New businesses entering community
Threats	•Increased government regulation •Excess bed capacity in area •Negative reactions to health care cost increases •Increasing competition •Increasing expectations of patients and physicians •Increasing costs •Increasing expectations from businesses

Fig. 5-1   SWOT analysis.

ethical behavior discussed earlier. Information gathering can be performed in an ethical manner, but CEOs must set the tone and nature of ethical behavior.

THE SWOT ANALYSIS

Once the data have been gathered, the next step is to analyze the information so that problems can be diagnosed and opportunities identified. An external and internal profile of the health care organization can be developed with each item evaluated and weighed in terms of its significance. Care must be exercised so that undue importance is not attached to small differences in numerical weights that may be assigned. Recall that we indicated that there are qualitative aspects of the situational analysis, as well as quantitative.

One approach that many find useful is to identify the **s**trengths and **w**eaknesses of the organization (internal environment) and **o**pportunities and **t**hreats (external environment). This is usually referred to as the SWOT analysis. An illustrative SWOT analysis is presented in Fig. 5-1. Once the strengths, weaknesses, opportunities, and threats have been determined, the objective is to relate, insofar as possible, the (1) opportunities with strengths and (2) threats with weaknesses, to exploit the former and eliminate or reduce the impact of the latter. Usually various alternatives are determined, such as acquiring other related health care organizations, increasing emphasis toward becoming a specialty hospital, incorporating as an HMO, eliminating the old section of the hospital, or acquiring or merging with another health care organization. The best or combination of the best solutions is agreed on and a strategy, strategies, or a business plan is agreed on for the health care organization. Of course the approach requires much concentrated attention to be successful.

STRATEGIES

Why do organizations initiate strategies in the first place? Shortell et al.[9] suggest the following four reasons (pp. 226-227):

1. The perception of performance gaps. If a health care organization perceives there is a difference in its performance compared with others or in terms of what realistically could be expected, this discrepancy creates an incentive for changing strategy.
2. The perception of dissonance gaps when an organization believes its view of itself or its identity is being threatened, the result is a recognition or a conclusion that there is a need for a strategy change. For example, how much diversification of activity is needed before a hospital ceases to be a hospital, but perhaps a conglomerate business organization with multi-independent units or businesses?
3. Changes in the external environment. Changes in the environment such as population changes in the catchment area or financial or government changes (DRGs for example) can necessitate a change in strategy.
4. Changes in organization leadership. A new chief executive officer is more likely than not to cause strategy changes, either because that person was hired to change the operation and/or because new leaders usually bring new strategies.

Once the data have been analyzed, the next objective is to develop a strategic plan for the organization that will emphasize objectives to be achieved and a plan or strategy to describe how the objectives will be achieved.

THE STRATEGY PLAN

Today, increasing numbers of health care organizations are developing strategic plans. An example of the table of contents of such a plan is presented in the box on page 77. In addition, a similar plan may be developed for each strategic service center or department. This is a form of management by objectives whereby objectives are jointly agreed on by the CEO and staff with supporting units so that there is mutual understanding of the expectations regarding each unit. The strategic service center, such as a laboratory or department, then develops a report, usually annual, outlining the course of events in achievement or nonachievement of the plan with recommendations for the next year.

GRAND STRATEGIES

A number of terms have been used by various authors to describe the long-run strategic thrust of the corporate entity. There is a tendency to group corporate grand strategies into a relatively small number of categories or grand strategies.

STRATEGIC PLAN OUTLINE

I. Executive summary
II. External environment/industry outlook
   A. Analysis
   B. Conclusions
III. Competitive outlook
   A. Analysis
      1. Opportunities
      2. Threats
   B. Conclusions
IV. Internal environmental outlook
   A. Resources
   B. Weaknesses
   C. Strengths
V. Marketing plan
   A. Utilization forecast
   B. Target markets/segments
   C. Objectives
   D. Strategies
VI. Clinical operations plan
   A. Capacity—utilization, efficiency, cost
   B. Operational capacity/capacity expansion
   C. Objectives
   D. Strategies
VII. Financial plan
   A. Past performance
   B. Objectives
   C. Strategies
   D. Pro forma income and balance sheets
VIII. Organization/evaluation/control
   A. Who will do what? When?
   B. Who will monitor the plan? Why?
   C. How will deviations from the plan be detected?
   D. Who will take corrective action?

Our plan is to discuss the various grand strategies used at the corporate level, utilizing the following categories that we believe are most appropriate for health care organizations:

- Stability

- Internal growth

- External growth

- Turnaround

- Retrenchment

Stability

Navy people would conceive of the stability group of strategies in terms of "steady as she goes." This phrase suggests movement but no unusual positive or negative motions or swings in the progress of the ship of enterprise.

Incremental growth is one of the stability strategies. Quinn,[10] in his research relative to strategic planning of General Mills, Inc., Pillsbury Company, Exxon Corporation, Continental Group, Xerox Corporation, Pilkington Brothers Limited, General Motors Corporation, Chrysler Corporation, and Volvo AB, found that managers move forward incrementally instead of following formal planning practices. He suggests that "managers in major enterprises tend to develop their most important strategies through processes that neither formal planning paradigms nor power-behavioral theories adequately explain." Quinn[10] suggests that such managers *consciously* and *proactively* move forward *incrementally* (p x):

1. To improve the quality of information utilized in corporate strategic decisions.
2. To cope with the varying lead times, pacing parameters, and sequencing needs of the subsystems through which such decisions tend to be made.
3. To deal with the personal resistance and political pressures any important strategic change encounters.
4. To build the organizational awareness, understanding, and psychological commitment needed for effective implementation.
5. To decrease the uncertainty surrounding such decisions by allowing for interactive learning between the enterprise and its various impinging environments.
6. To improve the quality of the strategic decisions themselves by systematically involving those with most specific knowledge, by obtaining the participation of those who must carry out the decisions, and by avoiding premature momenta or closure which could lead the decisions in improper directions.

We do not want to imply that they do not engage in other grand strategies. The important point is that there is a preference for incremental growth, probably because it is easier to manage and more appropriate to a successful health care organization. This list is useful to managers of health care organizations.

Internal Growth

Internal growth as a strategy places the emphasis for growth on internal development as opposed to external growth by means of acquisitions. Generally managers tend to view growth as desirable and equate it with personal success.

Innovation is generally a basic internal growth strategy. In many situations innovation is the way of life and without such a strategy a firm will not survive. For example, one notes significant emphasis on (1) innovation in HMOs, laboratories, and pharmaceuticals and (2) the use of computer and electronic equipment. However, it is well known that many innovations are never recognized or are not accepted by the public. Nonetheless, few organizations, if any, have successfully reduced research and development and managerial improvement and still remained viable in the industry.

Service market development is a competitive strategy that tends to be internal to the organizations but is designed to meet competition. It is a competitive strategy.

Porter[8] identifies five competitive forces that impinge on the enterprise. These are (1) threats of entry from competitor firms, (2) intensity of rivalry among existing competitors, (3) pressure from substitute products, (4) bargaining power of buyers, and (5) bargaining power of suppliers. To cope with these competitive forces, he suggests the following three generic strategies mentioned earlier in this chapter:

1. Overall cost leadership
2. Differentiation
3. Focus

Cost leadership involves aggressive construction of efficient facilities, utilization of cost reductions from experience, tight cost and overhead control, and cost minimization in areas where returns may be low. Differentiation aims at creating something that is unique. In health care organizations, the emphasis is on patient treatment relative to disorders and patient care. The generic strategy of focus requires zeroing in on a narrow segment of the market. In health care organizations, an example is the development of a hospice or eating disorders clinic.

A large group of theorists are convinced that the basic explanation for progress in the United States is the growth objective of managers. Without this goal as a motivating force, it is doubtful that as much could have been achieved. On the other hand, there has been undue exploitation of resources in many instances to achieve this growth goal. Achievement of internal growth requires great expertise on the part of management. However, as an alternative to internal growth or in addition, the health care organization may also engage in external growth. We turn our attention now to that subject.

External Growth

External growth strategies have been common during recent decades. The idea is not new and was practiced by many of the very early trading companies, such as the Hanseatic League and the East India Company.

External growth through a merger is when two or more organizations combine and one acquires the assets and liabilities of the other in exchange for stock or cash, or both. The merger may be horizontal: the organizations are in the same business or production/service process. As was the case in internal growth, external growth may involve a concentric merger: organizations are acquired externally that are in the same product or service. Mergers are generally thought of under the more general term *acquisitions*.

Related to mergers and acquisitions are other growth strategies. One of these is the joint venture. A joint venture involves the formation of a temporary partnership or a consortium. This situation exists because the organizations do not wish to merge or are not legally permitted to do so. Joint ventures between a hospital and medical staff are particularly relevant, such as for an HMO.

Mergers, acquisitions, and joint ventures may also be viewed from the perspective or horizontal and vertical integration. Horizontal integration involves the combination of organizations in the same stage of service or marketing. For example, in the health care industry several hospitals may agree to integrate their resources through merger or a joint venture arrangement, such as purchasing supplies. Vertical integration involves companies that serve as outputs for the base company's products or services. Because there are risks associated with any type of acquisition, the organization would be wise to consider the long-run impact of integration, especially as it relates to diversification.

A major factor that must be considered in acquisitions and mergers is the effect on employees, especially upper management personnel, as well as the service needs of the population served. Will these people be offered a position in the new arrangement, or will they leave? Unfortunately, in most cases the persons who have the most to contribute to the new organization are, generally speaking, the most likely to leave. Their reputations are usually such that they can easily and successfully enter the labor market. Thus what was a very effective and productive organization before a merger may not continue in the same successful mode. The solution to these kinds of potential problems involves strategic wisdom on the part of managers. We believe that there will be an increase in mergers, acquisitions, and joint ventures in the health care industry.

Turnaround Strategies

Turnaround strategies are generally identified as those coming as a result of a decline in the economy or internal hard times. It is necessary to determine the current operating health of the health care organization before making turnaround strategic decisions. For example, the financial strengths and weaknesses, market and service position, and technology must be carefully ascertained. The stage of the service/market evolution should be a part of the analysis. The six stages are development, growth, shakeout, maturity, saturation, and decline. Depending on the relative competitive position of the organization, different strategic concentrations are advisable. For example, if the competitive position is very weak and community needs are not adequately met, liquidation may be the best strategy. However, at the midpoint of the service/ market evolution stage, new strategies to serve unmet community needs are in order. If the competitive position is strong, the service/market stage is less significant in affecting turnaround strategies. A growth grand strategy with careful consideration to changes in the health care environment should be considered in such situations.

Retrenchment

The retrenchment grand strategies may be followed by organizations to stabilize their position or to avoid further loss. Divestment and liquidation are the usual retrenchment strategies, although turnaround may be the beginning of retrenchment.

Divestments may occur by selling the unit to another health care corporation, establishing the unit as an independent company, or liquidating (including the sale of assets and selling the unit to employees). No manager is enthusiastic about the retrenchment strategy of liquidation. However, in the situation of a declining community or depressed economy it may be the only recourse open to management. Thus it is the strategy of last resort and often an admission of failure.

We agree that decline is usually caused by a combination of factors, although incompetent management might be a precipitating factor. In the final analysis, however, the decline continues because of inadequate or inaccurate response of the organization to the environment. One could expect, however, that most if not all all communities would resist the dissolution of a health care organization in the community. Numerous issues are involved relative to health care organizations that must be considered, such as changing technology toward ambulatory care, addressing community needs, and addressing needs of the disadvantaged. Detailed consideration of these factors is beyond the scope of this book, although references are made to them in earlier chapters.

SUMMARY

There are two basic sets of relationships involved in strategic planning. First are the relationships between different units within the industry on a geographical basis involving competitive actions between units. The second set of relationships are internal to the health care organization and involve cooperative actions on the part of the units. These two sets of relationships obviously require different attitudes and approaches. Because both relationships are required in today's activities, the overall purpose of strategic planning is to reconcile these relationships so that the mission of the organization is achieved in terms of quality, effectiveness, and efficiency.

Some health care organizations have discovered that it is more meaningful to focus on a problem or an issue than on the "big picture." This approach no doubt permits better concentration and easier implementation. However, all problems tend to be interrelated, and at least from time to time it is necessary to review these interrelationships so that the coordinated effort is maintained.

For some organizations, strategic planning will be a new venture. In these situations it is probably advisable to hire a facilitator or consultant. There are many reasons for this, but the most important is that the first approach is likely to set the stage for future planning actions. If the first attempt is judged a failure, parties will be less interested in participation in the future. Furthermore, the strategic plan must be implemented, rather than filed for future reference.

Cohen[11] reports a number of strategic planning activities in various hospitals. For example, the Henry Ford Health Care Corporation in Detroit has taken steps to formalize its strategic-planning process, and these are described as follows (p. 17):

> With 1300 acute-care beds at three sites, the organization has established an elaborate system of encouraging and improving the planning process, according to . . . President Stanley Nelson. A corporate planning office provides data analysis, research and long-term planning services; a planning committee reviews new projects; a finance committee studies the cost, and a management committee gives final approval to projects. "It's a bottom-up process," said Nelson. "New ideas and programs can originate anywhere in the organization."

As mergers and acquisitions continue in the health care industry, it will be increasingly necessary for organizations to become involved in strategic planning. The complexities involved and the increased number of relationships will necessitate a more formal and detailed approach.

One final observation is appropriate. It has to do with the nature of the composition of hospital boards. People with the necessary skills and interests must be elected to boards so that the board can properly encourage strategic planning and management, appreciate the efforts of the top management group, and review the strategic plan, as well as encourage its formulation and implementation.

REFERENCES

1. Cannon JT: Business strategy and policy, New York, 1968, Harcourt Brace & World, Inc.
2. Weintraub AE: Health planning programs: the past suggests the future, Health Care Strategic Management 4(12):15, 1986.
3. Ansoff HI: Corporate strategy: an analytical approach to business policy for growth and expansion, New York, 1965, McGraw-Hill, Inc.
4. Cyert RM and March JG: A behavioral theory of the firm, Englewood Cliffs, NJ, 1963, Prentice-Hall.
5. Barnard C: The functions of the executive, Cambridge, MA, 1938, Harvard University Press.
6. March JG and Simon HA: Organizations, New York, 1958, John Wiley & Sons, Inc.
7. Wartick SL and Cochran PL: The evolution of the corporate social performance model, Acad Manage Rev 10(4):758, 1985.
8. Porter ME: Competitive advantage: creating and sustaining superior performance, New York, 1985, Free Press.
9. Shortell SM, Morrison EM, and Robbins S: Strategy making in health care organizations: a framework and agenda for research, Med Care Rev 42(2):219, 1985.
10. Quinn JB: Strategies for change: logical incrementalism, Homewood, IL, 1980, Richard D. Irwin, Inc.
11. Cohen P: Strategic planning: a new twist gets results, *Health Week* 2(2):17, 1988.

6
Implementation Processes

Our experiences and those recounted by others tell us that it is far easier to formulate plans than it is to implement or execute them. Who hasn't formulated an elaborate approach to requesting a special concession from a professor, such as taking a test late, getting into a course that is filled, or extending the date a paper is due, only to have the plan fail because of improper execution? The same can occur when approaching a superior for a salary increase or a job change. On the other hand, if our strategy is sound and effectively implemented, we have properly anticipated the implementation process.

A primary reason for the failure of implementation is that the motives of the various parties involved are not the same. In other cases the strategy involves change, and there is a natural aversion to change, at least initially. This chapter explores these and other significant factors associated with the implementation of strategy.

CHANGE

A major reason for lack of proper implementation of plans is because the implementation almost always requires change. It is the purpose of this section to examine the nature of the change process. There are many departure points for a discussion of the change process. However, because resistance to change usually is a factor, it is appropriate to begin with that subject.

Resistance to Change

First, a few comments about the nature of change are in order. According to a typical dictionary definition, change involves an alteration, substitution, movement from one condition to another, transformation, or modification.

Cooke[1] sees change in an organization as a modification in the tasks, technology, and structure of the organization and in the roles of employees. When we discuss resistance to change, we are referring to employees as members of the organization. Inanimate objects, such as machines or equipment, cannot by definition resist changes, although anyone who has found difficulty in starting an automobile might disagree.

The automobile engine seems to prefer a state of nonfunctioning as opposed to the changed running stage. We are not talking basically about alienated workers and medical staff, although some suggest that all workers are alienated from managers and owners and that a perpetual state of conflict and animosity exists. However, we will assume that there are no overt manifestations of employee conflict that will interfere with change.

Usually the true nature of resistance to change is not technical. That is, if a new method or technique is introduced into the work task, to implement this change or strategy there is usually a training program for employees so that they can qualify for the job. Some readers might dispute this, but an organization would be in desperate straits for it to not train present employees. This is not to say that such situations never occur, but the repercussions on the remaining work force may be so great that productivity declines and turnover increases, especially among the better employees, who can more easily find employment elsewhere.

If the true nature of resistance to change is not technical, one should ask what it is. We suggest that there are psychological, social, and economic components of employee and staff resistance to change. These may all be present in a given situation, but we will discuss each separately.

From a psychological point, most workers tend to develop an equilibrium within themselves and relative to their job with the organization. If the work expectations are perceived to be too difficult, one either asks for more recognition, probably in terms of pay, or reduces the work effort. If the work effort does not produce the expected recognition or pay, an effort is made to reach a point of acceptable equilibrium. This equilibrium point is perceived from the employee's perspective and may or may not be the same as the employer's expectation. At any rate, the employee feels comfortable. Of course, the longer the period of comfortable or satisfactory perception, the more attached the employee becomes to the situation. This kind of analysis can also apply to a work team or a department, but the larger the number of employees, the more likely it is that individual deviations will occur.

Social aspects of change can also be disconcerting to people. Most of us develop working relationships with fellow workers. There are very few jobs that are actually "lone wolf" positions. We know that some employees will leave and others will retire. These actions are usually almost imperceptible in comparison with change in the total work group. However, innovative changes may disrupt the entire work group so that new relationships must be achieved. Perhaps the informal group leader is displaced but that person still attempts to rally people. This is likely to divide the group and cause even greater disruptions. In fact, the change may have been instigated to break up established informal work groups. This is often dangerous, and most managers would avoid doing so unless the original group relationships are unproductive.

Finally, the social group may have well-established behavior patterns. Any attempt to interfere with these is likely to be disruptive. Wise managers are, as we have stated, reluctant to make these changes. However, in a retrenchment grand strategy situation, such changes are necessary. This is probably why most managers dislike this grand strategy, are not very adept at its implementation, and anticipate that the results are often far less favorable than originally expected.

From an economic perspective, resistance occurs because of a real or expected loss of earnings either at the time of change or in the future. Sometimes changes call for a reduction in employee wages, as occurred in many organizations during the early 1980s. The problem is always (1) to recover this loss and (2) for those who continue to work to decide whether the loss in wages is offset by having a job at all. Ordinarily the answer to this question would be that the job is preferable. However, because of unemployment compensation systems and the effect of income taxes, the employee may well ask if the job has sufficient economic reward at a reduced wage.

Another economic issue is how the change might interfere with career plans. As professors, we encounter many people who return to the universities for graduate programs because changes in their organizations caused a change in long-range career development plans—in most cases, the change ended such plans. Graduate education is a means of entering a different profession. Often it may be the only way people can develop a different career pattern. Naturally, changes that are perceived as affecting those career patterns should be resisted. We believe that the presentation of information on resistance to change results in a positive understanding that should be pursued. We believe that a discussion of resistance to change provides a base for reviewing approaches to implementation of changes relative to strategies and therefore it explains why certain approaches tend to be more effective than others. We turn now to the general approaches useful to managers in implementing change and hence strategy.

Facilitating Change

Over the years many theories of change were proposed by management scientists. Because each may be useful in a given situation, they will be briefly reviewed. An early theoretical framework focused on the problem. It was proposed that the problem must be defined accurately; analytical techniques were recommended, especially in problem definition, and optimal solutions were sought. A second set of theories can be classified as personality-centered. Hammond[2] suggested that personality differences between managers and employees tended to obstruct change. Zand and Sorensen[3] point out that theories set forth by behavioral scientists indicate the complexity of change and the many subactivities involved.

A final but important theory is the process theory, first proposed by Lewin.[4] He begins with a condition of social equilibrium, or state of balance. Change is accomplished by altering either the driving force or the resisting force to achieve a new level of equilibrium. Three phases are involved in the process: (1) unfreezing, (2) moving, and (3) refreezing. The unfreezing stage calls for activity that increases the receptivity of the people involved. Moving involves changing the direction, strength, and/or number of driving or resisting forces. Refreezing, the third stage, involves the reinforcement of the new equilibrium position so that the newly established balance is stabilized and maintained.

More recently, attention has been directed to the interaction of technical, political, and cultural pressures in the increasingly turbulent world of management. These three pressures can be interpreted as design problems that require continuous attention by managers. Tichy[5] states that the "key to managing strategic change and making an organization effective is to align an organization's structure, and its human resources—within these the three technical, political, and cultural systems and to align each of these systems with the others" (p. 66). For example, health care organizations were generally in strategic alignment before the development of DRGs. However, changes in reimbursement policies by the government, coupled with technological advances in the delivery of health care and cultural changes enhanced by consumer expectations, as well as cultural changes stemming from different organization relations both internally and externally, call for a different approach in managing change so that the relationships between the three pressures and the strategic management process itself can be in synchronization.

Beer,[6] as a result of his studies regarding change, concludes that there are three conditions that must be managed in corporate transformations. They are the following (p. 52):

1. *Dissatisfaction* with the status quo among employees who must change their behavior
2. The need for a *model* or vision of the future, which will guide the redesign of the organization
3. The need for a *well-managed process* of change to help employees modify their attitudes and behavior

It should be noted that the majority of situations calling for change in recent years stem from external forces usually necessitating cultural changes. Among the tools available to managers in managing cultural changes are the following:

- Philosophy definition activities
- Structural change
- Education and training
- Multimedia communication
- Pay system change
- Replacement and promotion
- Attitude surveys for unfreezing and monitoring
- Consultants
- Leadership by executives committed to change

Probably the last item in this list is the most important. The words of James J. Renier, president and CEO of Honeywell, Inc., lend credibility to this statement (p. 54):

. . . actions speak louder than words. Chief among them is the example that is set by he who is promoted and why. In setting the stage for our new corporate culture, we have been very careful to promote those managers who are comfortable in a particular milieu and to remove those who are not. This takes a lot of courage. You can't achieve an atmosphere of trust if anyone in the top management structure behaves in an inconsistent manner. I believe that this is why many turnaround situations fail.

Managers in change situations need to recognize the specific social arrangements that will be sustained or threatened by the introduction of change. This is of even greater significance for staff specialists (computer specialists, for example) who are often in positions of initiating change in technology or procedures. These people sometimes bring to work blind spots, such as "self-preoccupation" with their technology, so that they fail to recognize the social aspects of change. CEOs can counter specialists' self-preoccupation by broadening their interests and understanding of staff people, using understandable terms, viewing resistance as an indicator of unclear problems as opposed to something to be overcome, and redefining the staff person's job so that it includes not only generating new ideas but also getting the new ideas operationalized through the implementation stage. This of course will involve more coordinating skill by top management so that staff and operating people can work together as a team. A key to implementation of change among physicians and other professionals, such as nurses, is to gain commitment by participation in the decision for change. Underlying this process is also the need to be opportunity seeking, as well as problem solving. Isenberg[7] concluded from his research that "what managers need is a synthesis of rationality and entrepreneurial (or opportunistic) resourcefulness. Strategic opportunism is a way of approaching the complex, uncertain task of management, both creatively and rigorously" (p. 97).

It is usual to use the term *change agent* to refer to the person who is the facilitator of change. In this context, all managers, especially the CEO, are change agents in the modification of existing situations—the process we refer to as change in the implementation of strategies. A number of initiatives or management style approaches are open to managers. These are reviewed next.

MANAGEMENT INITIATIVES/STYLES

Successful managers develop a style that suits their particular experiences and their overall situation. Management style involves being an entrepreneur—initiating and controlling change in the organization. It involves leadership. Delegation of authority to subordinates is another aspect of style as is the supervision of these people so that they too can be innovators but not at the expense of failing to implement objectives that have been established for the organizations.

The manager needs to develop a style or an approach that provides motivation for the employees of the health care organization to achieve its mission and objectives. From time to time conflicts will arise, and the strategic manager must resolve them in a way that results in equity and fairness. Finally, the strategic manager must provide the resources so that employees can perform effectively.

Brodwin and Bourgeois[8] set forth five approaches or styles appropriate to the implementation of strategy. These are: (1) commander approach (application of rigorous logic and analysis dictated from on top); (2) organizational change (CEO utilizing steps such as structure, incentives, new personnel); (3) collaborative approach (enlists help of senior managers in the development of managers); (4) cultural approach (extension of collaborative approach to middle and sometimes lower levels of the organization); and (5) crescive style (the CEO approaches strategy planning and implementation simultaneously—growing strategies from within the organization).

Although we do not disagree with these approaches to implementation, we believe that there are others that are more appropriate to health care organizations relative to the implementation of strategy. We will now examine the following initiatives or management styles:

Type A: Business manager

Type B: Coordinator
Type C: Corporate chief
Type D: Management team leader

All are considered related to the environment, organizational characteristics, and the characteristics of the board, medical staff, support staff, and management team (Table 6-1). Of course, examples of each can be found in a given period if one examines the various kinds of health care organizations.

Type A: Business Manager

The business management approach was typical in hospitals before the 1950s, relative to managerial tasks and relationships with the board and medical staff. *Administrator* was a common title or in some situations *superintendent*. He or she was clearly under the direction of the board of trustees, who had the responsibility for external affairs, raised and controlled funds, and set policy. Trustees were also more involved in internal matters, such as personnel relations and building plans. Thus the trustees dominated the health organization. When specialization increased, individual physicians became more dominant, either because of their specialties or as members of the board, or both. The purpose of the agent or business manager was to supervise acquisition of supplies and personnel resources needed by individual physicians and to manage scarce funds and facilities within policies set by the board of directors.

Such a situation is still prevalent in some situations. For example, some medical group practice CEOs function in this way although others function as management team leaders. In some university hospitals where the medical school administration and faculty also function as the board of trustees, the role of the CEO could be that of a business manager. We know of a person who developed the type D role, but later the position returned to a type A situation because the medical school administration and some faculty believed that his position had become too powerful.

The organization itself in the business manager relationship setting is informal, with the individual physicians dealing directly with individual trustees. Historically, nursing dominated the administrative team, because there were few other employed health professionals. Because the CEO is less influential in this model or approach than in others, it is unusual to find strong functional specialists. Trustees and individual physicians tend to deal directly with administrative team members rather than through committees or an hierarchical structure with levels of managers.

Type B: Coordinator

Environmental and organizational factor changes usually call for more coordination. Hospital services and community relations have become more complex, and the physician's autonomy has declined in many settings because of increased specialization and stricter requirements for accreditation. Historically, with the decline of dependency on fund raising and increasing external influences, such as the JCAHO, came a decline in the board of trustees' role. Employee relations also became more critical because of increasing employee specialization, scarcity of skilled personnel, and the threat of development of collective bargaining. The CEO in these kinds of developments was the logical and necessary coordinator for employee, medical staff, board, and external agencies, as well as manager for the employee organization. A type B CEO is often in a boundary position, serving as a catalyst or referee. These CEOs also gain in influence as information systems improve, particularly if they keep information to themselves and serve as communicators or negotiators with external forces, such as the JCAHO and third-party payers.

In the type B model, the organization becomes more formalized, with the CEO serving as a link between medical staff, board, and managerial committees. Functional managerial specialists, such as controllers and systems engineers, begin to develop, usually coming to the organization, for example, directly from industry and needing the CEO as communication intermediary with the professional groups. This is a role that is found today in some nongovernmental, not-for-profit, short-term hospitals, as well as HMOs and other health care organizations. Many, however, have moved into a type C style.

Type C: Corporate Chief

During the 1970s and 1980s the chief executive's position changed quite rapidly to what is best described as *corporate chief,* similar to the role of president of a private corporation. Indeed, most CEOs now receive the title of president and are elected to board membership.

The American College of Hospital Administrators (ACHA) has supported a more dominant or authoritative role for the hospital administrator as CEO. Indeed, as early as 1973 the ACHA Task Force V[9] recommended and its board of governors endorsed the following role for the CEO (pp. 32-33):

> The hospital chief executive officer is the person basically responsible for skillfully leading the hospital toward securing and maintaining health for the people it has chosen or been mandated to serve.

> The chief executive officer's responsibilities are comparable to those of the president of a business or industrial service corporation which is labor intensive with a high degree of professional input and which requires extensive capital investment. In many communities, the hospital is the largest employer in the area.

> The chief executive officer, in effect, could be called a "social change agent." As a professional, he or she should view the hospital as a social instrument for change. The chief executive officer is responsible for planning policy and program development subject to approval by the governing body, so that the organization, in cooperation with other organizations, contributes its share of the total response required by community needs. The chief executive officer may also manage the hospital so as to execute approved plans, or may delegate authority for this responsibility to another hospital administrator in the organization.

> The chief executive officer's responsibilities are analagous in the world of music to a combination of those of the composer and the orchestra conductor, and in the world of drama to a combination of the playwright, the producer, and the director.

Table 6-1   CEO styles and characteristics of the organization, board, medical staff and administrative team

Style	Organizational characteristics	Board characteristics*	Medical staff characteristics	Administrative team† characteristics
Type A: business manager				
Responsible for procuring supplies and personnel for physicians and conserving limited resources	Informal	Board holds hospital in trust for donors to hospital Wealthy trustee may be important funding sources Board may be primarily influenced by individual physicians who bring in paying patients	MDs with most patients have dominant influence MDs function individually with board, administration, nursing, etc., rather than collectively through a staff organization	Few functional specialists Nursing dominates employee staff, and they relate directly with individual MDs
Type B: coordinator				
Boundary spanner Develops external role and becomes more influential as he negotiates for resources	More formal lines of communication CEO begins to serve as major source of communication	Board serves more as a representative link to the community	MDs begin to function collectively through medical staff organization rather than individually	Functional specialists begin to develop

Type C: corporate chief				
Relies on formal authority for influence and functions more like a private corporation president. Controls management information	Hierarchical—classical organization	Board is used to obtain community support as well as communicate community expectations to hospital	Medical staff organization bargains collectively with administrator and board	Stronger functional specialists who provide information to and help support the administrator
Type D: management team leader				
Functions as a partner with board members, medical staff, director of nursing, and other administrative team members. Relies more on knowledge, attitudes, skills, and sharing information than on formal authority and control of information to move the hospital toward desired goals	Matrix—open systems organization Project managers	Board is increasingly concerned about internal matters to cope with optimal regulation and scarcity. Board has more internal members Board sets objectives and evaluates total operations with information systems	Medical staff is actively involved and shares accountability for management decisions	Strong administrative team, which relates directly and in partnership with CEO, board members, medical staff, and other employees

*These are characteristics that relate to the manager's style; we do not suggest they affect ultimate legal responsibilities of boards, which have been increasing in recent years.

†Administrative team is defined, for example, as functional specialists (such as controller, personnel director, and director of systems engineering) and directors of nursing service and pharmacy.

Reference is made in the above section to the "corporate role." This is the corporate organization of business and industry in which the chief executive officer (president) is a dominant figure on the board of directors, which is usually headed by a chairman. When "corporate role" or "corporate organization" is applied to the hospital field, the implication is that the hospital chief executive officer should have broad responsibilities and accountability paralleling those of the corporate chief executive officer.

The type C role is more authoritarian and closer to the classical theories of bureaucratic hierarchical management espoused by Weber,[10] Fayol,[1] Davis,[12] and others. The ACHA task force calls for "administrative skills in participative management," which to us suggests a manipulative use of participation.

In many situations the medical staff plays a bargaining rather than a participatory role. Consistent with the type C role is the medical director reporting to the CEO. Increasingly, larger hospitals are establishing full-time service chiefs as well. As early as 1974, the AMA expressed concern and warned of the dire consequences of continuing these trends[13] (p. 4):

> In some institutions, the situation has become so grave as to create a line of authority that goes from the attending staff to a salaried medical hierarchy which in turn is responsible to a hospital administrator, often styled as president of the hospital and frequently not only chief hospital executive, but the dominant voice on the hospital governing board. In the institutions where the hospital administrator occupies the role of hospital president and chairman of the hospital governing board, the only line of communication between the governing board and medical staff is through him. This is lay domination at its zenith and is a trend that should be aborted as early as possible.

Such trends are not being aborted; on the contrary, they are growing. However, mistrust and concerns are promoting the development of physician unions and collective bargaining, which further separates medical staff and health care organizations. An ultimate result of this hierarchical arrangement may be the establishment of a physician as CEO in an effort to integrate the medical staff and hospital administrative organizations. In other hierarchically organized systems, such as hospitals in other countries, a physician frequently serves as CEO.

The governing board in a type C situation has a diminished influence in the hospital. With increasing external control and regulations, such as price controls, DRGs, labor negotiations, and area-wide plans, the influence of the governing board has decreased in recent years. This may result in boards being used to manage the organization's environment as if they were instruments of corporation executives, as has been found in for-profit industries.[14]

Under the type C management role, the management team becomes stronger, but in a classical line or staff relationship to the CEO. The increasing complexities of the organization and its negotiation function require CEOs to have better management information systems. Control of information is recognized as an important source of power. Strong functional specialties providing information to the CEO help support his or her power and the hierarchical arrangement.

Type D: Management Team Leader

As a management team integrator and leader, the CEO functions in a participative management role—more as a partner with, for example, the board, medical staff, and nursing staff. Type D is a proactive leadership role rather than a reactive, coordinative role, such as type B. It assumes that to develop a more effective team approach at the patient care level, a team should be developed at the top management level. CEOs bring the management team to consensus and coordinate decision making. The type D CEO promotes responsible management at all levels of the organization by sharing information openly, working with the management team to define objectives and problems, and letting the team either make decisions or determine who should be involved in making them; he or she uses management by objectives and other behavioral principles, rather than authoritarian techniques. The goal is to integrate the medical staff into major governance and management decisions through participatory practices rather than to rely on line authority through a medical director.

The role calls for team decisions but does not relieve the administrator of the responsibility to see that decisions are implemented. Behavior of the CEO outside of the management team would be more situational. A type D role is based on strong group process and interactive skills. It assumes a confident CEO who relies on management for results based on agreed-on goals. The difference between types C and D lies more in the approach than in the objectives of the role. Both types C and D call for a performance rather than symbolic orientation. However, type D de-emphasizes the CEO's legitimate authority and accentuates team accountability and responsibility in achieving goals. Participative management in other settings has been found to increase the influence of the manager in achieving proper institutional goals. And if participative management is used properly (not manipulatively), it may help remove some of the adversary roles and resolve excessive conflict in hospitals. It emphasizes administration in the broadest sense to include nurses, physicians, and others in the hospital who in fact manage services as a part of administration.

In the type D model, the board takes a more active role in establishing objectives and evaluating operating results against explicit objectives. It would be logical in this model for the board to include the CEO, the chief of staff, the director of nursing, and possibly other key administrative heads, while still retaining a majority of community representatives.

Type D CEOs de-emphasize their executive role to serve as integrators and leaders for consensus management by a team to deal with increasing external demands and more limited resources. The management team may vary from a limited partnership between the chief of staff and CEO to preferably a larger team that might include the administrator, chief of the medical staff, the director of nursing, the financial officer, and/or others. The team would have responsibility for determining objectives, establishing priorities and allocating resources, formulating policies, and setting standards, all of which would be submitted to the board for approval. The board must ensure that they fulfill these responsibilities; it also holds the team accountable for measurable agreed-on results. The manager still has the leadership role of seeing that decisions are based on the best available information and that they are executed. Staff specialists, although reporting to the administrator, would function in a more collegial relationship to health professionals, providing information directly to departments and to the management team as in a matrix organizational structure. It is important to repeat that although these are collegial involvements in problem solving and the development of decisions under type D, implementation of decisions and accountability for results are still centralized under appropriate administrative heads. For example, the director of nursing is accountable for nursing to the management team and governing board.

One might expect that under this arrangement, the CEO would have less control over nurses, medical staff, and fiscal matters. However, experience with a number of hospitals has shown that in practice, except for budget control, many CEOs exercise little effective control over the efficiency and effectiveness of nursing care or medical care. With a team approach and mutual trust, evaluation and accountability for results by each of the team members could increase the real influence of the CEO over quality and efficiency of professional services. The CEO should have responsibility for the management of patient care, and we suggest it could be exercised most effectively in a team system.

A number of points can be argued against a management team approach in addition to the expectation that some hospital CEOs will fear it. For example, the training and orientation of physicians is the antithesis of training for management. Medical training develops physician behavior of independence rather than cooperation. However, it should be noted that many examples of effective physician managers can be found.

Another argument against the management team concept is that consensus management inherent in a management team approach fosters conformity, which is a barrier to creativity. However, a counterargument is that heterogeneous groups have proved that they can develop creative solutions, although interpersonal cooperation is more likely with homogeneous groups. Another argument against a team approach is that it may handicap cost control. Participation by physicians, nurses, or other professionals may result in higher expenditures for esoteric programs or unnecessarily high staffing. Another argument against a type D team is that it is like a committee. Who really is in control; who will accept accountability and responsibility; can all, or will it be none of the team?

Looking at these four roles, we conclude that there is no "role for all seasons," but that each is appropriate for a certain time and environmental interaction. The type A role was appropriate for a certain time and environmental interaction. The type A role was appropriate for the laissez-faire era of the past, or at present for certain organizations where there is close board supervision of operations. Type B was and still is appropriate in community hospitals where there is a balance of power and need for coordination by a boundary spanner. The type C role appears viable in a rapid growth situation where resources are abundant and the CEO can negotiate for them to build a larger and higher quality institution, meeting most of the desires of physicians, nurses, and board members. Moreover, a type C role is common in a highly regulated, bureaucratic environment—one in which hospitals find themselves. We believe, however, that a type D manager may be an effective alternative, because the era of scarcity of resources needs far more integration and accountability in medical and nursing services relative to the technological, economic, political, and hospital objective changes projected in the introduction of this book.

TRAINING

A major part of change involves change in attitudes. A usual approach to changing attitudes in organization is training. A key question is how people learn. There are different ways to learn, and these have significance for the training method used. There are three possibilities: trial and error, modeling, and use of intermediary processes. Trial and error basically involves self-discovery and may be the most effective, since it involves full initiative by the learner but is also likely to be the most costly in terms of positive results and quality. Modeling involves imitating the behavior of others and the reinforcement of positive responses. The use of intermediary processes refers to the help the learner is given, such as written instructions, graphic displays, and demonstrations. People can effectively learn new behavior by exposure to a proper role model. In fact, the role model provides the necessary reinforcement. All too often the impact of social learning is lost in social situations where the attitude is one of doing what I say, not what I do. In such situations, what is often learned is what people see done because the communications network is such that the message is not received. However, the role model's behavior comes through loud and clear and tends to be replicated. Of course, management is concerned in such situations that change does not occur. Knowledge of social learning and the impact of the role model would explain why the learning did not take place and would necessitate changing the behavior of the role model.

An important part of training, especially relative to behavior change, in the achievement of organizational goals and objectives is that of attitude change. Campbell et al.[15] note that researchers have identified three components or elements that comprise an attitude. They are as follows:

1. *Cognitive*—intellectual knowledge or beliefs a person has about an object.
2. *Feeling or affective*—the emotions connected with the object and whether the object is viewed as pleasing or displeasing.
3. *Behavioral*—the action component.

The direction of the relationship between these three generally is cognitions-feelings-behavior. However, the opposite has been suggested, depending on the individual. The important point is that all three components are present and must be recognized in changing attitudes. Campbell et al.[15] summarize the methods used for changing attitudes under the following four headings:

1. *Communication of additional information.* That is, additional inputs are focused on the cognitive elements making up the attitude in hopes that the individual's beliefs will change.
2. *Approval and disapproval.* That is, making rewards or incentives contingent on a particular type, magnitude, and direction of attitude change.

3. *Group influences.* In general, what are the effects of interacting with group members whose attitudes are considerably different.

4. *Being induced to engage in discrepant behavior.* The individual may be *required* to engage in behavior which is contrary to his attitude (e.g., socialize with union officials even though he thinks they are bad.)

It is important to stress again the interrelationships between behavior change and attitudes. Most practical situations require both attitude and behavior change to be effective.

STRUCTURE

The structure of an organization is based on two concepts: (1) the delegation of authority and assignment of responsibility and (2) the establishment of relationships among people and various units. Organization structure has been of interest and concern for thousands of years. An early written example is found in the Book of Exodus in the Old Testament where Moses follows the advice of his father-in-law Jethro, who counseled Moses to teach the people statutes and decisions and delegate responsibility to be more effective, save the time of the people, and conserve his own energy:

> So Moses gave heed to the voice of his father-in-law (Jethro) and did all that he had said. Moses chose able men (trustworthy and who hate a bribe—verse 21) out of all Israel, and made them heads over the people, rulers of thousands, of hundreds, of fifties, and of tens. And they judged the people at all times; hard cases they brought to Moses, but any small matters they decided themselves (Exodus 18:24-26).

Over the centuries much has been written about organization structure. Chandler[16] was a researcher of note who related structure to strategy; that is, structure follows strategy as an implementing process. Chandler also identified four key growth strategies in large-scale organizations as a result of his research. They are (1) expansion of volume (increased numbers of patients treated and/or increased numbers of laboratory tests performed), (2) geographic dispersion (movement into other parts of a city, county, state, or nation), (3) vertical integration (pediatrics, acute care, geriatrics, long-term care), and (4) product diversification (additional services, such as drug abuse programs and outpatient treatment).

Chandler[16] conceives of structure as the design of organization through which the enterprise is administered. Also, the design, whether formally or informally defined, has two aspects: first, the lines of authority and communication between the different administrative offices and officers; and second, the information and data that flow through these lines of communication and authority (p. 14).

Chandler's thesis[16] that structure follows strategy suggests that every time important strategy changes are made, there will of necessity be a change in structure. This is important relative to earlier concepts that there is one best way to manage, as proposed by the scientific management group. What is supported by Chandler's thesis is contingency theory—the choice or structure depends on the objectives and needs of the organization. This is no doubt an uncomfortable proposition for many people who desire an exact prescription to follow. It does suggest that substantial time and thinking must be given to structure that is appropriate to the stage of development of the organization. For example, if two health care organizations are merged, one does not automatically conclude that all that is necessary from an organization perspective is to add another level of management. Because of additional costs and the possibility of continued and increased rivalry between the two merged units, a coordinated, effective, and efficient organization may never be developed. Because of the importance of organization, we devote several chapters to the subject, including organizational arrangements, governance, nursing, health professionals, and managerial functional specialists. Because of this heavy emphasis, we believe it would be redundant to devote more attention to the subject in this chapter.

RESOURCE DEPLOYMENT

Resources come in many forms, such as money, people, equipment, facilities, and materials. Unless resources such as these are provided for in the implementation of a strategy, there will be no change in operations. This is sometimes difficult for managers to understand, because they expect they can merely shift present allocations to attain new objectives. Of course it is not as simple as that. No one is going to change unless there is an incentive. Furthermore, when superiors appear to not really want the new strategies implemented or not be convinced of the need for new actions to implement the strategies, satisfactory implementation will not occur. There are numerous aspects and details associated with resource deployment, many of which can be understood fully only by specialists, such as financial experts, and often in the form of budgets.

Budgets

The budgeting process is an integral part of implementing strategies in terms of resource deployment. Beginning with objectives, strategic plans are developed to define what will be done and how the tasks will be accomplished. Budgets outline the resources dedicated to the achievement of the strategy—in other words, the costs that are expected to be incurred in the implementation of the strategy. Because firms have limited resources, the budgeting process becomes significant in implementing strategies. Budgeting is not only a planning approach to fund allocation, but also a valuable control approach in ascertaining which activities are on target and which are responsible for cost overruns. The budgeting process can be a sophisticated process, especially in the large organization. We cannot exhaust the subject in a book such as this, but we can summarize some of the significant aspects and note that more sophisticated treatment is available from courses and instructors who specialize in the budgetary process.

There are three distinct processes in budget preparation. They are (1) sales and volume budgets, (2) variable-cost budgets, and (3) overhead-cost budgets. The sales and volume budget forecasts the revenues and the quantities of services to be produced for the budgetary period, usually 1 year.

The budgeting process improves a communication pattern among various functional units in the company. Assume a goal of increasing revenue. The strategy to accomplish this goal is an increase in income. However, increasing income involves operations to provide the necessary services, as well as finances, to determine expenditures necessary and cash flow requirements. In fact, a cash flow budget may be established for the organization to ascertain whether sufficient funds will be available to pay for the operations as they proceed on a month-by-month operation of producing and selling.

The budget activity involves a variable-cost budget. This budget relates those costs that vary with the volume of services. The third budget (overhead) involves those costs that will be incurred in the short-run, regardless of what operation and service level is developed. They are the fixed costs of the operation. Overhead costs often pose a problem because they are often external to the firm, such as utility costs.

Another budget that could be of major concern, especially in the long run, is the capital budget. The concern here is almost always long run in nature and related to investment decisions, not financing operative decisions. Working capital decisions should also be included in the capital budgeting approach. With the increased number of mergers during the past 2 decades, capital budgeting has become important in such acquisition decisions.

Historically, budgeting has been done in a deterministic mode in that single value estimates are generally made. More recently the deterministic model has been upgraded by using mathematical models to show the relationship between variables, such as maintenance expense. The technology for the mathematical models is readily available; the problem is to determine the relationships without involving other variables that may remain unclear. More recently, probability theory has been introduced into budget preparation. In this approach, managers assign probabilities to a given event or to a set of relationships. Insofar as the assigned probability is realistic, the budgeting process can be made more accurate as a guide in the implementation of the strategies. These developments have permitted the introduction of flexibility into budgeting so that management can determine whether they are operating within the budget at various levels.

In a survey conducted by Daugherty and Donald,[17] five functions of budgets were identified by the respondents as follows:

1. Promotion of efficiency
2. Control
3. Planning, information, and feedback
4. Pressure exertion
5. Motivation

The authors also point out that the human component plays a major role in the budgeting process. Without proper attention to the human component behavioral patterns, dysfunctional consequences are possible. Among the suggestions made to overcome potential negative consequences were the following (p. 6):

- Active participation in the preparation of the budget
- An improved reporting structure (includes feedback)
- Increased responsibility and accountability for realistic objectives
- The use of positive motivators that appeal to higher level needs of organization members

Most managers of both for-profit and not-for-profit health organizations must become familiar with budgets and an implementation tool for strategies. Thus they are important processes for strategic managers to understand, both in their positive and dysfunctional aspects. The budgetary process will never be perfect, but it must be understood for successful implementation of strategies.

POLICIES

Policy is a very slippery concept. In its general, all-inclusive sense, policy is a guide to action. From this perspective any directive, statement, or gesture issued by a manager is a policy. In this sense a strategy can be conceived of as a policy and policy seen as an overall management responsibility. However, we will be using policy in a narrower sense to mean a guide to action on the part of managers and employees to implement the strategies determined by top-management personnel. In this sense, the strategy is what is to be accomplished and the policy is the how, when, and where the action will be completed, as well as the identification of who will do it. The purpose is to explain why certain actions are to be undertaken.

Policies, like so many other managerial tools and approaches, exist in hierarchies. Those developed at top-management levels are broad in scope, but the interpretation and policy formulation at lower levels become increasingly narrow. For example, it is probable that a broad, over-all policy of health service organization is that it will be an equal opportunity employer. As this general policy is interpreted at lower levels, it may mean a policy for a given department to hire only minorities until a certain percentage of the work force is reached. This hierarchy of policy concept or approach is also important in understanding the positive interrelationship between policies that must exist at the various levels of an organization. Obviously the lower-level policies must all be consistent with those developed by top management. CEOs relate strategic planning and top-level policies, whereas middle-management personnel develop policies, rules, procedures, and intermediate level budgets. At the lower levels of management, the chief concern is with schedules, programs, and short-run budgets. Policies are significant because they permit a rational and/or realistic approach to uncertainty situations. An uncertainty situation in this context refers to one where there is a disruption in the relationship between a person or organization and the environment. Given a severe disruption, the reaction is likely to be negative, such as trauma, inability to cope, frustration, and inappropriate behavior. Organizations try to prevent these kinds of negative reactions to disruption or problem situations by training and indoctrination, as well as developing policies and procedures as guidelines so that organizational managers can react in a positive manner.

Given the significant need for policies to guide behavior, the question should be raised as to how the policies should be formulated. This is largely a manner of style on the part of the manager as to how much other people will be brought into the policy-formulation process. It would be safe to say that top-management executives are very concerned about their ability to influence policy. Often, the ability to influence becomes a measure of the success of the executive, as well as his or her deferential treatment. The formulation or suggestion of the need for a policy often arises in middle- or supervisory-management levels and develops out of problems or needs these people see. Once this need is recognized by top management, a general policy could be established by top management. The key question, of course, is whether the disruptive situation is referred to that level or the policy is determined on an ad hoc basis (which eventually is formalized) at a lower level. Again, this depends on the executive's influence on policy and his or her leadership style in delegating problem situation resolution to lower-management personnel. It should also be noted that top executives usually are in a position to anticipate the need for policies and they are formulated and instituted on this basis.

Policy formulation may also be approached in terms of participative management. This approach involves managers at two or more levels in the organization or managers from two or more functional areas (patient care and marketing, for example) agreeing on a policy to guide the activities of both departments. This approach often ensures the proper execution of the policy, because the managers involved understand its need and feel that they participated in the formulation of the policy. In other words, it is their policy that is to be executed, rather than his or her policy, which "was not needed in the first place." Of course this procedure is likely to be time consuming, and sometimes the group cannot reach a decision. Then the superior-level manager must make the decision, which may cause greater negative reactions after the joint discussion.

On balance, however, it does seem that the participative approach has great advantages, especially when one considers that (1) a policy is a guide to action and (2) implementation of policies in health services depends on attitudes of professionals who have considerable autonomy.

Administration of Policy

The administration of policies has three major components: communication, interpretation, and control. Obviously, policies must be communicated to those who are going to use them. Because the communication task is often difficult, there is a tendency toward written policies. The problem with written policies is twofold: one is the difficulty of writing some kinds of policies and the other relates to the sheer volume of policy manuals (plural) that can be developed. A policy may be difficult to write and still protect the reputation of the organization and the needs of people. For example, an organization with a short-run cash flow problem may formulate the policy of no nonauthorized purchases over a given dollar limit. However, if such a policy is known outside the organization itself, it may cause negative reactions on the part of physicians (who may avoid the hospital) and/or consumers (who may join a competing HMO to be ensured of better [perceived perhaps] health care).

Attention also should be given to the dissemination of policy. Many organizations have policy manuals, some of which are voluminous. Another problem is that of encouraging managers to keep the manual current by inserting updated or revised policy. Usually the policy manuals become out-of-date, and a complete new volume must be distributed that supersedes older editions. This is usually costly but generally cannot be avoided if changes are going to be incorporated. Moreover, it is unlikely that many people will read such manuals, let alone retain the information if they do.

Other forms of written media include statements distributed to interested parties and notices on bulletin boards. Letters may be used, as well as pamphlets. There is a trend toward writing policy statements, as opposed to word of mouth dissemination. Generally, the written statement is more likely to be observed. In addition, the written statement is becoming increasingly important as evidence of compliance in such areas as discrimination. Also, more malpractice suits are being brought against management in various settings and situations. In some situations the written policy is useful as evidence in these malpractice suits and indicates management's intent to inform.

However, because a policy is in written format does not mean that it will be read, understood, and accepted. Training programs, indoctrination procedures, and personnel appraisal or evaluation programs may help ensure that the policy is not only understood but followed. Some care must be exercised, however, in these expectations, since most policies are general guides to action and not specific rules. Nevertheless, policy must be accepted by managers and employees in the organization. Otherwise it is impossible to be able to meet uncertainty situations and work together to achieve the goals and objectives of the organization in an effective manner.

A problem related to interpretation of policy is the possible conflict between policies. When policies are formulated at different times or by different people, conflicts are likely to occur. In these kinds of situations, the conflict is likely to be resolved by "referring the matter upstairs" to a superior. Sometimes this will result in yet a different or a third policy or interpretation. This certainly resolves the problem, provided that the two conflicting policies are rescinded and everyone knows this has happened.

As stated, policies are guides to action; they are not rules. Policies may be formulated at any level of the organization although they must be approved by higher authorities.

CULTURE

A key responsibility of the health care manager is that of establishing the managerial climate (culture). Health care organizations have personalities in the same way as people do. Their personality is not something tangible; it is composed of sensations and impressions of those who make up the work force of the health care organization. Such impressions are generated by the values held by those who govern or manage the organization, the physicians who use it, and the providers of patient care. Quite naturally, managers and other staff play a major role in the development of these values, since the organization tends to reflect those who govern and use it. On the other hand, Kets DeVries[18] suggests that "although the personality of the manager can vitally influence his/her organizations, a reverse relationship also exists" (p. 277). One cannot discount tradition or history, because usually managerial people must be compatible with each other and the organization. Despite this, the CEO manages change, and when a change in managerial climate is called for in order for the health care organization to present a different image, he or she must recognize the need and be capable of meeting it.

During the 1980s corporate culture has received increased attention. Culture has to do with the people in the health care organization and the unique quality of character of the organization. Qualities used to describe culture are psychological in nature and concern the ambiance of the organization, its unique atmosphere, the shared values, beliefs, attitudes, norms, ideologies, and behavioral patterns of employees. Although there are many definitions of culture, the simple statement by William B. Renner, vice-chairman of the Aluminum Company of America, is best for our purposes: "Culture is the shared values and behavior that knit a community (health care organization) together." Culture involves people, and where large numbers of people are involved providing personal services, their values must be important. Kilmann[19] suggests that culture is "most controllable through norms, the unwritten rules of the game." He suggests the following (p. 212):

> A good way to assess a health services organization's culture is to ask members to write out what previously was unwritten. . . . Members are willing and able to write out their norms under certain conditions: (a) that no member will be identified as having stated or suggested a particular norm (individual confidentiality), and (b) that no norm will be documented when one's superiors are present (candid openness). Furthermore, the members must have faith that the norm will not be used against them but will instead be used to benefit them as well as their organization.

When the guiding norms have been identified, the executives and planners are asked to identify any new directions and the norms associated with those new directions are determined. The difference between "what is" and "what is desired" is the culture gap. Even the identification of the gap together with the new norms often will cause change, provided of course that management is willing to change. Beyond this, agreements for change are usually required and new ways of behavior recognized and reinforced by managers and employees alike. Changing culture is a powerful tool but may require specialized consultants, at least initially. There appears to be no question that culture or the values of the health care organization can have a positive or negative impact. If the impact is positive, the entire work force assumes attitudes that, taken together, make the organization a good place to work, one that provides high quality of care. It is interesting how this attitude is communicated to visitors. One of the authors had an appointment with the CEO of one of the well-known hospitals in the nation. He stopped at the receptionist's desk to affirm his appointment at the scheduled time. The receptionist countered by asking that an appointment be made for *her* with the CEO, so that those at the working level could talk with him to resolve problems and improve quality of care. Her final comment was, "He never has time for the common worker, but hides in his executive suite." Obviously there were problems and a negative cultural attitude.

On the other hand, the same author visited a clinic and remarked to the receptionist how attractive the decor was and how pleasant the attitudes of workers were. He was treated to a quite lengthy report about how fortunate employees were to work there, how they participated in decisions affecting their operations, and how the employees had participated in choosing the color combinations in the office decor. The employee pointed out that all the employees in the office wore clothing that blended with the office. As a test, the author suggested that this was akin to wearing uniforms. The employee became quite agitated, and said she was misunderstood. In fact, she insisted that the clothing could not at all be considered a uniform but was quite the opposite—an individual expression of the positive attitudes held by the employees toward the organization. The author apologized, of course, thanked her for her information, and left with pleasant thoughts about the encounter and the hope that if he needed treatment in that city, it could occur in that particular clinic.

A key question is whether the culture of an organization can be changed. Some organizations have hired consulting "gurus" to change the attitudes of their employees. We hear stories about these attitude-change seminars causing more problems than solutions. If this is true, it is probably because there exists a basic mistrust of management that has been reinforced by years of experience. In such situations a seminar of a few days or a week that suggests "strategies" on conflict resolution (in terms of reacting to disagreement) has little long-run effect and probably the short-run effect is minimal.

What then can be said about changing the culture of the organization? First, it is necessary to evaluate the economic and service situation of the health care organization. Is the situation one of poor economic and service health—one requiring fundamental changes? If there has been a steady decline in positive attitudes over time, one can question the effectiveness of management. Also, has this decline had an effect on employees and their actions? Has there been an increase in turnover, especially among the more highly skilled employees? Has there been an increase in grievances and complaints? Has the quality of care declined? If answers to these kinds of questions are affirmative, there probably will be a degree of confusion on the part of management and the governing board. Management should be asked to bring forth a plan of action for change. If the plan is not acceptable, perhaps it is time to bring in a consulting firm or, in some cases, new management. No one likes to see anyone fired, but sometimes the health of the organization is at stake, to say nothing about the health of the patients. Fitzgerald[20] points out (p. 9):

> Although the management culture has been declared a needed instrument for strengthening organizational control and producing improvement, we can't talk intelligently about changing cultures until we understand how to change underlying values.

The CEO must know not only the value sets of his CEOs, but also his own. However, this knowledge will be insufficient unless the value sets are analyzed in terms of whether they result in an atmosphere that is considered to be valuable by patients and employees, rare, and imperfectly imitatable. Barney[21] points out that "without these three characteristics, organizations cannot expect their cultures to be the source of sustained competitive advantage" (p. 663). Each of us can think of health care organizations that have a unique culture that results in a unique environment and a resulting competitive advantage in providing health care for patients. (Examples include but are not limited to the Mayo Clinic, Massachusetts General Hospital, and Johns Hopkins Memorial Hospital.)

In most situations, fundamental changes or drastic actions are not necessary. Rather, the approach is incremental, calling for minor changes that will lead to a better understanding and a better working environment. In the negative cultural attitude situation mentioned above, a meeting with employees may resolve the problem, or the CEO and his or her staff could spend a few hours each week walking around—the "management by walking around" approach that Hewlett-Packard and other organizations follow. Usually this type of situation tends to be experimental in nature, with small changes introduced and observed to ascertain if subsequent developments are positioned in the desired direction. One might also ask how the culture is maintained, once it has been developed to a more desirable state. There are essentially three elements: selection of employees, training, and reinforcement. Selection is important in terms of hiring people with attitudes similar to those of the organization. One can argue that this will result in "group think" and no new ideas. Perhaps, but whether this is true depends on the training of new employees and reinforcement. Training is important so that employees know the nature of the organization and the expectations held relative to their job. Reinforcement is an ongoing activity. For example, innovative attitudes and actions can be reinforced or conformity stressed. Recognition via communication, promotions, and reward systems tend to be most significant.

We stress the importance of objectives in the acculturation process. The four objectives of community service, quality, and effective and efficient patient care should always be basic in the minds of managers so that employees have overall goals into which they can fit the individual service promised by them in the job they occupy.

SUMMARY

The focal point of this chapter has been the implementation of the strategic plan. Without implementation or execution of the strategies, the planning function is an empty exercise. This is a lesson that all planners must learn, and implementation suggestions must be included as part of the plan. At the very least, the CEO and his or her staff must be cognizant of the need to implement strategies.

This chapter summarized five major concepts associated with implementation as follows:

1. Change
2. Structure
3. Resource deployment
4. Policies
5. Culture

These are elements of the implementation of strategy process. We restate our opening proposition. Our experiences tell us, along with the experience of countless others, that it is far easier to formulate plans than it is to implement or execute them. The concepts in this chapter, however, will aid the manager in achieving the goal of putting strategic changes into action.

REFERENCES

1. Cooke RA: Managing change in organizations. In Zaltman G, editor: Management principles for non-profit agencies and organizations, New York, 1979, AMACOM, Book Division.
2. Hammond JS: The roles of the manager and management scientist in successful implementation, Sloan Manage Rev 15(2):1, 1974.
3. Zand DE and Sorensen RE: Theory of change and effective use of management science, Admin Sci Q 20(4):532, 1975.

4. Lewin K: Field theory in social science: selected theoretical papers, New York, 1951, Harper & Row Publishers, Inc. (Edited by D Cartwright).
5. Tichy NM: Managing change strategically: the technical, political and cultural keys, Organizational Dynamics 11(2):59, 1982.
6. Beer M: Revitalizing organizations: change process and emergent model, The Academy of Management Executive 1(1):51, 1987.
7. Isenberg DJ: The tactics of strategic opportunism, Harvard Business Review 65(1):92, 987.
8. Brodwin DR and Bourgeois LJ, III: Five steps to strategic action, California Manage Rev 26(3):167, 1984.
9. ACHA: Principles of appointment and tenure of executive officers, American College of Hospital Administrators Task Force V, Chicago, 1973.
10. Weber M: Theory of social and economic organization, London, 1947, (Translated and edited by Henderson AM and Parson T, 1921) Oxford University Press, Inc.
11. Fayol H: Industrial and general administration, London, 1930, Pitman.
12. Davis RC: The fundamentals of top management, New York, 1951, Harper & Row Publishers, Inc.
13. Anderson BJ: Hospital governance board and medical staff relations, Milwaukee Med Soc Times 47(4):April, 1974.
14. Pfeffer J: Size and composition of corporate boards of directors organization and environment, Admin Sci Q 17(2):218, 1972.
15. Campbell JP et al: Managerial behavior, performance and effectiveness, New York, 1970, McGraw-Hill, Inc.
16. Chandler AD: Strategy and structure, Cambridge, Ma, 1962, The MIT Press.
17. Daugherty W and Donald H: Some behavioral implications of budgeting systems, Arizona Business 20(4):3, 1973.
18. Kets DeVries MFR: Personality, culture, and organization, Acad Manage Rev 11(2):266, 1986.
19. Kilman RH: Management of corporate culture. In Fottler MR, Hernandez SR, and Joiner CL, editors: Strategic management of human resources in health organizations, New York, 1988, John Wiley & Sons, Inc.
20. Fitzgerald TH: Can change in organizational culture really be management? Organizational Dynamics 17(2):5, 1988.
21. Barney JB: Organizational culture: can it be a source of sustained competitive advantage? Acad Manage Rev 11(3):656, 1986.

7

Changing Roles of the Chief Executive Officer with Special Emphasis on the Evaluation/Control Process

If a health services manager were asked, "What is your role in the organization?" he or she is likely to respond, "To see to it that the organization meets community needs effectively and efficiently," or as one manager responded, "To manage 'my' institution and serve community needs 'better' than anyone else." If it were a for-profit organization, he or she would add "while earning a fair rate of return for the shareholders." These comments indicate the presence of a goal or objective (to meet community needs) and the competitive spirit (better than anyone else) that are present among health care CEOs today. We should note that there is not necessarily one best role for all health care CEOs; it will vary according to a number of environmental and internal factors. Roles are determined by others and by many institutional and environmental characteristics, such as size and control of the health care organization. The personal characteristics and style of the manager also affect roles. Moreover, managers have multiple roles to fill, such as task roles and social roles.

In spite of the difficulty in defining roles, it is important to attempt to examine them. A definition and classification of roles should help managers and board members to understand and improve relationships and responsibilities; it may also help to reduce conflict caused by role ambiguity and to select and train managers. Also, we suggest that roles change as the environment changes, and a classification of roles should help to evaluate the effects of such changes.

In the first section of this chapter we examine roles in light of published research. The second section considers what we will call roles/processes. A third section reviews

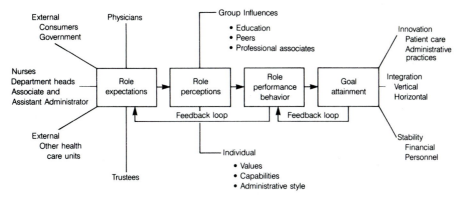

Fig. 7-1   Hospital CEO role model. (From Johnson, AC, Forrest CR, and Mosher J: An investigation into the nature, causes and implications of the future role of the health care administration, US Department of Health, Education, and Welfare, Public Health Service, Health Resources Administration, Bureau of Health Manpower, Washington, DC, 1978 DHEW Publication No (HRA) 78-33, p. 122. Adapted from Katz D and Kahn RL: The social psychology of organizations New York, 1966, John Wiley & Sons, Inc.)

some recent changes in organizations. The chapter ends with a summary of evaluation/control factors relative to strategic management.

We will use the term CEO to refer to the general manager. Aguilar[1] offers an action/oriented definition of the general manager as follows:

> The general manager is the person in charge of an enterprise (a relatively autonomous operating organization) with responsibility for the timely and correct execution of those actions promoting the successful performance and well-being of the unit.

ROLE MODELS—AN OVERVIEW

Johnson, Forrest, and Mosher[2] developed a role model of the health care CEO, which we will use in our examination of role models (Fig. 7-1). Beginning at the far left in Fig. 7-1, the typical role-set encountered by the CEO is identified. These are the role senders who set forth their role expectations of the CEO. Internally they consist of physicians, trustees, vice presidents, associate and assistant administrators, department heads, and nursing personnel. External to a hospital they are consumers, government laws and regulations, and other health care units, such as other hospitals in the community.

Role expectations are sent (communicated) to the CEO, who translates the messages into role perceptions. It is indeed possible that the CEO's role perceptions do not coincide with the role expectations because of misinterpretations or the impossibility of achieving the role expectations. Role perceptions can be considered as intervening variables between role expectations and role performance behaviors.

The degree to which a person's behavior conforms to the expectations held for him or her at one point in time will affect the state of those expectations at the next point. For example, if the CEO's response to the role sender is hostile, the role sender is likely to behave toward the CEO far differently than if the response were positive. An example of a role interaction situation between a physician and the CEO might be as follows. The physician, in requesting a new service for the hospital, might "expect" the CEO to be resistant because the physician perceived the CEO to be concerned primarily about costs. The physician under these circumstances may send an intimidating role message: "You better get this service or I'll take my patients elsewhere." The CEO perceives that the physician will expect more concern about costs and that the physician indeed will take patients elsewhere. Consequently, to avoid risk and conflict, the CEO could respond by submitting to the request. Feedback of this to the role sender might change the physician's expectations and/or reinforce future intimidating behavior on the part of the physician.

Role perceptions on the part of the CEO may be influenced by various groups, as well as the personality and experience of the CEO. Group influences as indicated in the model include educational experience, the peer group of CEOs in other hospitals, and local, state, and national professional associations.

However, there are other factors involved in establishing and perceiving roles. For example, organizational factors, such as a very strong board organization in a competitive hospital community environment, combined with open staffs, a surplus of beds, and low occupancy can affect both the role senders and the perceived role of the CEO. This situation would permit a physician to make a threat with some likelihood that it will be carried out and have an impact on the CEO.

The third major variable in the model is that of role performance behaviors. Role performance behaviors include overall role patterns, such as business manager, coordinator, corporate chief, or management team leader (discussed in Chapter 6). Subcomponents would include managerial role-behavioral patterns or process activities, such as strategic planning, negotiating, and evaluating the managerial performance of other administrative personnel. Role performance has been defined also in terms of the functions of planning, organizing, assembling resources, staffing, and control. In other situations, role performance has been analyzed in terms of the tasks or activity behavioral patterns of the CEO.

The output or dependent variable of the model is goal attainment. The concept of goal attainment is defined in terms of innovation, stability, and integration as the goals of the CEO for the health care organization. Innovation is important in terms of introducing new ideas, procedures, and knowledge. Stability is the attempt to control, order, and maintain the system. Cost effectiveness is sometimes a part of this goal.

Vertical integration refers to serving a series of different kinds of patients or clients. Examples can be found in the combination of group practice clinics, ambulatory care facilities, long-term care units, apartments for senior citizens, and community health education units, all associated with an acute, general care hospital. Sometimes the arrangements are rather loose in nature, but in other situations, such as mergers, a formal relationship is entered into by the various organizations, and all operate under one board of directors. If this approach improves patient care and also results in economies of scale through reduced administrative costs, for example, more and more of these types of combinations are likely to occur.

Horizontal integration refers to the combination of similar type organizations, such as acute or general care hospitals. The kinds of horizontal mergers range from the sharing of services, such as laboratory facilities, to affiliation agreements to mergers involving centralized management operation. CEOs may report to a local board, which is primarily advisory, and to a centralized management operation. In the case of investor-owned hospitals, the CEO of the local hospital would report to a system executive. Another intermediate arrangement is that of the consortium where organizations share services and facilities and a combined board of trustees is involved, with representatives from the affiliated hospitals whose function is to foster integrated activities.

Note that there are two feedback loops included in the model. One of these relates goal attainment to role performance, and a second refers back to role perceptions from role performance, as well as relating to role expectations. These account for learning by both the CEO and the role senders, perceptual errors that can be corrected, and changes in expectations that could occur as goals are attained. Role behavior of the CEO will ultimately affect his or her attributes, for example, if the CEO continually reacts defensively to threats, his or her personality will change over time and this will also affect interrelationship factors.

We suggest that this role model can be helpful to readers in diagnosing problems in role relationships and behavior. Note the impact of external factors on the role of the CEO. Not only are governmental factors involved, but also local environmental elements. Is this a wealthy suburban area that has expectations and resources available to develop a powerful and prestigious medical center? If so, it probably has a powerful and prestigious governing board and organizational strategies will be affected accordingly.

Environmental values and expectations influence the values and actions of the manager. He or she will probably hold or adopt many of these environmental values and expectations. Roberts and King[3] suggest a stakeholder audit (1) to determine who they are, their expectations, and the relevance of these expectations and (2) to form the basis of new strategies appropriate to the external environment and the capabilities of the organization.

The purpose or mission of the role of the CEO is to help move the organization to meet the health needs of the community and society, that is, improve health, improve access to health services, improve quality of service, contain costs, and achieve institutional objectives in relation to these output objectives. What managers perceive as needs will affect their personal attributes. Are the values of the manager and the environment, for example, circle of friends and community power groups, to improve health or to build the prestige of the organization and the manager? Although these are not mutually exclusive, there is evidence of conflict between values and objectives of and for the organization and the CEO. For example, a CEO of a hospital might argue that a second open heart surgery program in the community (at his or her hospital) is important for comprehensive services to patients. However, the underlying purpose may be to bring prestige to the hospital and the CEO that open heart surgery brings and that an outreach home care service may not bring, even though it might improve the general health of the community more effectively. We of course suggest that although general managers will reflect the values, expectations, and resources of the environment, their purpose is to identify needs of the community and to help influence values, expectations, and resources of the environment to meet community needs. This latter concept refers to leadership, and we will talk more about this subject later in the chapter.

ROLES/PROCESSES

Fayol,[4] an early observer of managerial activity, concluded that there are five major identifiable processes: planning, organizing, commanding, coordinating, and controlling. It was generally accepted doctrine that these were universal processes, regardless of the nature of the organization.

The American College of Hospital Administrators has identified four major areas or "domains" to encompass tasks performed by hospital and health services administrators. These domains were identified as governance and control; resource acquisition and management; service delivery; and environmental relations.[5] These are the major components of a task delineation, which is "a listing of the tasks, knowledge, and skills which are necessary for professional functioning in the field of hospital and health services administration" (p. 44).

In 1973 Mintzberg's book, *The Nature of Managerial Work,*[6] was published, which increased interest in the roles that were performed by managers. Included in his study was the CEO of a hospital. Ten roles were identified and associated with the three board classifications of interpersonal, informational, and decision roles. The descriptors of these ten roles are presented in the box at right. Johnson, Forrest, and Mosher,[2] as part of their study of health care administrators, asked administrators in hospitals (755), long-term care facilities (148), and clinics (31) to indicate the importance of ten managerial roles identified by Mintzberg.

The entrepreneur, leader, and monitor roles ranked among the three most important roles for all three groups (Table 7-1). The executives indicated a congruence with the importance of the various roles. There were minor differences among the groups for the entrepreneur and monitor roles, but a significant difference among the groups, and in particular, between the hospital administrators and the long-term care executives for the leader role. Note that in this section the words manager, executive, and administrator are synonymous. The long-term care executives rated the importance of the leader role higher than either of the other groups, suggesting that this role of interpersonal relationships and motivation is more crucial in the long-term care facility than it is in the hospital. A number of other significant and interesting differences were between the groups in the negotiator, spokesman, disturbance handler, and figurehead roles. The negotiator role was reported as significantly less important in long-term care facilities than in the other two settings. The spokesman role was significantly more important to the hospital administrators than to either of the other two groups. The hospital administrators further reported on average that the disturbance handler role was less important in their settings than in long-term care facilities or clinics. Finally, clinic administrators assigned a significantly lower importance to the figurehead role than did either hospital administrators or long-term care facility administrators.

In a similar but unrelated study, Kuhl[7] and her colleagues elicited responses from

MANAGERIAL ROLE DESCRIPTIONS BASED ON MINTZBERG, 1973

Interpersonal roles

The figurehead role   The chief executive is a symbol required by the status of his or her office to carry out a variety of social, legal, and ceremonial duties in which he or she represents the organization.

The leader role   The chief executive has interpersonal relationships with is or her subordinates; as he or she hires, trains, and motivates them, he or she must essentially bring their needs in accord with those of the organization.

The liaison role   The chief executive has interpersonal relationships with people outside of his or her own organization and spends a considerable amount of time developing a network of high-status contacts in which information and favors are traded for mutual benefit and through which the chief executive exerts community leadership.

Information roles

The monitor role   The chief executive continually seeks and receives information about his or her organization in order to understand changing situations and his or her organization's environment.

The disseminator role   The chief executive shares some of the environmental information with his or her subordinates.

The spokesperson role   The chief executive informs outsiders about the progress, problems, and activities of his or her organization

Decisional roles

The entrepreneur role   The chief executive continually seeks and receives information about changes in the organization, looking for problems and opportunities, and then initiating projects to deal with them.

The disturbance handler role   The chief executive takes charge when the organization faces a major disturbance or crisis and deals with the resulting problems.

The resource allocator role   The chief executive decides who will get what in his or her organization, establishing priorities, designing the organization, and authorizing all important decisions.

The negotiator role   The chief executive takes charge whenever the organization must enter into crucial negotiations with other parties; his or her presence is required because he or she has the information and the authority to make the decisions that difficult negotiations require.

From Johnson, AC, Forrest CR, and Mosher J: An investigation into the nature, causes and implications of the future role of the health care administrator, U.S. Department of Health, Education and Welfare, Public Health Service, Health Resources Administration, Bureau of Health Manpower, DHEW Publication No. (HRA) 78-33. Washington, D.C. 1977, p. 224.

Table 7-1 Managerial role descriptions: ranking of importance

Role	Hospital administrators		Long-term care administrators		Clinic administrators		F ratio	Significance probability
	Mean	Rank	Mean	Rank	Mean	Rank		
Entrepreneur	3.951	1	3.778	2	3.760	2	1.59	.206
Leader	3.942	2	4.299	1	4.074	1	6.37	.002†
Monitor	3.331	3	3.363	3	3.654	3	1.90	.152
Resource allocator	3.275	4	3.258	4	3.038	5.5	.86	.424
Liaison	3.137	5	2.864	6	3.038	5.5	2.92	.055
Negotiator	2.900	6	2.624	7	3.074	4	4.70	.010†
Spokesman	2.675	7	2.388	9	2.200	9	7.46	.001†
Disturbance handler	2.610	8	3.016	5	2.920	7	9.21	.000†
Disseminator	2.525	9	2.573	8	2.720	8	.68	.508
Figurehead	1.751	10	1.992	10	1.480	10	3.72	.025*

From Johnson AC, Forrest CR, and Mosher J: An investigation into the nature, causes, and implications of the future role of the health care administrator, US Department of Health, Education and Welfare, Public Health Service. Health Resources Administration, Bureau of Health Manpower, DHEW Publication No. (HRA) 78-33, Washington, DC, 1977, p. 176

Responses were scaled: 1—Least (time consumed, importance, anticipated importance); 2—Below average (time consumed, importance, anticipated importance); 3—Average (time consumed, importance, anticipated importance); 4—Above average (time consumed, importance, anticipated importance); and 5—Most (time consumed, importance, anticipated importance).

*.05 level of significance

†.01 level of significance

149 hospital CEOs concerning the activities, roles, and skills required to meet the responsibilities of their positions. Four major-component categories were established: internal management, organizational development, external relations, and environmental surveillance.

Related to internal management were organizational design, personnel management (staffing, labor negotiations, recruitment and training, promotions and dismissals, and evaluation), financial management (cost containment, cost accounting, billing, fee determination, budget determination, and fund raising), logistical management, and service delivery (management, evaluation, and improvement). In larger hospitals, many of these tasks would be delegated by the CEO.

Organizational development related to planning and external relations included community relations, organization relations, and government relations. Environmental surveillance referred to market research.

It should be noted that there are considerable similarities between these two studies. However, neither is directly concerned with the relationship between the performance of the various activities and managerial effectiveness.

It is interesting to relate Mintzberg's ten roles to the strategic management process. We suggest that the liaison, entrepreneur, and negotiator are involved with planning. The figurehead, leader, disseminator, spokesman, and resource allocator roles relate to implementation, and monitor and disturbance handling to evaluation/control. More will be said about evaluation/control later in this chapter, whereas the planning and implementation were discussed in Chapters 5 and 6.

Kleiner[8] in his study of the role of 42 hospital administrators in 11 different multihospital systems found that there were similarities and differences in role performance. The administrators viewed the "functional areas of planning, policy making, financial management, human resources management, organization design, and clinical services as most important" (p. 29). In addition to general agreement on these functions, the following areas showed a high frequency of personal involvement by the respondents (p. 28):

- Creating plans and policies to assure long-term viability
- Overseeing the major financial decisions regarding hospital operations and capital expenditures
- Creating a work environment through human resources management and organizational design that enhances worker satisfaction and productivity
- Maintaining close relationships with members of the clinical staff

There were also differences in the personal involvement of the administrators in performance of roles and tasks. Differences included the following:

- Local versus corporate responsibility for hospital operations
- Extent of corporate guidance
- Response to community needs
- Concern for long-term and operational viability
- Approval by regulatory agencies
- Maintenance of competitive salary structures and union or employee relations
- Concern for future physician recruitment

More recently, Zuckerman[9] concluded that an increasingly uncertain and turbulent environment, coupled with growing organizational complexity, suggests greater centrality of the role of the CEO. He suggests the following three categories of roles:

1. *Perimeter player*—the concern here is with the adaptation of the health care organization to its external environment
2. *Interior designer*—the CEO must include in his overall responsibilities the internal operations of the organization including tasks such as "management of costs and quality, maintaining requisite communication, coordination, and information flow, managing conflict, allocating resources, and managing human resources" (p. 26)
3. *Leader of the band*—involves developing and keeping corporate values and providing strategic vision and direction to the organization; the CEO must assure "that the organization remains true to its mission and responsive to its key influential constituencies (p. 26)

The 1980s have seen many changes in organizational relationships in health care. There have been various mergers, as well as other arrangements that can be described as "quasi firms." Luke, Begun, and Pointer[10] comment on these organizational arrangements as follows (p. 9):

> Significant political, socioeconomic, and governmental changes are causing health care organizations to configure and restructure in innovative ways. Some health organizations have merged with others in tight bureaucratic structures. Others have entered more loosely coupled multiorganizational arrangements, which, although created to function as interdependent wholes, maintain each organization's separate legal identity. These loosely coupled forms are linked in a number of ways, including by subcontracts, leases, interlocking boards, and marketing agreements.

Various reasons lie behind the development of these quasi firms. Often there is less risk involved than in acquisition or mergers. At the same time, efficiencies are present, as well as greater legitimacy for some participants.

D'Aunno and Zuckerman[11] discuss the importance of the organizational federations that recently developed as a form of multiorganizational collaboration. These federations involve no change in corporate ownership but do provide advantages to the members, as well as cause a change in the role behavior of the CEO as a key actor in continued relationships. Examples include the American Hospital Association, the Voluntary Hospitals of America, and many regional federations.

A key question is the impact these multiorganizational changes have on the role of the CEO. Hoare[12] suggests that "managing a multiunit system entails balancing the need to differentiate activities and the need to integrate activities on a scale new to the private health care industry" (p. 424). Mintzberg[13] developed a useful way of looking at the parts of multiorganizational structures. He pictures an organization with (1) a strategic apex (CEO and his or her staff), (2) middle line managers, (3) the large operating core as a base and two support configurations, (4) the technostructure, and (5) the support staff. Hoare[12] uses this model to set forth the new challenges and new knowledge areas and skills for institution administrators, managers of alternative delivery systems, and product line managers, as well as regional office staff (middle

Table 7-2   Challenges of new roles in multiunit organizations

	New challenges	New knowledge areas and skills
Institution administrators	Oversee the downward implementation of corporate directives and the upward communication of the institution's needs; represent the system to the local community; balance the demands of personnel, medical staff, and community against those of the corporate hierarchy Manage relationships with other local facilities and services that form the vertically integrated system Monitor the local environment for the system	Negotiation, conflict mediation, communication with different constituencies inside and outside the system, constructive use of power, media relations
Managers of alternative delivery systems (HMOs, ambulatory centers, home health, SNFs)	Develop contractual relationships with a variety of service providers to produce services at the lowest cost per unit Market those services to a variety of purchasers Know the clinical factors that affect service delivery	Negotiation, marketing, contract development, utilization review, physican relationships, insurance
"Product line" managers of clinical services or related products	Of clinical services: analyze related clusters of services to develop more cost-effective subunits within the traditional hospital structure and in related satellite settings Of health care products or services: analyze and develop strong internal units into related products that increase revenues or produce system efficiencies by (1) synergies from forward or backward vertical integration or (2) economies of scale	Work analysis, cost accounting, utilization review, quality assurance, organization design, project management, team building, negotiation, medical staff communication skills, constructive use of power, entrepreneurial initiative "Brand manager" skills of marketing, cost accounting, project management, constructive use of power, entrepreneurial initiative
Regional office staff (middle line)	As need for vertical integration increases, tasks will shift from downward implementation of corporate policies, compliance monitoring, and helping administrators manage board relations to "system development" tasks, sensing the local environment, sponsoring innovation	Negotiation, conflict resolution, project management, systems analysis, incentive systems, organization design, managerial accounting, familiarity with all types of service units

Table 7-2   Challenges of new roles in multiunit organizations—cont'd

	New challenges	New knowledge areas and skills
Techno-structure staff	Design procedures that will aid the vertical integration of systems through standardization	Systems analysis and needs assessment, interorganizational relations, transfer pricing, market research, project or temporary task force management
Support staff	Assist in the development of the system of relationships that allows regional or local vertical integration to succeed Help change the "cultures" of hospitals as hospitals become diversified health care centers	Organization development often from a distance with episodic contact, inteorganizational relations, problem sensing
Strategic apex executives	Plan on a regional, national or international basis. Design and incrementally implement an organization structure that appropriately balances the need to differentiate units to match the demands of local service areas and the need to integrate corporatewide activities in a decentralized structure, which rewards local initiative while maintaining control.	Diversification strategy development, corporate policy making, organization design, executive incentive systems, influencing government policy

From Hoare G: New managerial roles in multiorganizational systems: implications for health administration education, J Health Admin Educ 5(3):429, 1987.

line), the technostructure staff, support staff, and strategic apex executives. Table 7-2 outlines these positions, the new challenges involved, and new knowledge areas and skills required. In many instances these various units will require the skills of the general manager, who will operate as the CEO of the unit. Hoare suggests the need for new skills to meet changing roles associated with multisystem units. He suggests that these skills "involve the tasks of service or product diversification and integrated system development" (p. 435). These are related to the strategic management process we have discussed, developing a strategic plan, the necessity of evaluating the environmental situation, and identifying the necessary policies, structures and monitoring systems to implement and evaluate required strategies.

There can be a downside to the multiunit organizations. If CEOs concentrate on financing and marketing schemes, they may very well miss opportunities to improve the quality and efficiency of health care. Herzlinger[14] suggests that quality and efficiency can be improved by looking to the "key areas of administration of operations, management of human resources, management control systems, and the formation of a management philosophy" (p. 99) that is appropriate to the organization.

Goldsmith[15] also points out that large investor-owned organizations, such as the "Hospital Corporation of America, Humana, National Medical Enterprises, and American Medical International have divested marginal facilities and pruned shaky diversification ventures" (p. 105). He concludes that new organizations will develop with different organizational relationships as follows (p. 111):

> Increasingly, the chronically ill will be treated in the home or in settings remote from the traditional hospital facility. As technological advances continue to strike at disease, most illness will be associated with the infirmities of aging. The community hospital will decentralize its services and weave them into the fabric of the neighborhood and the community. The main role of most community hospitals will be diagnosis and treatment of the chronically ill. As the population ages, we will be reallocating resources from acute to chronic care. Those hospitals that recognize this shift in societal priorities can plan to adapt their programs and facilities to meet these new needs.

Shortell[16] concludes that economies of larger scale operations have not yet proven effective in hospitals. This no doubt is because personnel costs represent about 60% of total costs and many of the costs are associated with skilled professionals and technicians who are not necessarily attracted to multiunit organizations nor receptive to cost-containment procedures that may at least have the appearance of lower-level care for their patients. We should also add that the general philosophy of Americans is changing from one of treatment of illness to prevention. This change, of course, has ramifications for the role of the CEO if the trend continues.

What does this all mean? We can infer from the research that there are differences in the attention given various roles and that these differences are specific to the health care organization. It should also be noted that all of the roles are present and that the source of difference is related to the degree of attention given to the specific role, as well as the specific involvement of the CEO. Similar to the impact of the external environment on the roles of CEOs, the local internal situation of the health care organization will affect the attention given to implementing roles/processes. However, these differences are not troublesome to the extent that one needs to focus on specific strategic management aspects relative to hospitals, long-term care organizations, or clinics. Rather, it is satisfactory and reasonable to discuss strategic management and the associated roles from a generalized perspective. Indeed, we know of people who have successfully met the responsibilities of managerial positions in different organizations. For example, one person has been a successful associate administrator of a hospital, a state government health system administrator, and a clinic (HMO) manager. He was able to understand the clinical/managerial situation and effectuate a successful approach to specific performance of roles appropriate to the situation.

MONITORING/EVALUATING/CONTROLLING

A role that requires more discussion is that of monitoring (see Table 7-1), leading to evaluation and control of strategies. Most health care organizations devote considerable time and effort to record, evaluate, and interpret a tremendous amount of information. Some of this information is required by governmental and regulatory bodies. Other information is used for managerial purposes and should be appropriate for the needs of managers at the different levels of the organization, with higher levels requiring broader and more integrative information. Although all information, in varying degrees of appropriateness, contributes to improved decision making, it does not necessarily provide useful feedback to top management regarding the performance of the organization in implementing strategies and achieving objectives. Thus CEOs need to develop information regarding progress toward strategy achievement performance relative to success factor measures that were established as a part of strategy and the implementation process itself. This is a strategic control system.

What top management needs is a system that will provide salient information on a regular basis. Rockart[17] says that there are "four main ways of determining executive information needs: the *by-product* technique, the *null approach,* the *key indicator* system, and the *total study* process" (p. 82). Under the by-product technique, the executive uses the information processed for other purposes, such as financial reporting. The null method argues that because of rapidly changing conditions it is impossible to predetermine what is needed; CEOs must deal with informal, word-of-mouth, ad hoc reports by knowledgeable employees. There are three aspects to the key indicator system: (1) the selection of key indicators relevant to the health of the organization; (2) exception reporting (reports involving situations where performance differs from expectations); and (3) information storage, processing, display, and charting using a computer. The total study involves sampling a widespread group of managers to determine the information needs of the organization. Rockart[17] notes that "the objectives of the process are to develop an overall understanding of the business, the information necessary to manage the business, and the existing information systems. Gaps between information systems that are needed and those currently in place are noted. A plan for implementing new systems to fill the observed gaps is then developed" (p. 84).

A group of researchers at the Sloan School of Management, Massachusetts Institute of Technology, suggests an information definition approach that they call the "critical success factors approach." Rockart[17] defines critical success factors that "are, for any business, the limited number of areas in which results, if they are satisfactory, will ensure successful competitive performance for the organization. They are the few key areas where 'things must go right' for the business to flourish. If results in these areas are not adequate, the organization's efforts for the period will be less than desired" (p. 85). Who defines the critical success factors? The CEO and his or her staff are best qualified to do this. Thus the system would be tailored to the needs of a specific health care organization. For example, if the goals of a government hospital are excellence of health care and meeting needs of the future health care environment, the critical success factors could be regional integration with other area hospitals, efficient use of scarce resources, and improved cost accounting[17] (p. 36). Under this system it is highly likely that similar organizations could have different critical success factors.

The critical success factors can relate to the industry (excellent medical staff, competitor health care organizations, patients' view of the clinic, or range of services offered), or environmental factors (suburban versus inner core city locations). The success factors may be internal, such as execution of the strategy or improving the cost picture of the hospital.

Once the standards or criteria have been determined and an appropriate information system established, it is then possible to make satisfactory evaluations of the performance of the organization relative to strategies and goals—in other words, the measurement of actual or predicted results against the standards.

If deviations are deemed significant, corrective action must be taken. This may involve a change in the original objectives, strategies for achieving the objectives, the implementation of strategies, or the information itself. Corrective action is an aspect of change, and the observations made in the chapter on strategy implementation are appropriate. Evaluation should also be an ongoing process and not something performed once or twice a year.

However, the more important aspect of evaluation and control of strategy is whether there are not better methods of effectuating the process than a hierarchical approach. In organizations where employees have close relationships with patients and other professionals and where many of these same employees are highly educated and trained specialists, a strong case can be made for employee self-control. We want to introduce this possibility and make some suggestions regarding the process of self-control.

What can be done to effectuate a worker-centered sense of responsibility for self control? W. Edwards Deming has spent a lifetime studying quality control, self-control, managerial methods processes, and philosophy. Basic to a system of self-control is the development of a selection that promotes coordination and cooperation. The following statement made by Deming quoted in Walton[18] sets the stage for our exploration (p. 32):

> How to improve quality and productivity? "By everyone doing his best." Five words— and it is wrong. That is not the right answer. You have to know what to do. Doing your best won't do it. We should be thankful that not everybody's doing his best. Look at the chaos that there would be. Held down to this and that, bumping into each other, working at cross purposes. Not knowing what to do. Just doing his best.

> The system is such that almost nobody can do his best. You have to know what to do, then do your best. Sure we need everybody's best—everybody working together with a common aim. And knowing something together with a common aim. And knowing something about how to achieve it. Not just with what seem to be brilliant ideas, but with a system of improvement.

The question is what is the nature of this system of improvement. There is a tendency among many managers that the answer is in a control system where human performance is controlled through work standards and rules, with inspection at the completion of the provision of service or development of a project. This attitude may be more prevalent in industry but is not unknown in the service industry, including health care organizations. In health care organizations this approach to control is more likely to take the form of the following: elaborate policy and procedures manuals, reports, and paperwork; creative accounting to make things look better; and maintaining a nonprofit status, numerous inconsequential meetings, and duplication of work assignments.

Deming argues that the work environment can be changed to bring about quality and productivity without centralized control. One of the basic concepts is for managers to recognize the existence and nature of variation. Walton[18] suggests the following conclusions based on her study of Deming's approach (p. 51):

- Variation is part of any process.
- Planning requires prediction of how things and people will perform. Tests and experiments of past performance can be useful, but not definitive.
- Workers work within a system that—try as they might—is beyond their control. It is a system, not their individual skills, that determines how they perform.
- Only management can change the system.
- Some workers will always be above average, some below.

The key problem with variability is to know when to act and when to leave the process alone—in other words, understanding what is merely random variation and what variability is such that general managers need to take action. The answer is statistical control. Unfortunately, statistics is a red flag word for many people. However, years ago Walter A. Shewhart, a statistician at Bell Telephone Laboratories in New York, pointed out that workers can be trained to chart variations in their job tasks and detect highs and lows that fall outside of acceptable limits. Statistical ability is not the problem; the problem is more likely to be that management is unwilling to change the system. For example, if the variations in a patient's well-being is caused by excessive room temperature and management refuses to install air conditioning, there is not much a worker can do. A similar situation may be the problem with the understaffing or overstaffing of the emergency room or with patients not receiving the correct diet that was ordered.

In the following quotation, Gartner and Naughton[19] point out the significance of the concept of variability to management theory and practice (p. 139):

The concept of variability is to management theory and practice what the concept of the germ theory of disease was to the development of modern medicine. Medicine had been "successfully" practiced without the knowledge of germs. In a pregerm theory paradigm, some patients got better, some got worse, and some stayed the same; in each case, some rationale could be used to explain the outcome. With the emergence of germ theory, all medical phenomena took on new meanings. Medical procedures thought to be good practice, such as physicians attending women in birth, turned out to be causes of disease because of the septic condition of the physicians' hands. Instead of rendering improved health care, the physicians' germ-laden hands achieved the opposite result. One can imagine the first proponents of the germ theory telling their colleagues who were still ignorant of the theory to wash their hands between patients. The pioneers must have sounded crazy. In the same vein, managers and academics who do not have a thorough understanding of variability will fail to grasp the radical change in thought that Deming envisions. Deming's propositions may seem as simplistic as "wash your hands!" rather than an entirely new paradigm of profound challenges to present-day managerial thinking and behaviors.

Are statistical tools difficult or complicated to master? For the average employee, the level of mathematics is probably no more than what a seventh- or eighth-grader may learn. The approach for them is primarily organizing and displaying data. Employees can collect data and often perform the interpretation, although expertise is

14 POINTS FOR THE GUIDANCE OF MANAGERS

1. Establish constancy of purpose toward service.
   a. Define in operational terms what you mean by service to patients.
   b. Specify standards of service for a year hence and for 5 years hence.
   c. Define the patients whom you are seeking to serve—those here, those that you seek, those that have been here only once.
   d. Constancy of purpose brings innovation.
   e. Innovate for better service for a given cost; planning for the future will require the addition of new skills, training, and retraining of personnel, satisfaction of patients, new treatments, new methods.
   f. Put resources into maintenance of equipment, furniture, and fixtures; new aids to production in the office.
   g. Decide whom the administrator and the chairman of the board are responsible to and the means by which they will be held responsible for working for constancy of purpose.
   h. Translate this constancy of purpose to service into patients and to the community.
   i. The board of directors must hold on to the purpose.
2. Adopt the new philosophy. We are in a new economic age. We can no longer live with commonly accepted levels of mistakes, materials not suited to the job, people on the job that do not know what the job is and are afraid to ask, failure of management to understand their job, antiquated methods of training on the job, inadequate and ineffective supervision. The board must put resources into this new philosophy, with commitment to in-service training.
3. a. Require statistical evidence of quality of incoming materials, such as pharmaceuticals, serums, and equipment. Inspection is not the answer. Inspection is too late and is unreliable. Inspection does not produce quality. The quality is already built in and paid for.
   b. Require corrective action, where needed, for all tasks that are performed in the hospital or other facility, ranging all the way from bills that are produced to processes of registration. Institute a rigid program of feedback from patients in regard to their satisfaction with services.
   c. Look for evidence of rework or defects and the cost that may accrue as a result—an incorrect bill, an incorrect or incomplete registration.
4. Deal with vendors that can furnish statistical evidence of control. This will require us to examine generic lowest-price buying; it will cause us to ask more penetrating questions about prospective colleagues regarding their interactions and the track record of their interactions with patients and with colleagues.

   We must take a clear stand that price of services has no meaning without adequate measure of quality. Without such a stand for rigorous measures of quality, business drifts to the lowest bidder, low quality and high cost being the inevitable result. We see this throughout the United States industry and government by rules that award business to the lowest bidder.

   Requirement of suitable measures of quality will, in all likelihood, require us to reduce the number of vendors. The problem is to find one vendor that can furnish statistical evidence of quality. We must work with vendors so that we understand the procedures that they use to achieve reduced numbers of defects.

Reprinted from Out of the crisis by Deming WE by permission of MIT and WE Deming. Published by MIT, Center for Advanced Engineering Study, Cambridge, MA 02139. Copyright 1986 by WE Deming.

Continued.

14 POINTS FOR THE GUIDANCE OF MANAGERS—cont'd

5. Improve constantly and forever the system of production and service.
6. Restructure training.
   a. Develop the concept of tutors.
   b. Develop increased in-service education.
   c. Teach employees methods of statistical control on the job.
   d. Provide operational definition of all jobs.
   e. Provide training until the learner's work reaches the state of statistical control, and focus the training to assist the learner to achieve the state of statistical control.
7. Improve supervision. Supervision belongs to the system and is the responsibility of the management.
   a. Supervisors need time to help people on the job.
   b. Supervisors need to find ways to translate the constancy of purpose to the individual employee.
   c. Supervisors must be trained in simple statistical methods for aid to employees, with the aim to detect and eliminate special causes of mistakes and rework. Supervisors should find causes of trouble and not just chase anecdotes. They need information that shows when to take action, not just figures that describe the level of production and the level of mistakes in the past.
   d. Focus supervisory time on people that are out of statistical control and not those that are low performers. If the members of a group are in fact in statistical control, there will be some that are low performers and some that are high performers.
   e. Teach supervisors how to use the results of surveys of patients.
8. Drive out fear. We must break down the class distinctions between types of workers within the organization—physicians, nonphysicians, clinical providers versus nonclinical providers, physician to physician. Discontinue gossip. Cease to blame employees for problems of the system. Management should be held responsible for faults of the system. People need to feel secure to make suggestions. Management must follow through on suggestions. People on the job can not work effectively if they dare not enquire into the purpose of the work that they do, and dare not offer suggestions for simplification and improvement of the system.
9. Break down barriers between departments. Learn about the problems in the various departments. One way would be to encourage switches of personnel in related departments.
10. Eliminate numerical goals, slogans, and posters imploring people to do better. Instead, display accomplishments of the management in respect to assistance to employees to improve their performance. People need information about what the management is doing on these 14 points.
11. Eliminate work standards that set quotas, commonly called measured day work. Work standards must produce quality, not mere quantity. It is better to take aim at rework, error, and defects, and to focus on help to people to do a better job. It is necessary for people to understand the purpose of the organization and how their jobs relate to the purpose of the organization.

---

14 POINTS FOR THE GUIDANCE OF MANAGERS—cont'd

12. Institute a massive training program in statistical techniques. Bring statistical techniques down to the level of the individual employee's job, and help him to gather information in a systematic way about the nature of his job. This kind of in-service training must be married to the management function rather than to the personnel function within the organization.
13. Institute a vigorous program for retraining people in new skills. People must be secure about their jobs in the future, and must know that acquisition of new skills will facilitate security.
14. Create a structure in top management that will push every day on the above 13 points. Top management may organize a task force with the authority and obligation to act. This task force will require guidance from an experienced consultant, but the consultant cannot take on obligations that only the management can carry out.

---

generally advisable for the latter. For management staff, for instance, Deming[20] states the following (p. 47-48):

> Education in simple but powerful statistical techniques is required of all people in management, all engineers and scientists, inspectors, quality control managers, management in the service organizations of the company, such as accounting, payroll, purchase, safety, legal department, consumer service, consumer research. Engineers and scientists need rudiments of experimental design. Five days under a competent teacher will suffice as a base.

Not only do managers need to learn how to deal with variability, but even more important, they need to employ principles and practices that stress cooperation. To accomplish cooperation, managers must eliminate practices that are divisive. Deming refers to them as deadly diseases, such as management by numbers (numbers with no meaning or understanding by employees), performance appraisals with no useful corrective suggestions, or management by objectives when such objectives are determined by managers without employee input.

To counter such diseases and related obstacles, Deming[21] has proposed 14 points to guide managers. He points out that "Dr. Paul B. Batalden and Dr. Loren Vorlicky of the Health Services Research Center, Minneapolis, have written the 14 points for medical services." Their statement is contained in the box on pp. 121-123.

The Deming approach involves recognizing the significance of variability and taking actions that will promote, not destroy, cooperation. In the foreward of Walton's book,[18] Deming summarizes this as follows (p. xii):

> Recognition of the distinction between a stable system and an unstable one is vital for management. The responsibility for improvement of a stable system rests totally on the management. A stable system is one whose performance is predictable. It is

reached by removal, one by one, of special causes of trouble. Best detected by statistical signal.

Returning to the broader subject of the managerial role of monitoring and evaluation and control, Bedard and Johnson[22] argue for organizational effectiveness evaluation. This process involves examining the strengths or weaknesses of each program in the organization to determine its effectiveness. The organization that is involved in continuous self-appraisal will be better off than one that is not. Furthermore, measuring operational effectiveness should result in service improvement, thereby placing the organization in a better competitive position and enabling an improvement in quality and the meeting of needs of the stakeholders it serves.

Lorange et al.[23] suggest that recent years have brought about a period of discontinuity in many sectors of the economy. The environmental discontinuities stem from social, economic, technological, and social forces. An organization must set forth its goals and systematically monitor its progress to those goals. They point out that planning and control are two sides of the same coin. "Strategic control provides comparisons, and comparisons provide learning. If the organization can absorb this learning, it then embarks on a dynamic, constructive change process" (p. 3). Organizations are constantly in a state of change, ending the present state, moving through a transitional period, and entering another beginning.

From a somewhat different perspective, Byrd[24] argues that in light of all of the changes occurring in organizations, such as deregulation and increased competition, a new leadership framework is needed. He proposes the following five key categories of leadership skills:

1. Anticipatory—scanning the horizon for potential risks—projecting consequences, trade-offs, and building trust and confidence
2. Visioning skills—development and presentation to employees of a vision for the organization that is persistent and consistent
3. Value-congruence skills—establishment of values in organizations and consistently applying the values set
4. Empowerment—sharing of power so that employees can share the satisfaction of achievement
5. Self-understanding—self-learning and development and an understanding of himself or herself relative to an understanding of others

In the final analysis, perhaps the ancient philosopher Laotzu's description of a leader is as accurate today as in the past:

A leader is best
When people barely know that he exists.
Not so good when people obey and acclaim him.
'Fail to honor people,
They fail to honor you.'
But of a good leader, who talks little,
When his work is done, his aims fulfilled,
They will all say, "We did this ourselves."

CONCLUSIONS

The objective of this chapter was to examine the changing roles of the CEO and the strategic management process of evaluation and control. The first section presented an overview of role models, including a model oriented to health care organizations. The original roles developed by Mintzberg from his research were related to health care organizations. Recent changes in roles and knowledge areas and skills were examined in light of changes in the environment and changes in multiorganizational arrangements.

The second objective of the chapter examined the roles of monitoring, evaluating, and controlling. A part of that discussion centered on the work of Deming concerning variability and cooperation.

Relating this chapter to the type D managerial style described in Chapter 6, one can conclude that the CEO will be much more of a change agent. He or she will have to earn status through knowledge, attitudes, and skills rather than through just legitimate power by virtue of his or her position in providing information and controlling funds. The CEO will have to be extremely objective and sensitive to changing needs and expectations to expedite accomplishment of proper goals efficiently and effectively.

Managers of health care organizations must continually be involved in the evaluation/control of strategies. Various approaches are available to the manager although he or she must determine the critical success factors and ascertain the information needed to determine progress or lack thereof in the strategic attainment of objectives. In health care organizations it is appropriate that specialists be permitted to exercise self-control over their activities. This concept requires continual examination of ways and means to not only permit self-control but also to encourage higher quality achievement levels.

REFERENCES

1. Aguilar FJ: General managers in action, New York, 1988, Oxford University Press, Inc.
2. Johnson AC, Forrest CR, and Mosher J: An investigation into the nature, causes, and implications of the future role of the health care administrator, US Department of Health, Education, and Welfare, Public Health Service, Health Resources Administration, Bureau of Health Manpower, DHEW Publication No (HRA) 78-33, Washington, DC, 1977.
3. Roberts NC and King PJ: The stakeholder audit goes public, Organizational Dynamics 17(3):63, 1989.
4. Fayol H: Industrial and general administration, London, 1930, Pitman.
5. Enhancing executive competence—educational and practice perspectives, American College of Hospital Administrators, Chicago, 1981.
6. Mintzberg H: The nature of managerial work, New York, 1973, Harper & Row, Publishers, Inc.
7. Kuhl IK: The executive role in health service delivery organizations, Association of University Programs in Health Administration, Washington, DC, 1977.
8. Kleiner SG: The role of hospital administrators in multihospital systems, Hospital Health Serv Admin, pp. 26-44, March/April, 1984.
9. Zuckerman HS: Redefining the role of the CEO: challenges and conflicts, Hospital Health Serv Admin, 34(1):25, 1989.
10. Luke RD, Begun JW and Pointer DD: Quasi-firms: strategic interorganizational forms in the health care industry, Acad Manage J 14(1):9, 1989.
11. D'Aunno TA and Zuckerman HS: A life-cycle model of organization federations: the case of hospitals, Acad Manage Rev 12(3):534, 1987.
12. Hoare G: New managerial roles in multiorganizational systems: implications for health administration education, J Health Admin Educ 5(3):423, 1987.

13. Mintzberg H: The structuring of organizations, Englewood Cliffs, NJ, 1979, Prentice-Hall.
14. Herzlinger RE: The failed revolution in health care—the role of management, Harvard Business Review 67(2):95, 1989.
15. Goldsmith J: A radical prescription for hospitals, Harvard Business Review 67(3):104, 1989.
16. Shortell S: The evolution of hospital systems: unfilled promises and self-fulfilling prophecies, Med Care Rev 45(2):177, 1988.
17. Rockart JF: Chief executives define their own data needs, Harvard Business Review 57(2):81, 1979.
18. Walton M: The Deming management method, New York, 1986, Dodd, Mead & Co, Inc.
19. Gartner WB and Naughton MJ: The Deming theory of management, Acad Manage Rev 13(1):138, 1988.
20. Deming WE: Quality, productivity, and competitive position, Cambridge, Massachusetts, Massachusetts Institute of Technology, Center for Advanced Engineering Study, 1982.
21. Deming WE: Out of the crisis, Massachusetts Institute of Technology, Center for Advanced Engineering Study, Cambridge, Mass., 1986.
22. Bedard JC and Johnson AC: The organizational effectiveness paradigm in health care management, Health Care Manage Rev 9(4):67, 1984.
23. Lorange P et al: Strategic control systems, St. Paul, MN, 1986, West Publishing Co.
24. Byrd RE: Corporate leadership skills: a new synthesis, Organizational Dynamics 16(1):34, 1987.

III

HEALTH SERVICES ORGANIZATION ISSUES

8

Organizational Arrangements of Health Services Delivery Systems

In this chapter we examine organizational arrangements of health services systems. Trends toward increasing size of health services organizations, multi-institutional arrangements, needs to integrate physicians into managed care settings, and needs to bring together all services to focus on the whole patient argue for attention to organization design. Furthermore, to help prepare readers for discussions of intraorganization issues in the balance of this book, it is important to be able to visualize the different hospitals, physician group practices, and nursing home organizations. Because we are concerned about organizing systems, the chapter begins with an overview of systems theory.

HEALTH SERVICES AS COMPLEX OPEN SYSTEMS

The vast literature on management shows us that organizations have been pictured in a variety of ways. Whether managers recognize it, they too have theories about the nature of the organization they administer. Their theories may not be articulated; they may be biased or incomplete and may never be examined or revised in the light of new knowledge. If managers were to examine their theories along with others, this should provide them with new insights and knowledge.

In the early decades of the twentieth century we tended to view enterprises as formal organizations that provided a structure or cradle within which the various employees performed their tasks. The major concern was the formal design of the structure, which should let each person know his or her position and function. Rationality was emphasized, and an unemotional state was desired, even to the extent of viewing the employee as a predictable, self-motivated being who was given specific assignments. This has been referred to as the traditional or classical approach to organization. Because of the emphasis by health services on people, health services managers have not accepted this approach to the same degree as industrial managers in past years. However, there have been and still are autocratic managers, managers who adhere to Max Weber's seven rules of bureaucracy,[1] and a general tendency toward the proliferation of rules and regulations.

A second general theory views the employee as the key to the organization to the extent of believing that a happy, well-satisfied employee is a productive one. Hence, why not contribute to (manipulate) an employee's satisfaction and happiness to increase productivity? The relationship between job satisfaction and productivity has been questioned in a number of studies, and the possibility has been advanced that productivity itself causes job satisfaction. No one likes to be manipulated, and managers who continue to use this method are generally suspect so that productivity or effectiveness is hardly achieved.

More recently the behavioral model of the organization developed, with emphasis on interactions among employees, the behavior of the employees individually as group members, and the behavior of the total organization. Emphasis is on organizational development and change to bring about a better working environment to achieve sought-after synergy of $2 + 2 = 5$.

Attention has also been directed toward decision-making models, communication networks, and mathematical models in studying the organization. However, the important point is that all these approaches stressed the internal operations or relationships in the hospitals. In the 1960s it became increasingly apparent that the health service, like other man-made organizations, had external relationships. A systems theory or model was necessary to incorporate this development.

Two conclusions from this review of organizational theories require emphasis. The first is that a more comprehensive and accurate theory or explanation becomes possible as more is learned about management and organizations. However, despite the fact that much knowledge has been developed, we do not want to imply that a complete, widely held explanation is available to us. The second is that the manager is a creature of the period in which he lives. When production was praised as the worthwhile goal via the assembly lines of the automobile industry, emphasis was on efficiency, specialization, and hierarchical arrangements. During the depression of the 1930s when business and productivity appeared to have failed, emphasis was placed on the individual. Now, with increased concern about environmental pressures on organizational survival and the patient, consumer, client, customer, or recipient of goods or services, attention is directed outside the organization toward external relationships.

General Systems Theory

An encompassing and useful approach to organization is general systems theory (Von Bertalanffy,[2] Churchman,[3] Miller,[4] Kast and Rosenzweig,[5] and Katz and Kahn[6]). *Webster's New International Dictionary of the English Language* (Second Edition Unabridged) defines a system as "an aggregation or assemblage of objects limited by some form of regular interaction or interdependence" and "a formal scheme or method governing organization, arrangement, etc. of objects or material, or a mode of procedure."

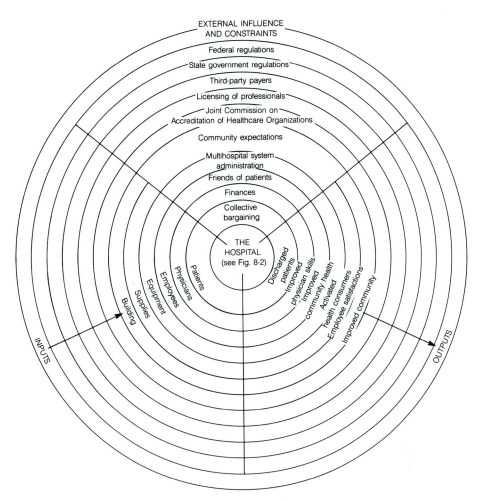

Fig. 8-1 A systems view of a hospital showing that external systems affect the hospital's inputs and outputs.

General systems theory may be seen as analogous to tossing a stone into a pool of water and noting the shock waves moving outward in ever larger circles. The hospital, for example, is at the impact point (Fig. 8-1). When a patient enters a hospital, a great many groups are involved, both inside and outside the hospital. Inside, the patient is concerned with admissions, doctors, nurses, dietetics, the business office, and housekeeping, to name only a few of the numerous internal relationships. Externally, the patient is involved with relatives, friends, and a third-party payer, and is influenced by government regulations, accreditation, and the community, to name a few.

What is most significant, however, is that the shock waves also work in reverse as far as the hospital is concerned. When the federal government changes its Medicare policies and procedures, these eventually reduce in concentric circles through various

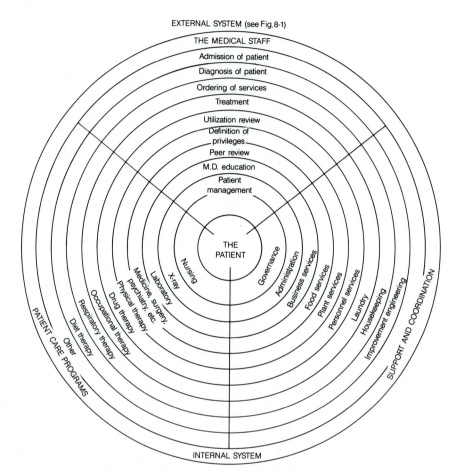

Fig. 8-2   A systems view of the internal organization of the hospital showing medical staff, patient care programs, and support and coordination services.

agencies to impinge directly on hospitals. Closer to home, the community, through a planning agency and fund raising, may or may not encourage a hospital to build an addition. Or, the multi-institutional system management will establish certain policies for the local hospital. The reader can no doubt supply additional evidence concerning forces that converge or impinge on the hospital.

Basically, a system converts inputs into outputs. In a hospital, the patient is the key input, but, for example, the skills and knowledge of the doctors, the equipment used, the nurses, and support people are all a part of the total input. This suggests that the manager would do well to consider the patient flow, or treatments to the patient, as his or her key or basic system. Consider, however, the many subsystems that affect the patient. Depending on hospital size and the needs of the patient, these include admitting, the medical staff, nursing services, laboratory, x-ray, surgery, central supply, dietary, purchasing, medical records, respiratory services, occupational or physical therapy, housekeeping, patient accounts, computer services, and volunteer services, to identify only a part of the many subsystems in the modern hospitals that relate to the basic patient system.

Figure 8-2 fits inside the previous figure, which portrayed the hospital's external systems. Figure 8-2 shows the internal systems of the hospital with the patient at the core. It identifies the three major components of the internal hospital system as follows:

1. The medical staff, who diagnose, admit, and treat patients and perform quality control procedures through their medical staff organization,
2. Programs for the direct care and cure of patients, such as nursing, x-ray, and laboratory
3. Support and administrative services, such as governance, administration, and business services

It is important to note again that these concentric circles move both inward and outward and affect each other as if a handful of pebbles were thrown into the water. Patient program departments, such as nursing, take orders from physicians and have line responsibility to administration, but all focus on patient needs. There are multiple lines of communication in hospitals; consequently, the traditional hierarchical organization chart is basically inappropriate for understanding relationships and influences in hospitals.

Thus we begin to see the advantage of the systems approach in the total picture aspect, as well as the complications of the maze of subsystem activities and internal and external relationships.

HEALTH SERVICE FUNCTIONS AND THE PATIENT CARE SYSTEMS

Systems exist to serve a function or functions.* Although the function of the hospital, for example, may appear to be obvious, in reality hospitals have multiple functions that are not only changing over time, but are in some respects conflicting. In this section we will explore hospital functions. We will then look more specifically at the patient, for whom the hospital really exists to serve, and then at some of the other functions or objectives that hospitals appear to be pursuing.

Changes in the functions of hospitals become evident from a historical review of their roles. The word *hospital* was derived from the Latin *hospitalis,* referring to a guest. Originally, hospitals were a place for the shelter or entertainment of guests or strangers. Historically, the functions of hospitals reflected their mission as charitable institutions for refuge, maintenance, or education of the needy, aged, or infirm, or of young persons. They had little to offer beyond custodial and comfort nursing care services. In fact, they provided a public health service to isolate the infirm from the rest of society as a nursing care service.

These functions or objectives persisted into the early years of the twentieth century.

---

*Functions are essentially synonymous with objectives. In systems terminology, they are frequently called *objective* functions.

McDermott[7] suggested that decisive medicine was not introduced until the 1930s when antimicrobial drugs became available. Although effective surgical intervention existed earlier, decisive medical intervention and surgical progress can be traced to that time. The principal function of most voluntary hospitals from the 1930s through the 1950s was to provide a workshop for physicians to practice decisive medicine.

During this period, knowledge expanded at an accelerating rate as did diagnostic and treatment services, and specialization proliferated. Beginning in the 1960s and continuing into the early 1970s, the community hospital emerged as a community diagnostic and treatment health center with a team of health professionals; it is no longer just a workshop for individual physicians. Into the 1980s it developed as a community health resource extending into the promotion, prevention, and rehabilitation areas. Future developments will depend on relationships with physicians and other environmental and behavioral systems affecting health.

Patient Care Function and Systems

At present, the primary function of the hospital and other health services is to treat the ill patient. (For purposes of this discussion, we will exclude obstetrical patients and worried well patients who may not be physically ill.) Just as the hospital is a complex system, so is the patient. Human behavior involves interactions between the individual's biological, psychological, environmental, social, cultural, and temporal systems. Table 8-1 lists human systems as categorized by Straus[8] and shows their relationships to illness behavior and treatment behavior.

In years past, a lack of biological knowledge resulted in hospitals concentrating on psychological and other nontechnical systems of care. Today biological systems and cure have become the focus of attention as the understanding and technological treatment of patients as biological beings have improved. Indeed, there is increasing concern that hospital and medical services are largely ignoring the other systems of man that also have an influence on treatment outcomes.

The importance of the psychological systems of man and the relationships of anxieties and stress to physical and mental health are well documented.[9] Moreover, the attitudes and behavior of health professionals are known to have an important influence on patient care[10] and quality of care.[11]

Environmental systems, such as air, water, and noise pollution, and demographic and physical factors were discussed in Chapter 1. The physical environment of the hospitals also affects patients' response to treatment. Jaco[12], for example, reported that patients and nurses were more satisfied with circular-designed nursing units for the more seriously ill patients but preferred traditional rectangular units for more mobile patients.

Social systems also affect illness behavior. Gonda[13], for example, found a relationship between age and family size and persistent complaints, with older people and those from large families more likely to be persistent complainers. Scheff[14] found social and demographic factors to be better predictors of the use of a college psychiatric clinic than the seriousness of the patients' illness. The social climate in the hospital, such as the attitude of the staff toward the patient, has an obvious influence on patient

Table 8-1 Human systems affecting illness and treatment behavior

Human systems	Relationships to illness behavior	Relationships to treatment behavior
Biological: Man the organism	Genetic, chemical, nutritional, functional adequacy	Organic responses to technical treatment
Psychological: Man the personality	Intelligence, anxiety level, stress	Responses to anxieties, stress, and other interpretation of behaviors of hospital staff
Environmental: Man in his physical milieu	Demographic, behavioral, and physical environment	Response to noise, aesthetics, comfort of the hospital environment
Social: Man's roles as a member of his society and various social systems	Relationships within his family, occupation, friends, and so forth	Response to dependency role, visitors, anticipated attitudes of his social system, relationships with the hospital staff
Cultural: Man responding to his normative and material culture	Customs, attitudes, values, expected way of behavior as developed from his religious, family, neighborhood, and other associations	Response to the hospital culture, culture of the hospital staff, and material culture of hospital equipment and supplies
Temporal: Man's orientation to dimensions of time	Time tables of age, rest, activity, eating, and so forth	Response to hospital schedules

From Straus R: Hospital organization from the viewpoint of patient-centered goals. In Georgopoulos B, editor: *Organization research on health institutions.* Ann Arbor, Mich., 1972, The Institute for Social Research.

care and progress. The change in status from an independent individual in normal life to a passive, partially clothed, dependent hospital patient is obvious to anyone who has been hospitalized.

Cultural relationships to illness behavior have been documented in studies by Zborowski[15] and Croog,[16] who demonstrated the relationships between ethnic background and pain and symptoms of illness. Italian and Jewish patients, for example, tended to exaggerate pain and to report more symptoms than others. Within the hospital, cultural differences have been shown to affect patient care; for example, lower-income persons have problems communicating with higher-socioeconomic-status physicans.[17]

The effects of temporal differences are reflected in the higher hospital occupancy in January through March, the higher incidence of disease among the elderly, and the cyclical differences in mental illness, births, and other factors requiring hospitalization. Within the hospital, the common complaints of patients about being awakened much earlier than they are accustomed and of having meals at the convenience of the hospital rather than at their own are evidence of the effects of time changes on patients.

Although the primary function of the hospital is to serve patient needs, seldom do we consider the patient as a whole person with complex needs; rather, the patient is treated as a biological system that must conform to effective and efficient medical and hospital technical services. Treating the patient as a whole person is a major challenge to physicians, nurses, and other professionals, and to trustees and managers who have ultimate responsibility to ensure that patient needs are met. Some hospitals have established patient advocacy—ombudsman or patient-care counselor positions to help overcome communication barriers between the less educated patients and the physicians and other professionals. Clergy, social workers, and consultant behavioralists might be utilized more effectively to help identify complex patient care needs and to propose improved patient care systems. Administrators, physicians, trustees, and others often gain new insights into and empathy for the broad scope of patient care needs after they have been patients. The complexities of human systems also underscore the importance of a team approach for identifying and meeting patient needs. Management, not just doctors and other health professionals, has primary responsibility to ensure these needs are met.

Other Functions of the Hospital

Providing a workshop for physicians is still a function of the hospital even though most hospitals view their role in the broader sense of providing care to patients. The traditional patient/physician relationship is still sacred and subject only to the surveillance of fellow physicians on the medical staff through peer review procedures. Even in government-controlled health systems, such as that of the U.S.S.R., the physician's right and obligation to treat patients according to what he or she sees as their best interests is inviolate. It is the physician who practices medicine; the hospital provides the resources to help the physician to diagnose and treat patients. Moreover, a primary function for the hospital is that of a *community health center* taking a proactive role to improve the health of the populations it serves, not just a reactive role of crisis care. As major community health centers, hospitals can sponsor programs, such as environmental and occupational health and home care services.

However, a primary operative objective of hospital management is to *serve the institution itself* by achieving perpetuation, growth, and prestige for the institution, its staff, and its community. In a number of communities, hospitals have been established to enhance the status of the community or of a particular sponsoring group. Moreover, it is not unusual for institutional objectives to take priority over community service objectives. A major problem in many communities is that of motivating hospitals to combine unnecessarily duplicated services while meeting unmet needs that may be unprofitable.

ORGANIZATIONAL DESIGN

The purpose of an organization is to bring together resources to perform certain tasks and functions. The organization should be arranged to perform the tasks and functions effectively and efficiently. Objectives of organizational arrangements are to facilitate coordination of efforts, communication among responsible parties, and accountability for results. Health services, and hospitals in particular, are complex organizations with a variety of technologies and goal priorities that must be coordinated.

Examples of Organizational Design in Health Services

There are a variety of organizational typologies proposed by organizational theorists. We summarize them within four models: functional, divisional, matrix, and team.

Functional. A functional organizational arrangement exists when labor is divided into departments specialized by functional area, such as nursing and purchasing. An example of a functional organizational arrangement of a 200-bed nursing home is portrayed in Fig. 8-3. This example is not unlike that of a traditional hospital organization, such as a smaller hospital. Individual medical staff members are autonomous except that they are accountable to the governing board for quality of care. A medical director may serve as liaison between the hospital or nursing home but does not have line authority over physicians. The actual numbers of functional departments will depend on the size of the organization. The functional arrangement enables decisions to be made on a centralized hierarchical basis.

A modification of the traditional hospital functional model is the independent corporate model. In this model the medical staff becomes a separate legal identity that negotiates with the hospital for its services in return for receiving the hospital's functional patient care and administrative support services.[18] The Kaiser Permanante organizational arrangement where physicians are employed by Permanente fits this model. If group model HMOs become more prevalent, the independent corporate model may become more common as a hospital/physician organizational arrangement.

Divisional. The divisional design, sometimes called the pavilion model if divisions are physically separated, might be found in an academic medical center, such as The Johns Hopkins Hospital, or a large multispecialty group practice. An example of a divisional model in a large multispecialty group practice is shown in Fig. 8-4.

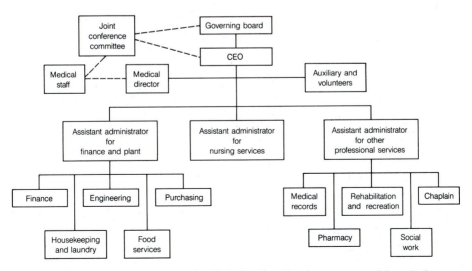

Fig. 8-3   Functional organizational design (nursing home or small hospital).

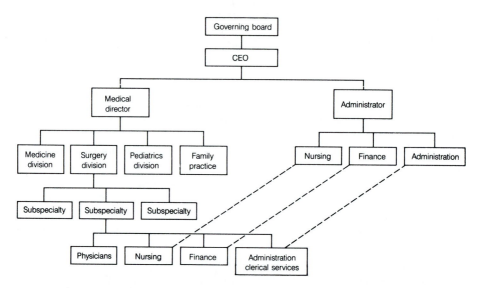

Fig. 8-4   Divisional organizational design (multispecialty group or academic medical center).

Divisions can center around traditional medical departments, such as surgery, medicine, and pediatrics. They can also be organized around organ systems, such as the heart (with cardiology and cardiovascular surgery as departments within the division), or divisions could be organized around specific target groups, such as women, cancer patients, or the elderly. This model decentralizes decision making to the service level, with each division having its own internal management structure. It places the clinical chief in a position of direct authority over all divisional activities. It is a model more closely centered on the patient service and/or academic unit.

Matrix Model. The matrix organization, originally developed in the aerospace industry, is characterized by a dual authority system as shown in Fig. 8-5. It is used in product-line management schemes, a relatively recent phenomenon in hospitals. Product-line staff are responsible to managers in their product line, such as substance abuse, cancer, or womens services, and to their functional authorities, such as nursing or finance. The matrix structure facilitates the coordination of a program or product-line team and allows team members to contribute their special expertise. It has the disadvantage of formalizing dual authority strains.

Team Model. Fig. 8-6 portrays the team model arrangement, which is common in other countries, such as West Germany. It requires consensus among the administrative, medical, and nursing heads for overall organization decisions. The team could be just two persons in a multispecialty group practice where nursing is not a large service, or the team of executive officers could be larger as it was in the British system. In the British National Health Service, the team model was expanded to six members, representing administration, nursing, finance, community health, consultants (that is,

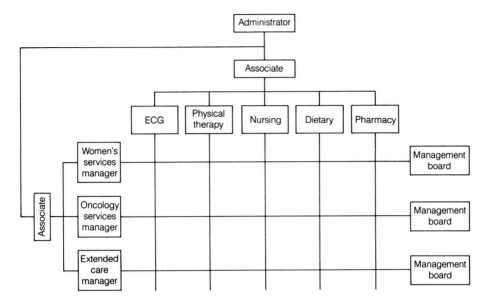

Fig. 8-5   Hospital matrix organization.

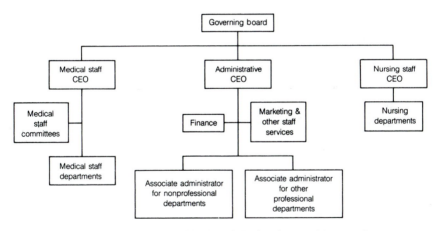

Fig. 8-6   Team organizational design (general hospital).

medical specialists), and general practice. This consensus model appeared to be an improvement in gaining commitment to management decisions among the various groups.[19] It was, however, superceded by a chief executive model, although most services retained the consensus model in practice. This team model has been adopted in only a few instances in the United States,[20] but it deserves consideration as a way to help achieve physician and nursing accountability and commitment to decisions, as well as coordination and perceived autonomy. It is, however, foreign to traditional United States' management traditions of chief executives.

JOINT VENTURES

While discussing organizational arrangements, note should be made of joint ventures, which developed rapidly in the 1980s. Hospitals that were otherwise unrelated formed joint ventures for expensive equipment that might be shared among hospitals in a community, such as nuclear and radiographic equipment and lithotripters. Equipment manufacturers might form joint ventures with hospitals or physician group practices, or group practices might form joint ventures for establishing a nursing home. There are many other combinations for joint ventures.

Purposes of joint ventures are to gain access to capital, share risks, expand referral networks, protect markets from others, gain experience from others, and gain economies of scale. An organizational structure for a joint venture might be for the joining organizations to appoint the joint venture board members in proportion to their investment in the venture. The venture board would then select their own CEO, or they could contract with another organization to operate the venture.

Although there are many advantages to joint ventures, they are not without risk and many have failed. Problems with joint ventures include issues of liability, control versus equity, venturing into complex services where neither organization is experienced (such as an HMO), lack of shared values, jeopardizing tax-free status, and the normal pitfalls of any new organization and venture.

CONCLUSIONS

It is important to note that the informal organization can be more influential than that documented as the formal organization. Legitimate authority as described in the organization chart is only one source of power in an organization. Other sources, such as expertise, control of resources, personal influence, and informal coalitions, might more accurately portray lines of coordination, communication, and control. In implementing change, managers need to recognize and utilize the informal, as well as formal, organization. The informal organization structure is frequently referred to as the political structure of the organization. Ideally the formal and informal structures would be identical, but there are usually some variations, particularly when dealing with professionals. Executives need to design organizations to minimize discrepencies between the two to facilitate implementation of change and accountability for results. Nevertheless, managers must recognize there are informal political structures, as well as formal structures, that are important to organizational performance.

Organization charts are important. They tend to comfort and assure people and to stabilize the organization. This includes the importance of defining titles and how they are determined. Organization charts along with job descriptions help to minimize role ambiguity and conflict. On the other hand, too much definition and creation of a rigid structure can be troublesome. Flexibility to focus on performance outcomes is more important than rigid adherence to organization structure.

When to change an organization arrangement can be quite controversial. Although stability is frequently a virtue, there are appropriate occasions for reorganization. First, when an organization or unit is experiencing severe problems, a reorganization with a change in personnel and responsibilities might give fresh breath and attention to needed improvements. On the other hand, reorganization may be just window dressing to show that something is being done, and this may or may not be an appropriate action depending on the situation. Second, when there is a change in the environment that directly affects internal operations, this may also be an appropriate time for reorganization. Third, when old programs or product lines are to be dropped or new ones added, this is an appropriate time to consider organizational changes that emphasize priority programs. Finally, organization design is an executive function. When there is a change in organizational leadership, the new leader has a fresh view of the organization. It is frequently a time for the new leader to put his or her stamp on the organization. Governing boards, however, need to approve organization design to ensure they recognize and support lines of authority and especially accountability.

The organization structure is not an end in itself. It is merely a mechanism to assemble resources to serve the outputs of the enterprise. On the other hand, peoples' positions in the organization are sensitive and can be sacred to the persons involved. Managers must be sensitive to the disruptions reorganization will create. Disruption can be beneficial in unfreezing the status quo, but skill is required in effecting changes. In a later chapter, we focus on implementing change.

REFERENCES

1. Weber M: Essays in sociology, New York, 1946, Oxford University Press, Inc (Translated by HH Gerth and CW Mills).
2. Von Bertalanffy L: General system theory, New York, 1968, George Braziller, Inc.
3. Churchman CW: The systems approach, New York, 1968, Dell Publishing Co.
4. Miller JG: Living systems: the organization, Behav Sci 17(1), Jan, 1972.
5. Kast FE and Rosenzweig JE: Organization and management: a systems approach, New York, 1970, McGraw-Hill, Inc.
6. Katz D and Kahn RL: Organizations and the systems concept, New York, 1966, John Wiley & Sons, Inc.
7. McDermott W: Demography culture and economics and the evolutionary stages of medicine. In Kilbourne E, editor: Human ecology and public health, New York, 1969, Macmillan Publishing Co.
8. Straus R: Hospital organization from the viewpoint of patient-centered goals, In Georgopoulos B, editor: Organization research on health institutions, Ann Arbor, Mich., 1972, The Institute for Social Research.
9. King SH: Social psychological factors in illness. In Freeman H et al, editors: Handbook of medical sociology, ed 2, Englewood Cliffs, NJ, 1972, Prentice Hall.
10. Rosengren WR and DeVault S: The sociology of time and space in an obstetrical hospital. In Freidson E, editor: The hospital in modern society, New York, 1963, Free Press.
11. Mechanic D: Correlates of frustration among British general practitioners, J Health Soc Behav 1, 2:87, 1970. 1 and 2, pp. 87-104, June 1970.
12. Jaco EG: Ecological aspects of patient care and hospital organization. In Georgopoulos B, editor: Organization research on health institutions, Ann Arbor, Mich, 1972, Institute on Social Research.
13. Gonda TA: The relation between complaints of persistent pain and family size, J Neurol Neurosurg Psychiatry 25:277, 1962.
14. Scheff T: Users and non-users of a student psychiatric clinic, J Health Human Behav 7:114, 1966.
15. Zborowski M: Cultural components in responses to pain, J Social Issues 8:16, 1952.
16. Croog SH: Ethnic origins, educational level and responses to a health questionnaire, Hum Organiz: vol. 20, pp. 65-89, 1961.
17. Roth J: The treatment of the sick. In Kosa et al: Poverty and health: a social analysis, Cambridge, Mass, 1969, Harvard University Press.
18. Shortell SM: The medical staff: replanting the garden, Frontiers of Health Services Management 1(3):3, 1985.
19. Schulz R and Harrison S: Teams and top management in the NHS, London, 1983, King Edward's Fund.
20. Danielson JM: Organized action: management advisory councils, JAMA 196:1062, 1966.

9

Governance of Health Services Organizations

As challenges to and opportunities for health services increase, the responsibilities and role of the governing board become more important. No longer is the role of the board member mainly honorific and philanthropic; holding the organization in trust in a turbulent environment is a heavy responsibility. To help meet increasing challenges, especially fiscal and competitive pressures, many boards have moved toward the business corporate form of governing structure. In this chapter we consider differences between voluntary-philanthropic and business corporate governing structures. However, we first consider the functions of governance. We then examine the voluntary versus corporate models. Finally, issues of control and consumer representation in governance are considered.

FUNCTIONS OF GOVERNING BOARDS

"To govern is to exercise continuous sovereign authority over; especially to control and direct the making and administration of policy."[1] As the policy-making body of the organization, the board is expected to play the key role in the strategic plan and its process.

The members of the governing board of any profit or nonprofit corporation are fiduciaries, and breach of a fiduciary duty can lead to personal liability. As fiduciaries, the members of a governing body have two paramount duties—loyalty and responsibility. Loyalty means that board members must put the interest of the corporation above all self-interest. For example, members and the board itself must guard against conflict of interest, such as a hospital board member selling goods or services to the hospital and thus reaping benefits to himself or herself that may not be in the best interest of the organization. There is also a fiduciary duty of responsibility, which means that members of the governing board must exercise reasonable care, skill, and diligence proportionate to the circumstances in every activity of the board. Trustees or directors must actually direct the organization; it is not enough merely to preserve the corporation as caretakers.

142

The governing board is accountable to the owners and must exercise authority to ensure that the organization carries out the mission of the owners, be they the government, citizens of the community or religious community, or stockholders. Most will agree that functions of a hospital governing board, be it a voluntary or corporate model, are to do the following:

1. Appoint a chief executive to execute board policy
2. Establish a long-range plan for the organization
3. Approve the annual budget
4. Appoint members of the medical staff
5. Monitor performance against plans and budgets
6. Have ultimate legal responsibility for quality of care to patients served

Although these functions will in general be similar for almost any health service, how board policies are developed and implemented will vary by type and ownership of the health service.

STRUCTURAL CHARACTERISTICS OF A GOVERNING BOARD

Structural characteristics of governing boards might be contrasted between the voluntary-philanthropic and business corporate models. Each type has certain advantages and disadvantages. Most health services will have some characteristics of each type. Drawing on research by Alexander, Morlock, and Gifford,[2] Delbecq and Gill,[3] and others, Table 9-1 summarizes differences between the voluntary-philanthropic and business corporate models.

The voluntary-philanthropic board has been a traditional model for the not-for-profit community hospital, nursing home, home care service, hospice, and others. Their development and effectiveness have depended on how well they met community needs and obtained resources to do so. Donations were responsible for the creation of most of these organizations, especially if they were created before World War II. Governing board structure and membership reflected the sources of support on which the health service depended. Health services owned by religious organizations had governing boards from the religious community that supported them.

The corporate model is taken from the business world. In the 1980s many not-for-profit hospitals restructured their boards, adopting features of the corporate model. In their 1985 survey of 5800 hospitals, Alexander et al. found that of the 55% who responded to the survey, more than one third had restructured their board organization along business corporate lines.[2] We compare the two on structure, size, homogeneity, inside versus outside directors, management as board members, focus, terms of office, and compensation.

Board Structure

Generally, voluntary boards will tend to be organized along functional lines. Fig. 9-1 provides a hospital example of a voluntary-philanthropic board. The hospital corporation may be a religious order, or it might be community citizens who contribute a few dollars, giving them the privilege of attending the annual meeting and voting

Table 9-1 Characteristics of governing boards in voluntary-philanthropic and business corporate models

	Voluntary-philanthropic model	Business corporate model
Structure	Functional	Divisional
Size	Large	Small
Homogeneity	Heterogeneous, generalists	Homogeneous, experts
Inside versus outside directors	Outside, representative	Inside
Management membership on the board	Ex officio without vote, adversarial	Membership with vote, consensual
Focus	Asset, acquisition, preservation, and operations	Policy and strategic plans
Terms of office	Unlimited	Limited
Compensation to board members	Volunteer	Compensated
Dominant power	Board	CEO

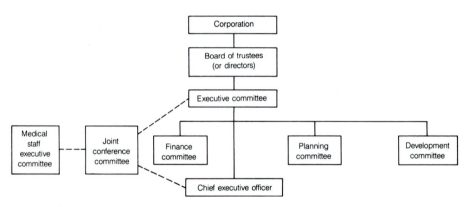

Fig. 9-1 Voluntary-philanthropic hospital or nursing home board structured functionally.

on a slate of board members nominated by existing board members. Boards are frequently large, and they meet quarterly. A smaller executive committee will act on behalf of the full board in the interim. Functions of trusteeship over investments, budgets, strategic planning, and development (that is, fund raising) are frequently organized around board committees. Board committees may include non–board members who are individuals being groomed for full board membership.

Figure 9-2 portrays a multi-institutional corporate board structured in a divisional model. The holding corporation in this example might be made up of the different organizations in the holding corporation. This corporate model can be applied to an individual hospital as well as to a multi-institutional system. Many larger hospitals have unbundled some of their services, such as the clinical laboratory, doctor's office building, or a fund-raising foundation. For example, the clinical laboratory might be

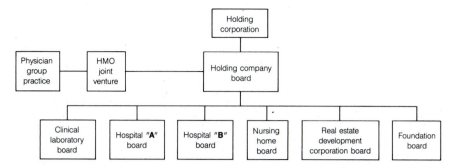

Fig. 9-2   Corporate multi-institutional system board structured divisionally.

a separate for-profit organization that has better access to capital and can sell services to other hospitals. It pays rent to the holding corporation and donates profits to the foundation, which might use those profits to provide charity care in the hospital. Although each divisional corporation has its own board, board members will usually overlap among the organizations. The holding company model enables the organization to have both not-for-profit and for-profit organizations, depending on which is most advantageous to the separate and holding corporations.

Board Size

Voluntary organizations tend to have large boards (12 to 30 or more members). Governing boards help to link organizations to the community they serve. Large boards broaden such linkages. Voluntary organizations usually seek donations. Board membership helps to gain potentially large donor commitment to the organization. Representatives of large employers, government officials, and other community leaders who control resources can be valuable linkages if they are on the board of the health service. Large boards broaden these linkage networks for health services. On the other hand, large boards are cumbersome.

According to corporate experts, seven is an ideal size for a policy board.[3] Smaller boards tend to come to decisions faster, and they are less likely to participate in tangential discussions. However, in their survey of hospitals that adopted features of the business corporate form of governance, Alexander et al.[2] found that size of boards in these hospitals was not significantly different from hospitals with voluntary structures.

Homogeneity

There are advantages to the voluntary organization that desires linkages to its community to have diversity among its board membership. Ewell[4] concluded from his study that there appeared to be a significant relationship between hospital program innovation and boards with a diverse occupational membership. Hospital boards that included more women, more representatives from minority groups, more members whose places of residence were closer to their hospitals, and more members from younger age groups tended to be more innovative. Ewell also concluded that boards with a more diverse membership appeared to have a higher level of concern for external environmental issues relating to community needs and cooperative health programs. However, surveys of hospital board membership from the 1960s into the 1980s show that most voluntary boards are not really very heterogeneous and that they tend to be dominated by representatives of the business community.[5-7] We return to this discussion of representation at the conclusion of the chapter.

The business corporation role model of a board member is a risk-oriented person recognized for an expertise that would be helpful to the corporate board.[8] On the other hand, a voluntary organization governing board member is more likely to be a generalist appointed as a representative of some segment of the population important to the health service. As a representative, the voluntary board member views issues from the perspective of the group he or she represents, not just the organization on whose board he or she serves. Moreover, as trustees for the donors, they are obligated to protect assets of the organization and may be less willing to take risks. The corporate board member by contrast is selected for the sole purpose of serving the interests of the organization. Because corporate board members have little obligation to protect any special interests, they can take somewhat greater risks in supporting and proposing strategies for the future of the corporation. Corporate board members are also selected for their expertise related to future strategies for the organization. If a health service follows the corporate board model, they might appoint a physician from another organization who would be considered an expert in the future directions of medicine, not primarily as a representative of the medical staff. They might also appoint persons expert in such areas as marketing and finance. Alexander et al.[2] found that hospitals that restructured along corporate lines were more homogeneous and had boards dominated by the corporate business community.

Inside versus Outside Directors

As suggested, voluntary boards tend to have governing board members who are outside the organization. External board members are consistent with voluntary organization needs to link into community resources and to assure that the organization is serving community expectations. Such persons external to the organization tend to be generalists rather than specialists commonly found on corporate model boards.

Corporate boards on the other hand tend to be dominated by people internal to the organization—again to assure that they represent organizational interests and to expedite actions. A physician group practice, which is likely to be a for-profit organization, usually follows the corporate model. Board members will consist of physicians from the clinic but may be supplemented by a medical leader from a noncompeting organization, a marketing expert, a banker, an economist, or an organization behavioralist. A hospital using the corporate model might appoint members of its medical staff, directors of nursing and finance, or others as internal members, in addition to external representatives. Internal members have the greater interest in the growth and survival of the hospital.

Before the 1970s physicians did not even attend board meetings in many hospitals, because it was seen as a conflict of interest—doctors on the board would have an unfair advantage over their colleagues, representing themselves or their colleagues and not the hospital or its constituents.[9] As late as 1970, 76% of the hospitals surveyed in Illinois and Wisconsin had no medical staff member participating in major board decisions relating to income and expenses.[10] Currently, however, most hospital voluntary boards will have at least the chief of staff as an ex-officio board member without vote. They may also appoint other physicians to the board with vote.

Management Membership on the Board

Although CEOs have always attended governing board meetings, only recently have they been given a vote on the board. In the traditional voluntary organization, the CEO is seen as executing board policy. The CEO in this model is the employee of the owners, not a representative of the owners. Governing board members represented the community, or church owners. The relationship is more adversarial; that is, the board protects the owner's interests in essence from the administrator and staff.

The corporate model by contrast is likely to have the CEO as a voting member of the board, and in many businesses the president also serves as chairman of the board. In the corporate business model, board members serve as resources to the CEO. In the corporate model the board's concerns are the organization and its stockholders, not any other organization or the community at large. Although board members and the CEO may differ on means, there is no question about ends as there may be in the voluntary organization. In their survey of restructured hospitals, Alexander et al.[2] found that most CEOs did have board membership with vote.

Focus

The voluntary board is likely to focus on the owner's mission as perceived from each board member's perspective. A church-owned hospital, for example, presumably will view the hospital from the perspective of the mission of the church. A community-owned hospital will view the hospital from a community perspective, which may not be in the best interest of the hospital as viewed by the CEO or medical staff. For example, a representative of a major community employer on a hospital board may argue for a merger with a competing hospital if it appears that it might reduce hospital costs in the community and to the employer. In contrast, in a corporate business model, the focus would be on survival and growth, which may not be in the community's best interests.

Voluntary boards also tend to focus on operations more than do corporate boards. In their role of protecting community or church assets and interests, voluntary boards tend to delve into operations. Moreover, with larger boards with a number of committees, operational issues tend to arise, which board members may want to pursue.

Corporate boards on the other hand usually do not have a conflict of objectives. An exception may be that in for-profit health services, such as an HMO or group practice, boards may be most concerned with annual profits, whereas management may take a longer-range view of profitability. Nevertheless, the board in the corporate structure focuses on success of the organization, not necessarily on whom it serves. As such it is concerned with policy and strategic plans for organizational success.

Terms of Office

Voluntary boards tend to be self-perpetuating; that is, board members serve for unlimited terms, and/or board members nominate similar persons to succeed them. The Wyatt study found an average of three 3-year terms for hospital board members, resulting in 9 years in office; less than 6 years was the average number of years in office in the for-profit hospital boards. In some voluntary hospitals, board members stay on indefinitely, especially if they are major donors or represent an influential segment of the population.

Compensation to Board Members

Seldom are voluntary board members compensated. The prestige and satisfaction of community service reward voluntary board members. Although the corporate board members may be compensated, they are not compensated at rates comparable with their salaries in industry; for example, technology industries report compensating their board members $5000 in retainers and $1000 per meeting plus expenses.[3] By contrast, Wyatt[11] found that less than 11% of health industry board members are compensated. Compensation of board members implies an obligation to contribute to the success of the organization. Some voluntary boards report that it is increasingly difficult to attract "the best" board members into an active role without paying them, because such persons are in great demand and they face increasing pressures from their own organizations.

Dominant Power

As the above characteristics suggest, the board is the dominant power in most voluntary health services, whereas the CEO tends to have more power in the corporate organizations. This is evident in the tenure of CEOs in the two types of organizations. In the voluntary organization, the CEO is the most expendable person in the tripartite relationship among the board, medical staff, and CEO, whereas in commercial corporate organizations, the CEO tends to have more tenure than board members.

In summary, we recognize that as the fiscal and market "bottom lines" become more important to health services, the corporate business model of governing board structure becomes more appealing. However, we tend to agree with Cunningham, who said, ". . . what I cherish is not the difference in methods (between the corporate business and voluntary board models), but the difference in goals: hospital boards are there to do good for others and business boards are there to do well for themselves. In this era of price competition in the market for medical services, I worry that the former may become more like the latter, and to my way of thinking that is all downhill."[12]

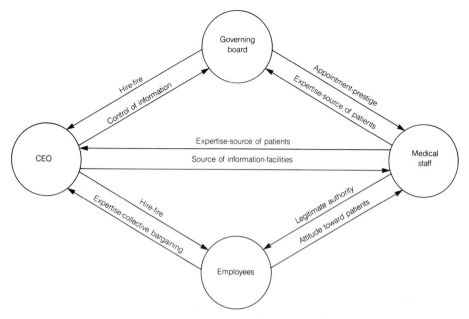

Fig. 9-3   Internal sources of influence.

WHO REALLY CONTROLS HOSPITALS AND HEALTH SERVICES?

Whereas physicians collectively control group practices, who controls hospitals? The hospital governing board has been charged legally, such as in the Darling case,* and traditionally as having ultimate responsibility and control. However, evidence on who actually controls or is the dominating influence in the hospital is contradictory.

It is evident that the traditional hierarchical organization chart with the governing board on top does not really describe relationships appropriately, that is, the varying amounts of influence wielded by the governing board, the CEO, the medical staff, and the employees. There is substantial agreement that ability to influence is derived primarily from: (1) legitimacy; (2) control of rewards and sanctions including money; (3) expertise; (4) personal liking; and (5) coercion.[13] Clearly, the CEO and medical staff have legitimate authority, although the trustees have the ultimate authority. Each group in the hospital has some base of influence over the others (Fig. 9-3). Trustees and the CEO control money and facilities. Physicians also exert some control over money by deciding when and where patients are admitted, particularly in communities where there are multiple hospitals and a surplus of beds. Physicians have used "heal-ins" in public charity hospitals and boycotts in private hospitals. Employees also have power through expertise and their attitudes in handling patients.[14] Moreover, employees can apply sanctions through collective bargaining or at least threats of it. Medical staff

---

Darling v. *Charleston Community Memorial Hospital,* 211 N.E. 2d 253 (1965) cert. denied 383 U.S. 946 (1966).

members, management, and employees have expertise in their profession and/or control of information.

We suggest therefore that external forces, the board, the administration, the medical staff, and the employees all have some influence or power. The traditional hierarchy, with a manager who hires, fires, and supervises, does not appropriately describe a hospital organization. Management should be a team effort.

HOSPITAL PERFORMANCE SEEMS TO RELATE TO ACCOUNTABILITY

We suggest that accountability rather than control is the important issue—accountability to consumers, individual patients, those who provide funds and other resources, regulatory agencies, sponsoring groups, and other members of the hospital family. Accountability should help provide justification for taking community resources to improve effectiveness and efficiency and to provide incentives for improved performance. Bowen[15] suggests the following ingredients for a system of accountability:

- A clear statement of goals and objectives with an ordering of priorities
- Allocation of resources toward maximum returns in relation to goals and objectives
- Cost and benefit analysis including allocation of costs and benefits to particular programs within the institution
- Evaluation of actual results
- Reporting on evaluation to all concerned

Shortell, Becker, and Neuhauser[16] refer to these as management practices that lead to "visibility of consequences." In their study of 42 general, short-term, nonteaching hospitals in Massachusetts, they found that visibility of consequences (measured in terms of the reports prepared, the number of reports sent to the governing board, and the degree of awareness of operating statistics) related positively to higher quality and greater efficiency. Presumably, when the governing board and management require accountability, that is, setting goals and making the consequences of operations visible, performance improves.

In prior years, when hospitals were symbols of humanitarian efforts for community welfare, accountability for performance was of little concern. Today, however, people are increasingly concerned about hospitals' performance because (1) hospitals use an increasing proportion of scarce community resources; (2) there is evidence of waste, such as unnecessary duplication of services, and (3) there are increasing questions about quality and effectiveness. It seems that in some hospitals, management clings to a symbolic orientation rather than focusing on performance.[17] In organizations structured to reflect societal beliefs, access to and stability of resources and autonomy is possible through a symbolic orientation and a lack of careful coordination or evaluation.[18,19] Examples of a symbolic orientation or evaluation would be where management focuses on and stresses physical facilities and equipment, reflecting societal beliefs that bigger and more luxurious or esoteric facilities are better, or focusing on anecdotal human-interest facets of the hospital, such as human-interest examples of saving lives. Though public relations efforts help a hospital to gain support for resources, they should not be used instead of performance measures. Performance evaluations might include cost-benefit or cost-effectiveness studies, staff and employee performance reviews, cost and quality comparisons with other instituions, and progress toward achieving explicit objectives.

HOW DOES CONSUMERISM RELATE TO GOVERNANCE?

In recent years consumer advocates have criticized hospitals for being unresponsive to their needs. Most of the criticisms stemmed from the fact that the urban poor had not received appropriate services, particularly in comparison with the services and amenities available to the middle and upper classes. The only services available to many of the poor were the large, public-charity hospitals. These public institutions were (and many still are) governed by individuals appointed by local governmental groups. In essence, they served the taxpayers of the community, and their implicit goals were to hold down costs rather than to provide superior service, the implicit goal of most community nongovernmental hospitals. However, when the urban poor attain more political power, board members become more responsive to the needs of consumers rather than just those of taxpayers.

The original intentions of Medicaid and Medicare were to provide the poor with health care funds so they could enter the mainstream (that is, the private sector) of health care. Access to and utilization of health care has clearly improved, especially for the poor, who have achieved utilization rates nearly the same as other income groups.[20] However, in the 1980s there were cutbacks in Medicare and Medicaid and if one bases use on need, the poor are still underserved.

As an alternative, the Office of Economic Opportunity (OEO) funded a number of community or neighborhood health centers to provide comprehensive health services to the poor with strong consumer involvement in governance. However, consumer representation or dominance in governance did not meet expectations in many of these centers. For example, dominance by consumers who had no previous experience in governing a complex health service reportedly contributed to the demise of several centers. On the other hand, consumer representatives can frequently be coopted so they no longer appropriately represent or appear to represent their constituency.[21] Studies in other settings show that group representatives play a rather passive role as board members and their communication and legitimacy with the group they represent gradually become weaker.[22] Wise[23] argues that in the ghettoes, community participation in health governance is not relevant because of the mobility of the population (about 50% turnover of residents every 5 years) and the lack of client participation in organized groups of any kind.

Bjorkman[24] notes the different forms and problems of representation, such as "descriptive representation," the most common form in which the representative "stands for" a larger group, such as a social classification. The problem is there is no guarantee that a socially descriptive representative will accurately mirror the interests of the larger group. A "substantive representative" on the other hand acts as a trustee or guardian for the group. The effectiveness of substantive representation can be determined only on the basis of evaluating the impact and results of the representatives actions for the group. Bjorkman also describes the problems of selecting representatives for a health service in terms of constituency, for example, the sick, or potential users, and the different expectations within groups to be represented.

It is not only difficult to find what might be considered broadly based consumer representation, but in our opinion it is also a fallacy to assume that consumers are the best judges of what are the best interests of the community. We have seen a number of situations where citizen groups have demanded construction of unnecessary facilities over the strong objections of physicians and/or administrators. It is important to note that management is supposed to work for the collective interests of all constituents in addition to the welfare of the institution.

Group Health Cooperative in Seattle, Washington, has a consumer-dominated governing board that successfully employs physicians and other health services personnel. However, it has leadership in its governance that is aware of the requirements for institutional success in an environment where there is considerable competition from traditional fee-for-service independent health services. It is also interesting to note that the highly successful Kaiser Health Plan is essentially provider-dominated in its governance.

To date, consumerism has not been an issue with middle- and upper-class segments of the population. Under the prevailing system of largely independent, fee-for-service, HMO, or PPO medical and hospital services, hospital providers must be responsive to individual paying consumers if they are to succeed. In most communities, therefore, individual consumers exercise control by selecting the physician and hospital plan that pleases them most.

It is important not to associate consumer controls only with the governance of health services. Other possible alternatives for consumer controls over medical services are as follows:

1. Market controls with consumers and providers having freedom of choice and each having resources needed by the other. This has worked quite well for the middle and upper classes. However, Medicaid, which was intended to accomplish this for the poor, has not worked as well as some had hoped, primarily because of underfunding, uninformed consumers, and the inaccessibility of private health services for the poor. The publication of physician and hospital charges and of utilization and quality indicators, and suggestions on how to avoid unnecessary surgery are among the current practices aimed at developing informed consumers.

2. Consumer dominance in the governance of health institutions. Lack of education and/or cooperation of the poor limits the effectiveness of this alternative.

3. Bargaining by groups of consumers with providers. This alternative may hold some promise if it can be made attractive to providers and if the consuming poor, as well as the providers, hold some sanctions.

4. Establishment of a nationalized system. Few are ready to overturn a traditionally private system that has been successful for most consumers simply because the minority are not reaping the same benefits. Experiences with nationalized systems in other countries indicate that even under conditions promoting equal access, the educationally advantaged have greater access.

5. Using group-process techniques to gain consumer input into the governance and management of hospitals.[25]

BOARD DECISION PROCESSES

Board decision processes are also important to the effectiveness of the governing board. Indeed, what is important for effective board processes is also appropriate to the many group decision processes throughout the health service. Principles of good meeting processes include the following:

- Hold prescheduled regular meetings (and cancel if the meeting is not really needed)
- Distribute an agenda and printed matter in advance
- Start the meeting on time
- State an ending time at the outset
- Determine in advance if an item is presented for information, for discussion and idea generation, or decision
- Use appropriate decision strategies for routine decisions, creative decisions, or negotiated decisions
- Facilitate discussions by the following:
  Asking for clarification if unclear about what is being presented.
  Encouraging more-or-less equal participation among group members
  Listening to others
  Summarizing what has been said
  Containing digression
  Managing time of each item
  Ending the discussion when there is nothing to be gained from further discussion
  Testing for consensus by summarizing the group's position or decision
  Evaluating meeting processes, for example, are we getting what we want from this discussion?

Group members, as well as the chairperson, have responsibility for effective meetings.

The chairperson of the health services board not only chairs board meetings but is in essence the spiritual leader of the organization. He or she articulates the values of the organization in setting expectations and the tone and pace of the organization. The CEO, as the name implies, executes to fulfill the values and meet expectations set by the board. The CEO, however, also has the responsibility to ensure that the board fulfills its responsibilities for setting expectations and holding the organization accountable. This calls for a close working relationship between the board chairperson and the CEO—and with the president of the medical staff if the organization's medical staff members are essentially guests. Informal weekly meetings among them is a common way to facilitate coordination among the three legs of the hospital management stool. Although the CEO needs to keep the chairperson and board informed of problems and to share major problem solving with them, the CEO has the leadership responsibility to bring solutions and implement them with support from the board and medical staff.

In the words of Robert Greenleaf[26]:

> The role of trustees (the governing board) is to hold what approximates absolute power over the institution, using it operationally only in rare emergencies—ideally never. Trustees delegate the operational use of power to administrators and staffs, but with accountability for its use that is at least as strict as now obtains with the use of property and money. Furthermore, trustees will insist that the outcome be that people in, and affected by, the institution will grow healthier, wiser, freer, more autonomous, and more likely to become servants of society. The only real justification for institutions, beyond a certain efficiency (which, of course, does serve), is that people in them grow to greater stature than if they stood alone. It follows then that people working in institutions will be more productive than they would be as unrelated individuals. The whole is greater than the sum of its parts. In essence, this view of the use of power holds that no one, *absolutely no one,* is to be entrusted with the operational use of power without the close oversight of fully functioning trustees.

CONCLUSIONS

Whether it is a voluntary or corporate model, we suggest that the primary functions of the governing boards are: (1) to control and maintain organizational effectiveness, (2) to be accountable to the region and its subgroups to ensure that community needs are met, and (3) to obtain support and resources from (or coopt) the environment. These three functions are not mutually exclusive, however. We suggest that a governing board can more effectively fulfill all three functions by carefully *defining objectives* in explicit terms and then *evaluating* the organization's operations.

Establishing objectives is not a simple task. An effective statement of objectives requires that a number of criteria be met:

1. Objectives should be based on a careful study of needs the hospital should exist to serve. Health planners, policy-makers, researchers, and consumers need to be consulted to determine needs objectively and knowledgeably.
2. In addition to administrators, medical staff members and key employees should be involved in formulating objectives.
3. Objectives should be explicit. Better patient care at lowest cost is a meaningless statement. Quality, cost, and other objectives should be defined in explicit, measurable terms so it can be determined whether they have been achieved.
4. Priorities should be identified, since objectives will often conflict.
5. Objectives should include explicit targets and time frames.
6. Objectives should be operational. Perrow[26] suggests that the actual objectives pursued by individuals in an organization (operational objectives) may be quite different from official or stated institutional objectives. It is essential that official and operational objectives be the same.

The governing board must regularly evaluate operations against objectives and the needs that objectives should be defined to meet. Management information systems should therefore be based on enabling management and the governing board to measure the performance of the hospital in achieving the explicit objectives.[27] Visibility of operational consequences is essential to ensuring accountability for meeting community needs. Without performance measures, representation is merely window dressing. With performance measures and visibility, concerns for representation are minimized. One of the primary benefits of multihospital systems is usually better information systems, closer scrutiny of performance, and holding system units accountable for achieving established performance goals. However, volume and fiscal performance goals are usually emphasized. Governing boards have primary responsibility to represent community performance expectations for really improving health while conserving community resources.

REFERENCES
1. Webster's New Collegiate International Dictionary, 1987.
2. Alexander JA, Morlock LL, and Gifford BD: The effects of corporate restructuring on hospital policymaking, Health Serv Res 23(2):311, 1988.
3. Delbecq AL and Gill S: Developing strategic direction for governing boards, Hospital Health Serv Admin 33(1):25, 1988.
4. Ewell C: What makes a board innovative? Trustee 33(9), 1980.
5. Goldberg T and Hemmelgard R: Who governs hospitals? Hospitals, p 72, Aug 1, 1971.
6. Berger I and Earsy R: Occupations of Boston Hospital board members, Inquiry 10(1):42, 1973.
7. Nigosian GL: New data on hospital governing boards, Trustee 33(9):5, 1980.
8. Gregory D: On the path to diversification: how to negotiate the direction your institution should take, Trustee 38(7):35, 1985.
9. MacEachern MT: Hospital organization and management, Chicago, 1946, Physicians Record Co.
10. Schulz R: Relationship between medical staff participation in hospital management and factors of cost of hospital care, doctoral dissertation, Madison, Wis, 1972, University of Wisconsin.
11. Wyatt Company Survey: Practices of boards of directors/trustees in the health care industry, Fort Lee, NJ, 1986, Executive Compensation Services.
12. Cunningham RM, Jr: Hospital boards are different—hallelujah! Frontiers Health Serv Manage 2(1), 1986.
13. Filley A and House RJ: Managerial process and organizational behavior, ed 2, Glenview, Ill, 1976, Scott, Foresman & Co.
14. Mechanic D: Sources of power of lower participants in complex organizations, Admin Sci Quart 7:349, 1962.
15. Bowen HR: Holding colleges accountable, Chronicle Higher Ed, March 12, 1973.
16. Shortell S, Becker S, and Neuhauser D: The effects of management practices on hospital efficiency and quality of care. In Shortell S and Brown M, editors: Organizational research in hospitals, Chicago, 1976, Inquiry Book, Blue Cross Association.
17. Schulz R, Greenley J, and Peterson R: Management cost and quality in hospitals, Med Care 21(9):911, 1983.
18. Meyer JW and Rowan B: Institutional organizations: formal structure as myth and ceremony, Am J Sociol 83(2):340, 1977.
19. Greenley J: Reciprocal selectivity between basic boundary personnel and clients in welfare institutions. Paper presented at OECD conference on Responsiveness of Public Services to Client Needs, Berlin, Germany, June 1978, from the Departments of Psychiatry and Sociology, University of Wisconsin—Madison.
20. Roemer MI: Optimism on attaining health care equity, Med Care 18(11):775, 1980.
21. Shostak AB: The future of poverty. In Kosa J, editor: Poverty and health, Cambridge, Mass, 1969, Harvard University Press.
22. Thorsrud E: Participation—industrial democracy. Presented at International (IUC) 17th Annual Con-

ference, Bergen, Norway, Aug. 23, 1970 (unpublished). Author's address in Work Research Institutes, Oslo, Norway.

23. Wise H: A closer look at community control, 4th Annual Report: Martin Luther King Health Center, Bronx, New York, 1971.

24. Bjorkman J: Citizen control of health services: an international perspective on participation, representation and social policy, Proceedings of 9th World Congress of Sociology, Uppsala, Sweden, Aug. 12-19, 1978.

25. Delbecq AL: Critical problems in health planning. Paper presented at 32nd Annual Meeting of Academy of Management, Cleveland, Aug. 13-16, 1972.

26. Greenleaf RK: Servant leadership: a journey into the nature of legitimate power and greatness, New York, 1977, Paulist Press.

27. Perrow C: The analysis of goals in complex organizations. In Hill WA and Egan DM, editors: Readings in organization theory, Boston, 1967, Allyn & Bacon, Inc.

28. Kovner AR: Hospital board members as policy-makers: role, priorities, and qualifications, Med Care 12(12):971, 1974.

10
Physicians

No group associated with health services is more important, frustrating, exciting, or unexpendable than physicians. Whereas some physicians are reactionary, others are very progressive. It has been our experience that in a partnership with trust and understanding, physicians can be very supportive of organizational goals and will work hard to achieve them.

Whether in management of an HMO, hospital, clinic, or even a home care service or nursing home, relationships between management and physicians will be a major, if not the most important, factor in the effectiveness and job tenure of health services managers. Unlike commercial enterprises where the CEO is most permanent, in the health service the CEO is often most expendable. The medical staff will not be changed, and short of a change in ownership, the board will not be changed. Health services are similar to football and baseball teams. Although wins and losses are hardly measurable in health services, if there is trouble, management goes out. Unlike baseball team managers, health services managers have the burden of convincing their professional planners that goals are the same and that management is interested in quality of patient care and not merely financial performance. Moreover, many professionals in health services cherish their autonomy, and the team, that is, institution, may be perceived as a threat to their autonomy.

The type of organization affects management/physician relationships. For example, it is hard for management in third-party payer organizations (Medicare, Medicaid, commercial carriers, and HMOs) to convince physicians that management does care about the quality, as well as cost, of care. Similarly, some physicians also perceive goal conflicts with hospital management. On the other hand, in clinic management where the organization is the physicians and the primary goal of management is to serve the physicians, trust and goal congruence are seldom problems. Speaking from personal experience, we suggest that managers of physician clinics may have more executive power than hospital managers because of goal congruence, trust, and physician respect for specialty skills, be they medical or managerial.

157

BARRIERS TO PHYSICIAN/MANAGEMENT RELATIONSHIPS

In the hospital, increasing competition and other external forces strain physician/hospital relationships. A recent survey by Hamilton/KSA of 623 hospital CEOs found that the CEOs reported the following factors to be causing conflict between physicians and hospitals: physician recruitment, competition for outpatients, PRO activities (that is, audit of medical practices), managed care, designation of priority programs, buying physician practices, and board representation.[1] In addition to these program forces, there are certain inherent barriers to management and physician relations.[2]

- Physicians and managers have differing orientations. A variety of impediments create conflict between physicians and hospital management. Some of the acknowledged ones are as follow:
  — The authority and power of physicians are based on technical expertise, whereas managers' authority and power stem from their position within the organization and to an increasing extent on their managerial style and expertise.
  — Distribution of authority within the medical staff is diffuse, with individual physicians having authority based on their specialized expertise, whereas management authority is hierarchically structured.
  — The orientation of practicing physicians tends to be cosmopolitan; that is, it is external to the hospital and directed toward professional specialties and individual patients; the orientation of management tends to be local—toward the hospital. However, with increasing competition, developing physician surpluses, and multi-institutional systems, some reversal of this trend is developing.
  — Clinicians' goals are directed toward treatment of patients; management strives for maintenance of the organization.
  — Physicians tend to be collegial and informal in their organizational relationships; administrators tend toward more formal organizational relationships.
  — Work of practicing physicians is more intensive, on a one-to-one basis, and decisions are authoritarian, independent, and based on more objective data. Management usually works with groups and depends more on others, and decisions are often negotiated, frequently involve compromise, and are based on subjective information.
- Medical staff members are typically busy, averaging a 52-hour work week in 1986.[3] They frequently resent spending time on administration.
- Largeness begets looseness. The medical staff is large and diverse and frequently does not take a uniform stand on issues. It is difficult to gain broad participation in joint efforts; moreover, physicians apparently see no need to agree with their professional colleagues on every issue when public pronouncements are not involved. Few representatives of the medical staff do, in fact, speak for a majority of the staff.
- Personal insecurities clash with institutional goals. Some managers and physicians are more concerned about their status and power than about the ultimate goals of the hospital or the community. Some managers are cautious about

sharing information and decisions openly; control over such factors represents a major source of their power.

Because they are such a crucial force in health services management and effectiveness, it is helpful to have some understanding of some general findings on backgrounds of physicians and their major professional organizations.

WHO ARE PHYSICIANS?

This section describes (1) the kinds of individuals who select and are selected for medical school, (2) medical education and its influences on physician behavior, (3) the profession of medicine, and (4) some of the behavioral characteristics and impressions of physicians as identified in behavioral research. Most of the data are drawn from the 1988 education issue of the *Journal of the American Medical Association*.[4]

WHO BECOME PHYSICIANS?

Career choices for the professions are frequently determined early in life. Medicine is a field in which an individual can contribute in a major way toward meeting social needs in addition to receiving other intrinsic rewards. Freidson,[5] however, suggests that there is little evidence that individuals aspiring to become physicians have a stronger service orientation than those aspiring to other occupations.

Competition for entry into medical school is severe. For the medical class entering during the 1987-1988 school year, there were approximately 267,000 applications from 28,000 applicants for approximately 17,000 actual positions. However, this represents a 31% decline in applicants from 1977-1978. Those who apply usually have substantial qualifications, for it is well known that only those students with a strong academic preparation and high grades will be admitted.

The "average" medical student represents less than 5% of American college graduates, with the average undergraduate grade-point average being 3.41 in 1987. Few drop out of medical school. An Association of American Medical Colleges report on a "Longitudinal Study of Medical School Graduates of 1960" suggests that medical school admission criteria might be counterproductive. "It may be that certain undesirable personality patterns are unwittingly overincluded contrary to long-term interests of both society and the profession."[6]

In 1971 only 11% of the entering class of future physicians were women. By 1987-1988 they represented 37% of the entering class. Although the percentage of women medical students is increasing, the United States still has one of the lowest percentages of women medical students and practicing physicians in the Western world.

Although black Americans constituted over 12% of our nation's population, only 6% of the nation's medical students were black in 1987-1988. The number of black and other minority group medical students has increased very slightly in the last few years. Only 3% of physicians in practice are black. Although we have a surplus of physicians in many communities, there is a severe shortage of physicians serving racial minorities.

WHAT IS THE CONDITIONING PROCESS OF MEDICAL EDUCATION?

From the first day of medical school through residency training, both favorable and unfavorable experiences mold the future attitudes and behaviors of developing physicians. These attitudes and behaviors, in turn, affect the role of the physician in relation to hospital management.

It has been suggested that medical education tends to reinforce aggressiveness, impersonality, and distance—complaints that are frequently directed against physicians. Rezler[7] suggests from a review of the literature that the medical school environment fosters cynicism.

One impression particularly relevant to the management of health institutions was stated in an address by James Dennis, M.D.,[8] when he was dean of the University of Oklahoma School of Medicine:

> As medical students, interns and house staff officers, we are exposed to a rigidly organized and structured discipline that provides no real opportunity to participate in or learn the democratic process. After 6 to 8 years of professional conditioning as the lowest man in a feudal (futile?) system, the M.D. is trained to quickly assemble some facts, promptly make his decision, and to stick to it. He learns to make a decision, then to think in terms of right and wrong, and not to compromise. Once in practice he must gain acceptance from his peers so he identifies with them and communicates with them almost to the exclusion of others—a process that guarantees the reinforcement of his own prejudices and fosters group bias, which is usually expressed in some form of "motherhood." The actions and reactions of organized professional groups, including medical school departments, usually reflect these ingrained characteristics by assuming a positive posture of being "right"—frequently with dedication. Since it is wrong to compromise on what is "right," we tend to deal from a position of all or none.

Friedson,[5] in summarizing data on the values of physicians, concludes that

> while physicians do not lack a service or collectivity orientation, it does not seem to be a very prominent value compared to others. Furthermore, the value is addressed to concern for helping individuals rather than serving society or mankind. Second, physicians have some intellectual investment in their work, everyday practitioners having less than others emphasizing instead practical knowledge and action. Third, physicians emphasize the value of the income and prestige connected with their occupation. And, finally everyday practitioners more than others emphasize the value of independence and autonomy. These values, I believe, stem from the social background of the practitioner more than from his work reflecting both the values of his bourgeois origins and special intent or career choice (p. 178).

Training to be a physician is a long, rigorous process. It has probably meant 4 years to obtain a bachelor's degree, 4 years of medical school, 8 years of residency, and some practice time before becoming certified as a specialist. Of course, physicians are delivering medical care at least after completing medical school. Some schools, however, accept students after only 2 years of college; the internship requirement has been eliminated by almost all specialty boards; and some boards have eliminated the practice requirement for certification.

Almost all graduates of U.S. medical schools pass state licensing exams on their first try, and few physicians' licenses are revoked. Moreover, once a physician is licensed, he or she generally does not have to submit evidence of continuing education.

With rapid advances in knowledge there have been efforts toward requiring continued medical education. The American Academy of Family Practice requires it for continued certification, and a few states require it for registration. Recertification and relicensure are current issues in organized medicine.

Almost all medical school graduates go into residency training. General practice, which most graduates went into after a 1-year rotating internship, has essentially been replaced by family practice, which requires a residency. About 9% of the residents in 1987 were in family practice, but another 30% were in internal medicine and pediatrics. A National Academy of Sciences Institute of Medicine study[9] recommended 60% to 70% of first year residents should be in primary care. However, subspecialty residents and residencies continue to expand, and surgery ranks behind only internal medicine in number of residents. Back in 1975, a study of Surgical Services for the United States (SOSSUS) by the American College of Surgeons reported there were already at least 20,000 to 34,000 too many physicians performing surgery. The number of surgeons continues to grow out of proportion to estimated needs. The tragic implication of having too many surgeons—or too many physicians doing surgery—is unnecessary surgery leading to unnecessary deaths, to say nothing of unnecessary costs.

THE PHYSICIAN SURPLUS

A short 30 years ago, it was assumed that the answer to America's health problems was to enlarge the supply of physicians. It was thought that with more physicians, access to medical care and consequently health status would improve; distribution would improve as more physicians filtered into rural areas; and medical charges would not rise because there would be more competition. With this in mind, the federal government poured billions into increasing the number of medical schools by more than 60%, expanding medical school class sizes, and developing physician extenders, such as physicians' assistants and nurse practitioners. However, by the 1970s it became evident that medical care per se does not improve the health status of populations, that increasing supply does not necessarily result in better distribution, and of most concern to the government that was now paying for health care, that increasing supply increases costs. It was found that when the supply of physicians increases, so does utilization of services. Moreover, fees tend to rise as physicians need to charge each patient more—and although not a conscious decision by most physicians—when they perform more services per patient, their income is not sacrificed should they be seeing fewer patients. Even though each added physician results in increasing health costs, over $1 million per year in terms of what they order and charge for their patients, it was difficult to turn off the spigot of producing more physicians, nurse practitioners, and physicians' assistants. In responding to national needs and incentives, medical and other health profession schools find the reversal in priorities and policies to be very painful.

A 1980 report of the Graduate Medical Education National Advisory Committee to the Secretary of the Department of Health and Human Services suggested there will be 150,000 too many physicians in 20 years unless steps are taken to reduce the production and importation of physicians and physician extenders.[10] They cited six problems in graduate medical education as follows:

- A substantial *imbalance* in some specialties
- A marked *unevenness* in geographic distribution of physicians
- *Too many nonphysician* providers in 1990
- The factors influencing specialty choice are *complex*
- The total cost of graduate medical education is *unknown*
- Economic motivation in specialty and geographic choice is *uncertain*

This projected surplus of physicians and their extenders is of great importance for hospital management and can be looked at as both an opportunity and a threat. It is an opportunity in that doctors should be more receptive to basing their practice in a hospital setting if doing so promises to facilitate their professional interests and security. Physician oversupply is a threat in that physicians are establishing competing services, such as surgical, renal, and other expanding ambulatory services. Hospitals and organized medicine also have to guard against unnecessary surgery, fad medicine, and gimmicks to attract patients in competition with other services. With fewer clinical options for physicians and increased importance of organizations, managerial positions are becoming become more attractive to them.

Another potential conflict exacerbated by manpower surpluses will be demands by limited licensure personnel, such as podiatrists, clinical psychologists, and chiropractors, for some type of medical staff membership. Though hospitals may be prone to bring in such persons to expand revenue sources, physicians will likely oppose such moves, just as they may also tend to limit privileges of other physicians, such as family practitioners. Limited licensure personnel may logically be excluded based on arguments for maintaining quality. On the other hand, bringing them in under hospital controls, education programs, and consultations can help to improve and integrate quality of care in the community.

More recent studies suggest an even larger surplus based on the assumption that competitive medical plans (for example, prepaid group practices and other managed care plans) will suppress demands for service. However, a minority view proposes there will be no physician surplus by the year 2000.[11] Projections of no surplus are supported by estimates of increased demand from technological advances, an aging population, needs to serve those who are currently uninsured and underinsured, desires for more leisure time by practitioners, and more physicians moving into non–patient care activities, such as management. Whether a national surplus will exist or not in the next decade, shortages will probably remain in some geographic areas and surpluses will continue to be evident in a number of cities.

ORGANIZED MEDICINE

The American Medical Association has long been the traditional voice for American physicians. In addition to its efforts to improve the quality of physicians' services, which it still pursues actively, the AMA has worked toward reforms in the delivery of health services. For example, in 1917 it endorsed the concept of compulsory health insurance. This resolution was based on an AMA report that included the following statement[12] (p. 2):

> The time is present when the profession should study earnestly to solve the questions of medical care that will arise under various forms of social insurance. Blind opposition, indignant repudiation, better denunciation of these laws is worse than useless. It leads nowhere and it leaves the profession in a position of helplessness as the rising tide of social development sweeps over it.

However, in 1920 the resolution to endorse compulsory health insurance was rescinded. Since then, the AMA has sought to preserve the independence and financial positions, as well as the technical competency and ethics, of the physician. Like most of the population during the Depression, physicians had problems obtaining work, that is, patients. Until the late 1960s, the AMA, the professional agency of physicians, was a major factor in restricting the number of medical school students.[13] Throughout the thirties and forties it opposed Social Security legislation and voluntary health insurance, since it did not want third-party intervention in medicine. In the late 1960s when both had come into effect, the AMA, faced with an attempt to institute compulsory national health insurance, argued for increased voluntary health insurance instead of government involvement. It took until 1980 for the AMA to give a qualified approval to HMOs, and it took legal pressure to permit physicians to refer patients to chiropractics and to advertise fees and services.

Over the years the power of the AMA has waned. In 1975 a little more than half of all physicians were members, but by 1987 42% were members. Perhaps the main criticism of the organization among doctors is that it does not represent the physician's interests vigorously enough. There are left-wing groups in medicine, such as the Medical Committee for Human Rights and the Physicians for Social Responsibility; however, their membership is small and is drawn generally from some of the Eastern cities, full-time employees of government agencies, and university medical schools. Much faster growing are the groups who attack the AMA from the right, such as the Association of American Physicians and Surgeons and the Congress of County Medical Societies. In the view of these and other physician groups who are unhappy with the "unprofessional" control over medicine, the answer is to unionize. Although AMA leadership remains opposed to true unionization, seeing it as a sellout of professional integrity, the physician's union movement has growing support.

Specialty boards, such as the American Board of Surgery, and specialty associations, such as the American College of Surgeons, have considerable influence on physicians and on the type of medical care received by consumers. The principal and almost exclusive objective of specialty boards and associations has been to upgrade the qualifications of specialists. Until recently, this has meant increasing the length of time needed for training and development of subspecialties, and sponsoring numerous continuing education programs and professional journals. Certification by a specialty board after rigorous examinations is indeed a recognition of professional knowledge. Fellowship in a specialty college is also a peer recognition of competence.

Incomes of physicians are at an all-time high. Incomes exceeding $200,000 before taxes are common. Although these are earnings after the deduction of business expenses, many doctors complain that their practice expenses have been rising faster than their incomes. Soaring costs and difficulties of obtaining malpractice insurance is an example. Percent of expenses to billings varies widely, from 15% to more than 50%, depending on a physician's specialty and office services. The average doctor today spends as much time on each patient as he did in 1950—approximately 18 minutes. Although a physician collects more than 91 cents of every dollar billed, the balance being bad debts or free care, the costs for high-profit office items, such as injections, x-ray studies, and laboratory procedures, have increased. Increasing burdens are also placed on physicians' time and energies by peer review requirements and the hospital utilization and quality review activities that are described in the next section of this chapter. Physicians could increase their productivity by delegating more tasks to other health personnel, such as physicians' assistants, or by working longer hours; the latter, however, places a strain on them and on their families.

Generally, a physician may earn more by working more, but earnings will not be proportionate to the additional hours worked. These diminishing returns are being discovered by doctors, and many are changing their ways of practice. Because of a desire to delegate responsibilities, such as finances, and to have more free time, doctors have been leaving solo practice and joining or forming more partnerships, expense-sharing group practices, and medical corporations. HMOs and other prepaid medical groups are becoming more common, as are salaried physicians who work limited hours. By 1986, 25% of all physicians worked as employees.[14] Nearly 40% of physicians younger than 36 years and not in residency training or in a federal service are salaried employees.

In spite of all the criticism that is heaped on organized medicine today, it is clear from the high regard patients have for "their physicians" (confirmed from many surveys) that by and large, doctors are dedicated to the welfare of their patients. At times expectations for the individual patient come into conflict with the organizational requirements of the large and complex hospital, hence conflict between physician and hospital ensues. The increasing demands of society at large for cost and quality controls over medical care are naturally viewed as a threat to the traditionally sacred physician/patient relationship, hence there may be conflict between organized medicine and the representatives of people—be they in government or from consumer groups.

HOSPITAL MEDICAL STAFF ORGANIZATION

The Joint Commission on Accreditation of Healthcare Organizations (JCAHO) states[15] (p. 101):

> There [should be] a single organized medical staff that has overall responsibility for the quality of the professional services provided by individuals with clinical privileges as well as the responsibility of accounting therefor to the governing body. There [should be] a mechanism to assure that all individuals with clinical privileges provide services within the scope of individual clinical privileges granted.

The JCAHO defines clinical privileges as "permission to provide medical or other patient care services in the granting institution, within well-defined limits, based on the individual's professional license and his experience, competence, ability, and judgement."

An example of a traditional medical staff organization of a hospital that has essentially autonomous medical staff and hospital organizations is portrayed in Fig. 8-3. In that model the medical staff is self-governing but accountable to the board for quality of care. The medical staff organization relates to the hospital through a joint conference committee composed of board and medical staff officers and the CEO. However, in many hospitals, joint conference committees are ineffective for communication between the governing board and the medical staff.[16]

Except where the medical staff is small, there will be an executive committee of the medical staff on which the hospital CEO or his or her designate serves with or without vote. Each clinical department or major clinical service (or medical staff in smaller hospitals) holds monthly meetings to consider findings from the ongoing monitoring and evaluation of the quality and appropriateness of care and treatment provided to patients. Chairmen of the clinical departments

- Are accountable for all professional and administrative activities with the department
- Provide continuing surveillance of the professional performance of all individuals who have delineated clinical privileges in the department
- Recommend to the medical staff the criteria for clinical privileges in the department
- Recommend clinical privileges for each member of the department
- Assure that the quality and appropriateness of patient care provided within the department are monitored and evaluated.[15]

Because of the effort required to fulfill these responsibilities, many larger hospitals employ full-time medical directors and department chairpersons. In 1985 nearly half of the hospitals of more than 200 beds reported having paid medical directors.[17] Paid medical directors and department chairpersons is just one example of the increasing integration of physicians and hospitals.

CORPORATE INTEGRATION OF PHYSICIAN SERVICES

Forces contributing to the integration of physician services include increasing competition, development of multi-institutional systems, rising costs of practicing alone, and a blurring of medical and business decisions. Increasing competition among physicians comes from a variety of sources. The growing supply of physicians has resulted in increasing competition. HMOs, PPOs, and other competitive developments make it increasingly difficult for the independent practitioner to retain patients without joining their colleagues and hospitals in such market-oriented systems.

In multihospital systems, decisions that affect physicians are made in corporate offices removed from the physician's practice site. To gain some control over such decisions, physicians are forced into formal decision development and implementation processes at the local level. They can no longer influence managerial decisions informally by dropping in to the administrator's office or influencing a board member at the country club. In vertical systems, such as HMOs, acceptable decisions require formal communication and negotiation among physicians and between them and their hospital to assure equity.

The costs of managing an office practice are rising rapidly, not only in dollars, but in strain on the physicians involved. Although physicians will frequently employ consultants to assist them in managing their practices, it can be frustrating and time consuming to employ, train, direct, and evaluate an office staff. Relationships among physician partners are frequently emotionally exhausting experiences. Rising costs of malpractice insurance and all office expenses are further burdens on physicians. In 1986 median practice expense was more than $72,000, representing 38% of gross income. Malpractice insurance has been rising rapidly. Although it represents only 2.1% of gross receipts for doctors in nonsurgical specialties, it consumes an average of 10% of gross receipts for neurosurgeons, thoracic surgeons, and OB/GYN specialists.[18] Physicians who are not trained for or do not have interest in business find such activities a major detraction from their primary interests of patient care. To avoid such hassles, many physicians are joining group practices, selling their practices to hospitals to take salary arrangements, or even leaving the practice of medicine.

The boundaries between business and medical decisions are becoming blurred. In the past, physician decisions were based solely on medical questions if the patient had full-coverage insurance. Today, however, third-party payers and hospitals place limits and decision requirements on physician diagnosis and treatment orders. Physicians naturally want to participate in making such decision rules and have a voice in their implementation. It may be easier to have an organizational role in such processes than to be an adversarial outsider to such organizational decisions.

Methods of Integrating Physician Services

There are a variety of ways to integrate physician services. Group practice is a common way to integrate physician and other outpatient services. Physicians and hospitals can be integrated by process means, such as appointing physicians to hospital governing boards, appointing physicians to hospital management committees, and/or appointing a medical director and salaried chiefs of services. Physicians and hospitals can be integrated through a number of structural means, such as divisional, independent-corporate, and team organizational arrangements, as described in Chapter 8. Physicians and hospitals can also be integrated by physician group practices taking over hospital ownership, or hospitals purchasing physician practices. A staff model HMO, such as Group Health Cooperative, is an example of total integration where physician services are combined with financing and hospital services.

Physician Group Practice

The group practice model was discussed previously, but it is important to highlight it as a growing model for the integration of physician office practices. Although new groups are being formed, expansion of existing groups accounts for much of the growth of group practice. The Mayo Clinic, for example, has not only enlarged in Rochester, Minnesota, but has established new groups in Florida and Arizona. In other communities, groups have merged and have added more physicians to their organization.

Physician/Hospital Organizational Integration

Although physician membership on hospital governing boards was a controversial issue just a few years ago, it is now a more tempered form of integration. Management-oriented medical staff committees, such as for planning or cost containment, are another way to formally involve physicians in hospital decisions. Participation can be fostered by appointment of physicians to management positions, such as medical director or department chiefs. The independent-corporate model, where physician and hospital management representatives form joint ventures for major hospital policy decisions, is another mechanism for integration. They may also form other joint ventures, such as an HMO or costly high-technology services. Team consensus management, such as in the British experience, is still another model for physician/hospital integration.

As external pressures continue, we predict that there will be more hospital/physician mergers. Such mergers can be created by hospitals purchasing medical practices, physician organizations taking control of hospitals, or merger with equal representation. For example, in 1987 more than 23% of hospitals reported that they had purchased physician practices.[19] Although employed physicians report earnings to be $38,000 a year less than self-employed physicians, they work fewer hours; consequently hourly pay is not that much less.[20] On the other hand, physicians are also taking over hospital operations. The Mayo Clinic, for example, has taken ownership of its primary hospitals St. Mary's and Methodist. We foresee other group practices acquiring ownership of their primary hospital to compete more efficiently with other providers and to help obviate perceptions of adversarial relationships.

Implications of Physician Integration

Over the years individual practitioners have lost considerable autonomy. Autonomy of physicians is likely to continue to decline with increasing external pressures from reimbursement sources, such as HMOs, Medicare, and Medicaid. Income of physicians may or may not decline. In 1986 incomes of physicians in solo practice averaged $115,000, whereas their counterparts in groups averaged $122,000.[16] Physicians in groups see fewer patients, but they usually participate in profits from ancillary services offered by the group. External forces, such as pressures for cost containment, uncompensated care, rising practice expenses, managed care plans, and a surplus of physicians, are likely to constrain physician earnings. Implementation of the proposed relative value scale for Medicare patients, which calls for reduction of physician fees in the process-oriented surgical specialties and increasing fees for the cognitive services of medical specialists, may also have an impact on earnings of individual physicians. Such fee schedules are likely to be utilized by other payers as well.

Integration of physician and hospital services may contribute to the rise in hospital costs. Studies by Alexander and Morrisey[21] reported a relationship between hospital/physician integration and costs. Although their conclusions might be questioned, it is not illogical to assume that physicians would argue for application of advanced technologies and patient care services that add to costs, as well as quality. However, in the long run with increasing external cost-containment pressures, integration of physician and hospital services can help to achieve efficiencies with economies of scale, less duplication of services, and more physician accountability for hospital costs.

There is no evidence that quality of care will suffer with the integration of physician practices or physician and hospital services. Studies that compared quality of care between staff and group model HMOs and fee-for-service found quality to be at least as high in the HMOs as FFS.[22] Group practices, such as the Mayo and Cleveland Clinics, are renowned as centers of excellence. One might also assume that formal physician participation in management decisions would contribute to a focus on individual patient needs within limited financial resources. Nonetheless, integration alone does not necessarily assure quality or efficiency of care.

Satisfaction of patients may not be as high with the larger integrated organizations as with the smaller solo practitioner model of personalized services. Physician characteristics themselves are likely to determine physician's satisfaction with integrated organizations. Physicians preferring the autonomy and independence of solo practice are likely to have more difficulty than physicians seeking professional stimulation from multidisciplinary integrated settings. Through participative and supportive communication practices, managers can have a substantial influence on physician satisfaction in bureaucratic settings.[23,24]

Paying Physicians

With take-home pay before taxes exceeding $100,000 for most doctors, they are in the top first percentile of the nation's income distribution. Physicians' pretax net income has been about 4½ times that of the average wage earner, averaging about $75 per hour in 1984.[25] Physician services represent nearly 20% of total medical care costs. In addition, physicians control about 80% of total health care costs because most services must be ordered by physicians. Methods of paying physicians are therefore crucial to incentives for physician earnings and total cost of health care.

Methods of paying physicians can be categorized on the basis of (1) procedures rendered, that is, fee-for-service (FFS), (2) case, for example, by diagnosis related group (DRG), (3) number of patients responsible for per year, that is, capitation, and (4) hourly rate or a salary basis. FFS, case, and capitation relate to physician productivity or output, whereas salary is an input method. There are obvious advantages and disadvantages to patients, physicians, and payers for each method. These are summarized in Table 10-1. Although FFS is currently the most prevalent payment method, it is declining in importance and will probably continue to decline as other methods have greater incentives for cost containment. Whatever method prevails in the future, there will most likely be more monitoring to ensure that quality is not sacrificed by monetary incentives.

MANAGEMENT AND PHYSICIANS

Just a few years ago it was inconceivable to think of physicians in the context of management. However, in an environment of managed care and integration of physicians into formal organizations, management must confront such issues. We examine management and physicians in the context of physician autonomy, changing physician behavior, and achieving physician satisfaction.

Table 10-1   Strengths and weaknesses of alternative bases for physician compensation

Base	Advantages	Disadvantages
Fee-for-service (individual procedure)	■ Automatic adjustment for case complexity ■ Provider's reward is closely linked to his/her output of services ■ Patients have economic clout over physician ■ Provides transparency of the physician's profile of practice ■ Widely used throughout the world and typically preferred by physicians	■ Provides incentive for overservicing per case treated ■ If fees for particular services do not stand in constant proportion to the cost of these services, fee-for-service compensation may tilt the treatment modality toward more profitable procedures ■ Inflationary tendency through ever finer decomposition of treatments into distinct, billable tasks ■ Difficult to budget *ex ante*
Diagnostic related groups (DRGs) (the medical case)	■ Logically the most compelling definition of the physician's "output" ■ Fairly good adjustment for variation in case mix (albeit not a perfect adjustment) ■ Provider's reward is fairly closely linked to his/her output of services ■ Provider has economic incentive to minimize the resource cost per medical case treated ■ Patients retain economic clout over physicians ■ Fairly good transparency of the physician's practice profile	■ It is technically difficult to force all cases into a finite list of DRGs ■ There may be a substantial variation of case complexity within a defined case category (DRG) ■ To the extent that case complexity varies significantly within DRGs, physicians may engage in adverse risk selection of patients ■ Physicians may underservice their patients for the sake of economic gain ■ Physicians may misrepresent diagnoses (DRG creep) ■ The method is relatively untried here or elsewhere in the world ■ Difficult to budget *ex ante*

Reprinted with permission of Williams and Wilkins. From Reinhardt UE: A framework for deliberations on the compensation of physicians, J Med Pract Manage 3(2):85-95, 1987.

Continued.

Table 10-1 Strengths and weaknesses of alternative bases for physician compensation—cont'd

Base	Advantages	Disadvantages
Capitation (no. of patients under continuing care)	■ No need to decompose physician's work into procedures or cases; therefore, administratively simple	■ Physicians have incentive for adverse risk selection and may dump patients with complex, costly conditions onto other providers
	■ Facilitates budgeting for health care *ex ante*	■ Physicians have incentive to underserve patients they do accept (to the extent that patients remain unaware of it)
	■ Provider's effort still somewhat linked to his or her effort	■ If average case mix varies greatly among physicians under one capitation system, capitation may be viewed as unfair
	■ Medical treatments are not influenced by the relative profitability of individual procedures	■ There is little transparency of the physician's practice profile
	■ Physicians have incentive to minimize the cost of medical treatments	
	■ Patients still have some economic clout over physicians if patients can change physicians from time to time	
Salaried practice (mo or yr)	■ Administratively simple	■ Unless salary can be linked somehow to output and patient satisfaction (as it is in group practices), patients lose economic clout over the physician who renders care as an act of noblesse oblige
	■ Medical treatments are not influenced by the relative profitability of individual procedures	
	■ Facilitates cooperation among physicians in treating complex cases	■ Physicians may underserve patients
	■ Facilitates budgeting for health care expenditures *ex ante*	■ There is little transparency of the physician's practice profile

Physician Autonomy

Autonomy is a hallmark of professionalism and almost a sacred component of physicians' care. To be autonomous is defined as being self-governing, but it is clear that individual physicians in the United States are not self-governing. As a collective group in hospitals, the medical staff is usually considered self-governing, but even this is open to question.[26] In his classic book, Starr[27] describes the rise and potential fall of the sovereignty of American medicine, Haug[28] suggests a proletarianization of American medicine, and Friedson[29] proposes that individual physicians will lose their autonomy to a medical elite. Although doctors are rarely able to articulate a definition of what autonomy constitutes,[30] Tolliday[31] defines it as "the right to practice free from hierarchical management, the right to refuse an individual patient, the right to lead and coordinate other health professions, and the right to regard medical knowledge as overarching that of other disciplines." Based on a survey of physicians, Schulz and Harrison[32] describe it in somewhat broader terms of freedom of choice of specialty and practice location, control over earnings, control over the nature and volume of tasks, control over acceptance of patients, control over diagnosis and treatment, control over the evaluation of care, and control over other professionals. Clearly, control over these facets by individual physicians or even physicians collectively is limited in organized settings. Nevertheless, perceptions of autonomy are cherished by physicians, and it is a challenge for managers to satisfy this need while managing health service organizations and patient care. Schulz et al.[33] propose that perceived physician autonomy does not necessarily relate to actual autonomy and that management can have considerable influence over perceived physician autonomy.

Autonomy to practice their skills is also important to nurses and other health professionals. Indeed, there is convincing evidence from research in other industries that worker autonomy is important to job satisfaction. Is autonomy a zero-sum game between physicians and nurses and other professionals, or can management contribute to perceived autonomy of all? We propose that it is not a zero-sum game and that management practices of participation in goal setting, information on organizational effectiveness, and role clarification can contribute to perceived autonomy of all. This is discussed in later sections and chapters.

Changing Physician Behavior

Managed care means changing the behavior of physicians who may be outliers to practices considered to be most effective and efficient for patients and payers. For example, unexplained practice variations, such as noted in Chapter 1 for hysterectomies, tonsillectomies, and prostatectomies, may require changes in physician practices. Physician behavior in making referrals, completing medical records, and handling of personnel, for example, may need changing. How might managers go about changing behaviors of physicians who cherish their autonomy and who are not accustomed to being told what to do?

Fineberg et al.[34] propose using cognitive, behavioral, and sociological theory in changing physician behavior. Cognitive theory treats the doctor as a processor of information. Physicians may have inaccurate or incomplete information about the values of certain procedures or needs of others. If inaccuracies and errors are major reasons for problems, the appropriate intervention would be to educate the physicians and to provide them feedback about differences between their behavior and optimal practices. Behavioral theory suggests that physicians respond to the stimuli that they confront. Behavioral interventions might include reimbursement or other incentives, instituting penalties, or trying to change expectations. Sociological theory suggests that professional peer group pressures be used to change an individual physician's behavior.

Eisenberg[35] suggests a combination of methods for changing physician behavior. These include education, feedback, participation in policy making, administrative rules, incentives, and penalties. He notes that each addresses different factors that govern medical decision making and behavior. Consequently, multiple interventions should be used.

Physician Satisfaction

The satisfaction of physicians is an important goal for managers of health services, just as job satisfaction of all workers is important. Physician satisfaction will be used by governing boards or to whomever a manager reports, as a measure of managerial effectiveness. Additionally, there is preliminary evidence that physician and patient satisfaction are related.[36]

In their survey of psychiatrist autonomy and satisfaction in organized settings in West Germany, Schulz and Schulz[37] found that management practices of goals for high performance, supportive communication practices, and participative decisions were significant in predicting physician perceptions of autonomy and their work satisfaction. Preliminary analysis of data from a companion study in England suggests similar findings. Although these findings are from other systems, they are consistent with investigations of job satisfaction in a variety of industries in the United States. We also hypothesize that the use of such management practices will contribute to perceptions of autonomy and satisfaction for both physicians and other professionals. We do not believe that solutions to doctor/nurse conflict over professional autonomy necessarily mean taking autonomy from one to give to the other.

In a recent national survey that asked 100 physicians what they really wanted from hospitals, responses included the following:[38]

- Good patient care
- Better communication
- Quality care measurement
- Recognition of the physician as a respected and necessary person to the hospital
- Mutual trust
- Increased interest in patient care

Steps to Building Physician/Management Teams

Building physician/management teams is not merely a matter of appointing physicians to managerial positions. Specific steps that management might consider to achieve physician support for health service organization goals and programs are as follow[2]:

- *Clarify goals*. Agreement may exist on general goals, such as quality of care and efficiency of service, but specific goals and priorities within this broad range seldom are agreed on or even understood. Formal definition of hospital objectives and goals including an outline of priorities, can provide a foundation for joint efforts among board, medical staff, and administration. Clarification takes time. Furthermore, it can occur only if it is accorded ongoing attention together with realistic expectations from everyone involved. In other words, do not expect too much too soon.
- *Specify responsibility in formal terms*. Cooperation and support will be increased to the extent to which responsibilities can be identified. One reason teams fall apart is a lack of clear understanding of the role of the CEO vis-à-vis the medical or nursing staff. Role ambiguity and conflict invariably follow. Many crises in hospitals actually are manifestations of goal and role ambiguities.
- *Establish task forces, project groups, coordinating committees*. Joint problem solving can be achieved through project groups created to plan for a new service, for example, or through task forces created to serve as search and screen committees for such key positions as director of nursing, medical director, or assistant administrator. It is unlikely that these short-lived groups will diminish the power and authority of the CEO. In fact, an open and supportive approach ought to enhance respect for him or her. Small project groups can generate ideas for institutional change. And the administrator must be willing to weigh these changes carefully. Sometimes staff members may want to initiate a totally new policy for the entire institution. One way to handle these situations is to field-test the policy or idea to determine to what extent it deserves broader application. If the staff is sufficiently interested in a proposal or venture, they will devote time and energy to putting it in motion—with the end result that teamwork becomes the natural way to achieve goals.
- *Lean on liaison personnel*. In addition to assuming certain executive responsibilities, the medical director should serve as liaison between the medical staff, the administration, and the board. The role of this individual is currently undergoing significant redefinition. Opportunities for persons who have had training in liaison boundary-spanning work (few have) are beginning to develop.
- *Appoint representatives in residence*. When members of the medical staff are permitted to serve on the governing board, the potential for team development is greatly enhanced.
- *Improve communication skills*. Some pointers in that regard are:
  - *Spring no surprises*. It is only human nature to be resentful when we are not consulted about decisions that affect us. If, for example, the medical staff is allowed to collaborate in identifying a problem and alternatives for solving it, the staff is more likely to help develop a good working solution. On the other hand, if the CEO or the board decides on a course of action and unilaterally announces it to the medical staff, the idea may never be accepted.
  - *Encourage closeness*. Common meeting areas, mutual involvement—these

are factors that can help to break down the distinctions that create conflict and mistrust. When management teams were being formed in Great Britain, sherry time and group meals helped promote understanding among administrators, physicians, nurses, and fiscal officers.

— *Focus on problems, not personalities.* It is critical to face the issues at hand rather than to point fingers of blame at individuals. Threatening language, aggressive postures, and certain physical gestures are manifestations of conflict that fade quickly when people sit down and talk rationally about the problem rather than about personalities.

— *Minimize power and status.* Cooperation among factions in hospitals will grow when it is recognized that each person or group has equal power to compete. It also should be recognized that instead of competition, cooperation should be the standard approach. Having the power to compete, coupled with the good sense not to use it, encourages joint efforts and accomplishments.

— *Make dissension work for, not against.* Research shows that cooperation is increased when persons who are on the same side are not afraid to disagree out in the open—in one another's presence. Cooperation and its resulting benefits to both sides are maximized when everyone agrees to talk out his differences together, focusing on problem solving and not just on maintaining a preconceived position.

— *Work toward personal and group goals simultaneously.* It is unrealistic and perhaps immoral to assume that people will compromise their own values and goals for the good of the organization. To encourage joint effort, methods must be devised to help each person obtain what he personally wants from a given situation while providing the organization with a measure of achievement toward its goals.

— *Share information.* Suspicion is implied whenever important information is withheld. Many times, when data are closeted, mistrust develops.

— *Send signals that say "You're okay."* It is only natural to be cautious about expressing approval of others, particularly in an institutional setting, but it is important to do so nonetheless. Taking time to demonstrate sincere interest in others (the administrator, for example, who joins a group of physicians or nurses at lunch rather than eating with other administrators or alone in his or her office) gets the message across that one is honestly interested in others. These caring attitudes open the way to honest and healthy communication.

To be sure, the illustrations cited here represent only a few of many ways to which joint efforts can be encouraged within hospitals. Too frequently, the tie that binds board, medical staff, and administration is one of avid competition with another hospital or regulatory bodies. This is a negative unifying force that can cloud the commitment to a hospital's goals, it also is counterproductive as far as meeting community needs.

A more positive technique that helps solidify cooperation is education in a team setting that includes management, medical, and nursing personnel. Getting away from the routine work environment and into a "vacuum" where objective thinking is made easier is one of the best moves hospital managers can make toward opening the doors to constructive change.

A discussion of the art of joint effort would not be complete without acknowledging that some hospitals appear to have more success at nurturing cooperation than do others. The reason: inevitably there is at least one individual on the staff who has a knack for bringing diverse groups together. It makes sense, therefore, to look around and pinpoint such talents—to exploit them to everyone's benefit.

Do not expect these staff members to be miracle workers, though. It may take 4 to 5 years before the mood of teamwork is instilled. But the wait and the work are worth it. Unquestionably, we must develop the ability to work as teams, or our health care system will lose that unique spark of altruism that is its major strength.

REFERENCES

1. *Hospitals,* p 32, Feb 20, 1989.
2. Schulz R and Detmer D: How to get doctors involved in governance and management. In The hospital medical staff: selected readings 1972-1976, American Hospital Association, p 8, 1977.
3. SMS Survey: MDs earning more, but working more hours too, Am Med News, p 13, Nov 20, 1987.
4. Medical Education Issue, JAMA, 260(8): 1988.
5. Freidson E: Profession of medicine. New York, 1972, Dodd, Mead & Co, Inc.
6. AAMC: Longitudinal study of medical school graduates of 1960, NCHSR Research Digest Series, DHEW Pub No (PHS) 79-3235, Jan 1979.
7. Rezler AC: Attitude changes during medical school: a review of the literature, J Med Educ 49:1023, 1974.
8. Dennis JL: Speech delivered while Dean, University of Oklahoma School of Medicine, 1967.
9. National Academy of Sciences: Institute of Medicine: A manpower policy for primary health care, Washington, DC, May 1978.
10. Report of the Graduate Medical Education National Advisory Committee to the Secretary, Department of Health and Human Services, Vol 1, GMENAC Summary Report, KGPO #1980-0-721-748/266, Washington, DC, 1981, US Government Printing Office.
11. Schwartz WB, Sloan FA, and Mendelson DN: Why there will be little or no physician surplus between now and the year 2000, N Engl J Med 318(14):892, 1988.
12. Somers HM and Somers AR: Medicare and the hospitals: issues and prospects, Washington, DC, 1967, The Brookings Institution.
13. Kessel R: The AMA and the supply of physicians, Law Contemp Prob 35(2):1970.
14. Marder WD, et al: Physician employment patterns: challenging conventional wisdom, Health Affairs, p 137, Winter 1988.
15. 1989 Accreditation Manual for Hospitals, Joint Commission on Accreditation of Healthcare Organizations, Chicago, 1988.
16. Harvey JD and Wallace ST: Are JCC's Effective Forums? Hospitals 46:49, 1972.
17. Physicians grapple with changing health care delivery, Hospitals, p 56, Dec 20, 1986.
18. Paxton HT: Why you're spending a lot more to earn your practice. Med Econ, p 170, Nov 9, 1987.
19. Survey spots the tight turns in MD-CEO Relations, Hospitals, p 48, Feb 5, 1988.
20. SMS survey: MDs earning more But working more hours too. Am Med News, p 13, Nov 20, 1987.
21. Alexander JA and Morrisey MA: Hospital-Physician Integration and Hospital Costs, Inquiry, 25(3):388, 1988.
22. Luft HS: Health maintenance organizations: dimensions of performance, John Wiley & Sons, Inc. New York, 1981.
23. Barr JK and Steinberg MK: Professional participation in organizational decision making: physicians in HMOs, J Commun Health, 8:160, 1983.
24. Schulz R and Schulz C: Management practices, physician autonomy and satisfaction: evidence from mental health institutions in the Federal Republic of Germany, Med Care, 26(8):750, 1988.

25. Reinhardt UE: A framework for deliberations on the compensation of physicians, J Med Pract Manage, 3(2):85, 1987.
26. Carlova J: Can a hospital board wipe out medical staff election? Med Econ p 27, July 4, 1988.
27. Starr P: The social transformation of America medicine, New York, 1982, Basic Books Inc, Publishers.
28. Haug MR: Deprofessionalism: an alternative hypothesis for the future. In Halmos P, ed: Sociology review, Monograph 20, professionalization and social change, p 195, Dec 1973.
29. Freidson E: Reorganization of the medical profession, Med Care Rev, 42(1), Spring 1985.
30. Harrison S, Haywood S and Fussell C: Problems and solutions: the perceptions of NHS managers, Hosp Health Serv Rev, 80(4), 1984.
31. Tolliday H: Clinical autonomy. In Jacques E, editor: Health services: their nature and organization and role of patients' doctors, and the health professions, London, 1978, Heinemann Educational Books, Inc.
32. Schulz R and Harrison S: Physician autonomy in the Federal Republic of Germany, Great Britain and the United States, Int Health Plan and Management 1(5):335, 1986.
33. Schulz R et al: Physician adaptation to health maintenance organizations and implications for management, Manuscript accepted for publication by Health Services Research, 1990.
34. Fineberg HV, Funkhouser AR, and Marks H: Variations in medical practice: a review of the literature. Paper presented at the conference on cost-effective medical care: Implications on variation in medical practice. Institute of Medicine, National Academy of Sciences, Washington DC, Feb 1983.
35. Eisenberg JM: Doctors' decisions and the cost of medical care, Ann Arbor, Mich, 1986, Health Administration Press Perspectives.
36. Linn LS et al: Physician and patient satisfaction as factors related to the organization of internal medicine group practices, Med Care, 23(10):1171, 1985.
37. Schulz R and Schulz C: Management practices, physician autonomy and satisfaction: evidence from the Federal Republic of Germany, Med Care, 26(8):750, 1988.
38. Omega Research Consultants: What do physicians really want from hospitals? Hospitals, p 46, June 5, 1987.

11

Nursing*

Nursing is a profession in transition. The trends and issues that underlie this phenomenon hold important implications for the management of hospitals and other health care institutions and agencies. Most important, nursing service is a critical component in fulfilling hospital, long-term care, and other health service organization objectives for patient care. Nurses constitute the largest single group of health professionals. Currently there are more than 2 million registered nurses in the United States.

The first section of this chapter will briefly explore nursing in transition as a background to current issues. The seocnd section will consider issues in nursing, and the third will explore implications for management of health services.

NURSING IN TRANSITION

In years past, nursing service comprised essentially the entire hospital staff; other hospital employees were there to help nurses, who in turn served the physicians and patients. Although nurses were subservient to physicians, they had an important healing role in a close working relationship with each physician.

The healing powers of nursing were perhaps more apparent before World War II and the advent of antibiotics and other technologies. It is speculated that many of the healing actions employed by nurses stimulate the immune system of the patient. The growing field of psychoimmunology holds great promise for explication of these actions. Nurses as healers function differently from physicians, who tend to use more invasive and expensive therapies. These two groups of healers can function in a complementary manner in illness. Since World War II, however, improvements in blood banking, surgery, and other technologies, and increased knowledge of physicians have resulted in physician dominance and control. The healing powers of nursing have suffered a concomitant decline in importance in hospitals. The art and science of nursing, which provides holistic care and puts ". . . the patient in the best condition

---

*This chapter was co-authored with Mitzi Duxbury.

for nature to act upon him . . ." (Florence Nightingale), is difficult to observe in some of today's hospitals. The mechanism of promoting healing is incorporated in the conceptual frameworks and theories of nursing today.

Profound changes in nursing began during World War II and have accelerated since then. After World War II, nurse shortages escalated when the supply of nurses provided by the Cadet Nurse Corp terminated in 1945. This shortage was qualitative, as well as quantitative. Inadequacies were identified in terms of curricula, faculty preparation, theory, and clinical preparation. Solutions to recruitment, preparation, and retention in the workplace included ". . . moving control of education from service to educational institutions, strengthening accreditation standards, and providing a more participatory role in hospital employment. . . ."[1] The professional nurse traineeship program addressed student recruitment and qualitative and quantitative aspects of education.

Concerns of the workplace were largely left unaddressed as the supply of nurses increased. This lack of attention to working conditions was responsible for the movement toward collective bargaining by nurses and is the major contributing factor to the shortage that exists today.

In the 1950s considerable unrest developed in nursing because of low wages, a long work week, rotating shifts, diminished authority, and the fact that other health professionals, for example, physical therapists, began doing tasks formerly performed by RNs. It became more difficult for the nurse to provide holistic care. Collective bargaining developed in a few locations, such as California and Minneapolis/St. Paul, but it was thwarted in many other areas because nurses and other hospital workers were excluded from national labor legislation until 1974. Other factors relating to collective bargaining are discussed in Chapter 17.

In the 1960s, hospital diploma nursing education programs began closing as a result of a number of pressures, among them the high cost of nursing education to hospitals, the pressures of the American Nurses' Association for baccalaureate and associate degree education, and the desires of high school graduates for a college degree. Although more than 80% of graduates from nursing schools in 1960 were from diploma programs, by 1985 only 15% graduated from such programs.[2] In addition to the increase in 4-year baccalaureate programs, 2-year associate degree programs emerged, along with the 2-year community college development in the United States. Today about half of the graduating nurses are from associate degree programs, which are usually based in community colleges. Table 11-1 describes the various levels and initial educational programs in nursing. The term *nurses* covers practitioners educated in all of these programs, yet there is a wide range in training and in roles. The licensing examination is the same for all registered nurses regardless of educational preparation (associate degree, diploma, and baccalaureate or higher). The examination for licensed practical or vocational nurses is different.

In the 1960s and 1970s trends toward (1) clinical nurse specialists, (2) nurse clinicians, and (3) nurse practitioners developed.

1. **Clinical nurse specialists.** These nurses have a master's degree with education in specialties such as pediatrics, obstetrics, or psychiatry. There is also a trend toward certification of specialists. Objectives of clinical nurse specialization are to return the

Table 11-1 Educational programs in nursing and related career opportunities (USA, 1985)

Programs in nursing	Usual length of study	Minimum educational requirements	Site of training	Degree awarded and license eligibility	Type of position occupied upon graduation
Practical nurse	1 year	High school diploma or graduate equivalent degree (GED)	Community college and clinical training in area hospitals	Certificate: eligible to take exam for licensure as L.P.N.	Bedside nursing (with supervision): primary care (with supervision)
Diploma (hospital-based)	2-3 years	High school or GED	Hospital and sometimes community college for liberal arts courses	Diploma: eligible to take exam for licensure as R.N.	Staff nurse: bedside nursing: primary care or in physician's office
Associate degree	2 years	High school or GED	Community college or 4-year college, and clinical training in area hospitals	Associate Degree in Nursing: eligible to take exam for licensure as R.N.	Staff nurse: bedside nursing: primary care, self-employed or in physician's office
Basic or generic baccalaureate	4 years	High school or GED	University or 4-year college, and clinical experience in area hospitals and agencies	Bachelor of Science in Nursing: eligible for Nursing licensure as R.N.	Bedside nursing: public health (PH) nursing: primary care, self-employed or in physician's office
Baccalaureate for R.N.	1.5-2 years beyond diploma or associate degree	R.N. associate degree or diploma in nursing	University or 4-year college, and clinical experience in area hospitals and agencies	Bachelor of science in nursing	Bedside nursing: PH nursing: primary care, self-employed or in physician's office: administration
Master's	1.5-2 years beyond baccalaureate	B.S. in nursing and R.N. licensure	University, and clinical experience in area hospitals and agencies	Master of science or Master of science in nursing	Bedside nursing: PH nursing: primary care self-employed or in physician's office: administrator: educator: supervisor: clinical specialist
Doctoral	3 years or more beyond baccalaureate depending on major	Baccalaureate degree in nursing	University and area hospitals if program requires	Ph.D.	All of the above for master's and researcher: higher education administrator

From Donabedian A et al: Medical care chartbook, p. 221, Ann Arbor, Mich, 1986, Health Administration Press. Data from Office of the Assistant Dean for Student and Alumni Affairs, School of Nursing. The University of Michigan, February 1985. Reprinted with permission from Health Administration Press.

nurse from administrative duties to direct patient care, to apply advancing nursing clinical knowledge, and to provide for greater comprehensiveness, continuity, and coordination of patient services. In such a role the clinical specialist functions as a partner with the physician rather than in a subservient role.

Clinical specialization often parallels the major medical services, such as medicine and surgery. It is the role that is receiving most attention in the larger hospitals; however, cost containment and nursing shortages have eliminated the role in some hospitals. Although the definition of clinical nurse specialization is somewhat unclear in terms of activities, based on a study by Hummel,[3] there is general agreement that it involves direct patient care, interdisciplinary activities, development of innovative and experimental approaches to patient care, consultation, and staff development.

Clinical specialization is acknowledged and accepted as an essential function in today's complex health care institutions. It appears from a review of the literature and from discussions with those closest to its development that the clinical nurse specialist is expected to do the following:

Help cope with advancing knowledge and technologies. New patient care services, such as cardiovascular surgery, renal dialysis, and neonatology, require advanced knowledge and skills.

Help return the nurse to the patient so he or she can focus on patient rather than just system needs. This means more accountability and responsibility to the patient and more independence from physicians and non-nursing duties. Accountability also means concerns for costs in relation to benefits.

Expand roles of nurses, particularly in ambulatory care settings, nursing homes, and other places currently significantly ignored by health professionals. The health of the consumer will be the focus of attention rather than just intermittent crisis care.

Function more in a collegial team setting as opposed to the current hierarchical relationships. Implied is the education of the clinical specialist in a team setting rather than the current isolation from medicine and other health professions.

Develop a more professional status for nursing within the mentioned criteria for a profession.

2. **Nurse clinician.** This term is used in some hospitals to define a middle-level position of nursing practice that is attained by demonstrating advanced clinical competence in providing leadership for the nursing team. There are no uniform educational requirements, and there is great variability between hospitals on the use of this title. The nurse clinician may function as a generalist or a specialist. She or he is usually prepared at least at the bachelor's degree level and often at the master's level.

3. **Nurse practitioner.** This term is frequently used to express the expanded nursing role, often in an ambulatory patient care setting. This nurse is usually prepared at least at the baccalaureate level and often holds a master's degree. In most cases she or he works closely with a physician. However, a few have "hung out their own shingle." Nurse practitioners tend to function in areas that overlap with traditional physician functions, for example, taking medical histories, doing physical assessment, screening patients, and managing long-term care. Some view this as expanded functions of nursing. Nurses have always taken nursing histories, done screening, performed

limited physical assessments, and assumed some primary responsibilities in the management of long-term care. In the next chapter nurse practitioners are discussed further in reference to physician assistants.

There has been renewed interest also in nursing administration. With impetus from the Kellogg Foundation, new nursing administration programs developed in the late 1970s at the master's level. Many of these have been established as joint endeavors between nursing schools and health administration programs. A trend today exists where dual or joint master's degrees in nursing and business administration are developing to better prepare nurses to manage complex health care facilities.

Nursing in ambulatory settings is also experiencing many changes, particularly in relation to nurse practitioners and extended roles. Nurses in community mental and neighborhood health centers and in family and pediatric office practices are providing services in ambulatory and home care and performing tasks that were formerly viewed by physicians as their role.

Changes in Organization of Nurse Staffing

Because nursing is the largest and probably the most important single department in the hospital and other health services, nurse staffing patterns are crucial to the organization's effectiveness and efficiency. Changes in the organization of nursing on the patient unit might be classified as (1) the care method, (2) functional assignments, (3) team nursing, (4) primary nursing, and (5) case method.

1. The care method was prevalent in the early part of the twentieth century. Nursing at that time was more like special-duty nursing, where the nurse provided all nursing functions for the patient. It was a one-to-one relationship concept of "my patient/my nurse."

2. With the shortage of professional nurses around World War II, the impact of "scientific management" from industrial models, and advancing technologies, functional nursing developed. Aides and licensed practical nurses (LPNs) were hired to fill nursing vacancies. Nursing personnel were therefore assigned to functions: for example, aides to maintenance duties, one nurse to medications, and another to treatments. As a result, care became fragmented and more impersonal.

3. Team nursing was developed in the 1950s to coordinate activities more effectively. It was a method of assigning groups of patients to a team of nursing staff members headed by a registered nurse called a team leader, who was primarily responsible for planning and evaluating nursing care. However, in some settings, short staffing, inadequately prepared auxiliaries, and poor communication led to fragmentation and nonpersonalized care. Frequently the team leader served more as a nurse who administered medications.

4. In the 1960s primary nursing was developed. It began to be adopted in the 1970s, especially in the last half of the 1970s. In most cases the primary nurse assumes 24-hour accountability (although in some institutions it is only for the time on duty) for the care, planning, and evaluation; and when on duty, the nurse assumes responsibility for providing the total care of the patient. Coor-

dination of activities with the patient's physician and other health professionals is also a function of the primary nurse. In such arrangements the clinical nurse specialist (CNS) may serve in a staff-consulting arrangement with the primary nurse, or the CNS may serve in a line managerial role, having overall responsibility for the unit.

5. The case method is a more recent development in nursing service task organization. It is a modification of both the primary and care arrangements. In the case management system, the nurse is responsible for developing and administering the nursing care plan for the patients he or she case manages. The case manager nurse is also responsible for coordination of all services to the patient, serving as the patient's advocate in this case management role. The case manager role is discussed further in the next chapter.

ISSUES IN NURSING

In 1970 a National Commission for the Study of Nursing and Nursing Education, Lysaught[4] called nursing a "troubled occupation." There is little evidence that troubles have dissipated since then. Indeed, nursing shortages today appear to be traceable to problems evident since the 1960s. There are many issues and pressures on nursing, both on the professional and health services levels. Included in the professional issues are environmental pressures, and ambiguities related to nursing roles, education, and their professional organizations. Organizational issues mirror these pressures and ambiguities, along with managerial issues related to increasing intensity of patient care coupled with requirements to control quality and costs. Overriding and perhaps reflecting both professional and organizational issues is a severe shortage of nurses.

Professional Issues

The environment within which every organization functions is more stressful than it was in the past. Nursing, traditionally an occupation for women, faces additional pressures from the changing opportunities and expectations for women. Nursing, as the largest health profession, has probably received the brunt of the rapid changes in health care services.

As noted in the previous section, other health professionals have absorbed parts of the roles previously performed by nurses. On the other hand, physicians delegate more responsibility to nurses, yet in the hospital setting at least, nursing autonomy to fulfill their responsibilities has been eroded. Nurses' responsibilities must be coordinated with many other professions. Moreover, organization management is much more aggressive in monitoring and controlling patient care practices.

One of the most persistent problems faced by nursing is that of defining what nursing is and what is distinctive about it. Although nurses understand nursing and perhaps most physicians understand nursing, the difficulty in translating nursing to hospital managers remains an enigma, and both nursing and patient can suffer. This of course stems from the close historical relationship between medicine and nursing and their joint involvement in the clinical care of the patient. In trying to define the nurse's role in relation to the physician's role, some have suggested nursing's primary emphasis is concerned with care while medicine is concerned with cure. Donna Diers[5] suggests:

> There are fads and fancies in the way we define nursing. The latest is "caring." Now that goes back a long way to the distinction between nursing and medicine—a political difference, not a practice one. Medicine "cures;" nursing "cares." Since challenging the right to cure is treading on tender toes, nursing claimed "care" as exclusive territory. Well, nonsense. Caring is not all there is to nursing.

Many physicians and nurses dispute such a discrete separation, noting current overlaps in both areas. Some physicians and administrators see nursing in a dependent role, carrying out the orders of the physician and fulfilling "discrete tasks" designed to help and comfort patients. Some treatments may be done by either a physician or a nurse, and some feel that there appears to be overlap in roles.

Nursing care is not a series of tasks provided to, at, or for someone, but represents holistic care individually rendered and based on needs of the patient and family. Such nursing output is not easily measured. This lack of quantification can be a source of frustration for some managers. Long-term patient/family outcomes may be the ultimate evaluation of nursing care. But institutions generally are not geared to either short-term (or, much less, long-term) patient outcomes. Further, the financial incentive to the institutions is not directed to improved patient outcome; indeed, the converse may be true; for example, under fee-for-service reimbursement systems, there are additional financial rewards for complications, such as infection.

Another model suggested by nursing groups emphasizes a decision-making role for nurses. Although it designates a separate domain of expertise and practice, this approach views nursing interacting with the physician and other health workers. It sees nursing as separated into professional (decision-making and leadership) and technical (cure and care services) activities. This approach stems from increased emphasis on the behavioral sciences. It also represents a determined effort by the profession to develop a science of nursing that will permit accurate prediction and control of the outcomes of nursing intervention.

Educational Issues

Both the American Nurses' Association (ANA) and the National League For Nursing (NLN) have formally adopted the position that a baccalaureate degree is the minimum qualification to become a "professional registered nurse." They propose that an associate degree or diploma in nursing be designated as "technical nurse practice." However, as of 1989 only one state (North Dakota) requires a baccalaureate degree for licensure as an R.N.

Not only has there been confusion in roles of nursing and different educational routes for nursing positions, but within the collegiate schools, there is no common agreement on what constitutes the content of the "long and disciplined educational process." Perhaps the most ubiquitous criticism of the present state of nursing education as a professional discipline is the lack of research in that discipline and the institutional system providing it. Nursing research explicates the body of knowledge on which nursing practice rests. Without a scientific body of knowledge, the quality of nursing care and the movement toward professional practice will not improve. A major impediment in facilitation of clinical nursing research is lack of control over a clinical laboratory where new scientifically based nursing practice and new methods of delivery can be studied and evaluated. Unlike most other professional practice disciplines in universities, nurse faculty in general have no laboratories that they control. This lack of control and its concomitant autonomy have seriously retarded the ability of nursing to address the major practice issues. In short, then, there are difficulties in nursing education that stem from the location, the content, and the development of content. Furthermore, these problems stack up against nursing in its efforts to satisfy the professional characteristics of a long and disciplined educational process. Clearly the trend is toward a greater utilization of institutions of higher education; the trend is less clear when we examine the need for rapprochement between education and service that will strengthen meaningful research in the nursing practice.

Collegiate nursing also has the burden of providing clinical training within the normal baccalaureate curriculum. Almost all other occupations/professions are introduced into the real world of practice via apprenticeships or internships. In spite of efforts on the part of nurses, they have not gained this advantage.

Professional Issues

It would seem that the ANA should meet criteria of self-governance, source of professional self-discipline, standards, ethics, and cohesiveness. Here again, nursing is struggling toward but not yet attaining a completely successful professional association that is characteristic of other disciplines. In 1967 only 25%, or just over 200,000, of the registered nurses in the nation belonged to the ANA. By 1977 the percentage of total registered nurses employed in nursing in the United States that belonged to the ANA declined to 14%. Membership as a percent of total working registered nurses continued to decline, reaching only 9.5% at the end of 1988. Dues of more than $200 annually for state and national memberships, lack of tangible benefits in relation to costs, and ANA stands on controversial issues, such as a baccalaureate degree for an R.N. and collective bargaining, are some of the reasons attributed to declining membership.

Nursing encompasses large numbers of auxiliaries and paraprofessionals who may or may not share nursing's professional concerns, but who are ineligible for membership in the ANA. Beginning with the first course in practical nursing in 1890, there has been a struggle over the roles, the education, and control of various aides to nursing.

Nursing also has a unique situation to consider: the existence of another national organization that appears to serve many of the same functions as the ANA. The NLN is an organization that includes representatives from registered nurses, practical nurses, aides, orderlies, allied health professions, and lay bodies. Accreditation, one of the prime functions of most professional bodies, has resided traditionally with the NLN, rather than the ANA. Most professional organizations also have a major role in achieving prestige for their members and in determining to some extent the distribution of rewards within the profession. In recent years the ANA has become much more militant in matters of salary and benefits and has used a number of tactics to apply pressure on hospitals and administrators who fail to meet satisfactory conditions of work. In some cases, the points of argument covered nursing service and the conditions of patient care, as well as basic monetary concerns. This forceful approach to pay and working conditions has not always found favor with those in and out of nursing. Some find it closer to the work of a labor union than a professional group, but this tactic has succeeded in improving salary levels.

Whether nursing enjoys professional status is not the only issue. It is obviously faced with serious problems that affect the major functions of the health service institution, especially the hospital and nursing home.

Institutional Issues

The knowledge explosion has affected nursing as it has other disciplines. However, in addition to the need to know more, nursing faces the stresses of (1) caring for sicker patients in shorter lengths of stay and (2) staff shortages, both within an increasingly complex environment.

Patients undergoing cardiovascular surgery or renal dialysis or those in coronary care units and other specialized services require specialized nursing care. The knowledge explosion has been along clinical lines, resulting in creating clinical nurse specialists similar to the increasing specialization of physicians. At first physicians opposed clinical nurse specialization and increased nursing knowledge. However, after being exposed to the capabilities and performance of such persons, most physicians support such developments. The knowledge explosion has also affected nursing education, resulting in increasing numbers of master's and doctoral programs.

Average length of stay in nonfederal, short-term, general hospitals has declined from 8.4 days in 1968 to 7.2 days in 1987.[6] Meanwhile the volume and intensity of services to patients has increased. When length of stay was longer and patients recuperated in hospitals, the pace was slower and the nursing staff had more time to provide optimal nursing care and patient education. With the implementation of the prospective payment system (PPS) and diagnostic related groups (DRGs), Medicare patients and other patients are discharged from hospitals earlier and admitted into nursing homes, placing burdens of sicker patients on already strained nurses in those organizations. The increased intensity of service without concomitant increases in resources and rewards takes its toll on nurses in terms of stress and burnout.

Cost and Quality Control

All health professionals (including nurses) and health institutions are under increasingly stringent cost and quality controls. One method receiving attention today is patient classification and/or acuity systems. A major challenge for nursing and administration is to identify and provide for the true cost of nursing services. Hundreds of thousands of dollars is spent each year attempting to quantify measures of nursing services. Numerous patient classification systems have been developed over the past 30 years. Many of the systems have attempted to measure tasks performed (the old industrial model), and these systems have been directed toward staffing concerns and not patient outcomes. Attempts have been made to correlate nursing intensity and DRGs. The literature is not uniform in these relationships, with some authors reporting extreme heterogeneity. Some methods hold greater promise for improved quantification of nursing services. Those using the patient as the unit of analysis, rather than the task, may be able to provide more realistic data congruent with the goals of nursing practice.

Investigators are beginning to be more attentive to measurement of patient outcome, at least short-term outcome. For example, in the carefully done study by Knauss et al.[7] of 5030 patients in 13 hospitals' intensive care units, using Acute Physiology and Chronic Health Evaluation (APACHE) to estimate the pretreatment risk of mortality of these very ill patients, the mortality ratio ranged between .59 and 1.58 for predicted mortality. That is, some hospitals had significantly less mortality than predicted and some significantly more. Closer examination of these extremes (lower than predicted mortality and higher than predicted mortality) of the hospitals revealed major differences between hospital 1 (much lower mortality than predicted) and hospital 13 (much higher). Hospital 1 gave more "daily therapeutic intervention" (40 points more), but there were not additional invasions. Indeed, hospital 1 had "one of the lowest utilization rates of pulmonary artery catheters." Hospital 1 had many clinical nurse specialists with intensive ICU experience. Communication and coordination between nursing and medicine were described as excellent. Nurses were respected and appeared to have considerable control and autonomy. For example, major elective surgery could be cancelled if "adequate unit nursing staff was not available—a decision that could be made by the unit nurse in charge." This hospital also had an extensive and comprehensive nursing education support system.

Although the patient outcome measures, other than mortality, are more difficult to ascertain, greater attention must be given to other short-term patient outcomes and both the quality and quantity of nursing care. Some of these measures are use of drugs, indwelling bladder catheters, invasive hydration, and restraint to substitute for minimal nursing care. Other physiologic measures include delayed wound healing, vascular disorders, gastrointestinal obstructions, bleeding, shock, pneumonia, and other complications, or iatrogenic effects that may be associated with poor nursing care. Cognitive and psychosocial patient outcome measures are being explicated as measures of quality nursing care, as well as length of stay and readmission to the hospital.

Nursing Shortage

Although the number of registered nurses in the United States is now estimated to be 2 million, a 35% increase from 1977, demand grievously exceeds supply today. Part of the shortage was a result of a large number of RNs employed part time. The labor participation of RNs has increased also from 72.7% in 1977 to 78.7% in 1984.[8] More nurses remain in practice than teachers, for instance.

In 1988, in response to the growing shortage of nurses, the Secretary of the U.S. Department of Health and Human Services established the Secretary's Commission on Nursing to examine these shortages. This 25-member advisory committee was charged with addressing four questions:

1. Does a shortage of RNs actually exist?
2. If a shortage exists, what is causing it?
3. What are the effects of the RN shortage?
4. What are the implications for the future?

The commission reported that the shortage indeed exists. It is primarily the result of increased demand. There are also supply-side considerations, and these include the following:

- Expanding career opportunities for women
- Declining student populations
- Decreased subsidies for education
- Problems with retention
- The effect of AIDS
- The image of nurses

The final report of the Secretary's Commission on Nursing to address the nursing shortage recommended actions to be undertaken and stated, "the health of this nation will be at risk if the changes suggested in these recommendations do not occur." These recommendations are in the box on p. 188.

Although virtually all studies of nursing and nursing shortages have concluded that nursing must have greater participation in decision making in hospitals, to date this has remained elusive.

In response to physician concerns about nursing shortages, in February 1988, the American Medical Association (AMA) Board of Trustees approved a proposal to develop a technical bedside caregiver called a registered care technologist (RCT). The AMA intention was to provide support services for nurses, coordinate education of hospital-based technicians, and develop hospital-based apprentice and in-service programs. There were three post–high school levels: assistant (2 month training); basic (an additional 7 months of training and eligibility for licensure); and the advanced care technologist (an additional 9 months of training, which would provide for certification). The RCTs would be licensed under the state medical board. This program would target recruitment to low income groups, and educational programs would be carried out in hospitals cooperatively with community colleges or vocational schools.[10]

The ANA house of delegates unanimously opposed the AMA proposal. Other nursing organizations and allied health groups have also vigorously opposed this proposal. Concerns of these organizations focused on safety issues, duplication, cost, and fragmentation of services. A fundamental underlying issue is threat to nursing control. As stated by the president of the ANA, Lucille Joel," one of the primary effects of the proposal will be to enhance the monopoly power of physicians in the health care market. Nursing will not let this happen."

IMPLICATIONS FOR MANAGEMENT

One of the most important and challenging responsibilities of health services managers is to achieve and maintain a high level of nursing performance and satisfaction. Nurse satisfaction is critical to other essential elements of health services performance,

Utilization of nursing resources

- Nurses' time should be spent on nursing, for example, providing direct patient care; adequate staffing levels of clinical and nonclinical support services are required.
- Staffing patterns should appropriately utilize levels of education, competence, and experience among RNs.
- Automated information systems and other labor-saving devices should be developed and utilized.
- Costing, budgeting, reporting, and tracking nursing resource utilization should be developed and implemented.

Nursing compensation

- RN compensation should increase; innovative compensation should be pursued based on performance, experience, education, and merit. Also, RN long-term career orientation should improve by providing a one-time adjustment.

Health care financing

- The government should reimburse efficiently organized health care delivery organizations not able to support the compensation suggested above.

Nurse decision-making

- Policy-making and regulatory and accreditation bodies that have an impact on health care should foster greater representation and active participation of the nursing profession.
- Employers should ensure active nurse participation in governance, administration, and management.
- Employers of nurses and the physicians should recognize the appropriate clinical decision-making authority of nurses in relationship to other health care professionals, foster communication and collaboration among the health care team, and ensure that the appropriate provider delivers the necessary care; close cooperation and mutual respect between nursing and medicine is essential.

Development of nursing resources

- Financial assistance to undergraduate and graduate nursing students must be increased.
- Nonfinancial barriers to nursing education—both for those entering and those wishing to upgrade—should be minimized.
- Curricula must be relevant to contemporary and future nursing practice, must prepare nursing for a variety of settings, and must provide the foundation for continued professional development.
- The nursing profession must promote the positive and accurate image of the profession and the work of nurses.

Maintenance of nursing resources

- The Department of Health and Human Services (DHHS) should establish a commission to monitor these recommendations.
- DHHS, private foundations, and employers of nurses should support and carry out research on the effects of nurse compensation, staffing patterns, decision-making authority, and career development on nurse supply and demand, as well as health care cost and quality.
- The federal government should develop data sources needed to assess nursing resources as they relate to health planning and manpower.[9]

such as patient and physician satisfaction, recruitment and job turnover, marketing, and collective bargaining. Although there is little empirical evidence in the industrial setting linking job performance to job satisfaction, there is some evidence that nurse satisfaction relates not only to patient satisfaction, but to patient compliance.[11] When asked what contributes to quality of hospital care, 97.3% of hospital CEOs surveyed ranked nursing care among the top three factors, 96.4% ranked clinical skills of the medical staff, and 93.3% ranked employee attitudes.[12]

First, it is important to stress that in spite of "troubles in nursing," most nurses find great satisfaction in direct patient care. Studies confirm the intrinsic rewards in nursing. However, satisfaction in nursing workplaces varies widely. There have been many studies of determinants of nurse satisfaction. Most of the variables relating to job satisfaction concern management. Included among these are such factors as task autonomy, nature of supervision, relationships with physicians, remuneration, and educational activities.

A relatively recent survey of both large and small "magnet" hospitals that have been particularly successful in recruiting and retaining professional nurses is enlightening to ways health services managers can help to achieve nurse satisfaction.[13] This study was patterned after the Peters and Waterman study of factors related to excellence among successful corporations in the United States.[14] Elements of "magnetism" were found to be the following:

Management style of participative management. Nursing is involved at all levels of committee work, nursing is informed, and nursing has considerable contact not only at the level of the CEO, but some contact with board members.

Quality of leadership. That is, that there is a recognition of an unbroken chain of qualified leaders at each level of the organization from the board to head nurses. The quality of nursing managers is pivotal, especially head nurses who are clinically competent and directors of nursing.

An organizational structure where the director of nursing is at the executive level, reporting to the CEO. A number of the magnet hospitals had a decentralized departmental structure whereby departments had both control and accountability for their performance.

Adequate staffing with favorable nurse/patient ratios. Many of the hospitals had large numbers of baccalaureate prepared nurses and employed clinical nurse specialists.

Personnel practices included salaries and benefits at least competitive with others in their communities. Attention was also paid to scheduling hours of work, with attempts to minimize shift rotation. There were also efforts for career ladders that rewarded clinical expertise with both title and salary changes.

Quality of patient care. That is, that nurses believed they were providing high quality care. There were a variety of nursing delivery models, such as primary nursing and holistic nursing, but the major thrust was to give the nurse the responsibility and related authority for care of a group of patients. There was also the ability to establish standards, set goals, monitor practice, and measure outcomes, and there was availability of consultation and resource personnel.

Image of nursing is high in the institution.

Education is important, starting with orientation of new staff, an active inservice education program, and financial support for formal educational opportunities. It was also evident that nurses themselves were active in teaching.

These findings are also very consistent with sound management practices for other health professionals in health services. We would add good physician/nurse relationships to the list. Management can do much to facilitate both a formal and informal culture for good relationships between nursing and the medical staff and between nurses and physicians in a joint practice setting. A major part of the strategic plan can focus on characteristics of magnetism. We also address these and other management practices to achieve a culture for satisfaction and performance in later chapters.

REFERENCES

1. Brown, EL: Nursing for the future, New York, 1948, Russell Sage Foundation. Cited in Secretary's Commission on Nursing: Interim Report, Department of Health and Human Services, Washington, DC, 1988.
2. Aiken LH: Nurses. In Mechanic D, editor: Handbook of health care and the health professions, New York, 1983, Free Press.
3. Hummel P: Identification of different approaches to clinical specialization in graduate education in nursing, University of Wisconsin-Madison, 1977.
4. Lysaught JP: An abstract for action, National Commission for the Study of Nursing and Nursing Education, Lysaught, JP: Director, New York, 1970, McGraw-Hill, Inc.
5. Diers D: On clinical scholarship–again, Image 20(1):2, 1988.
6. American Hospital Association: Hospital statistics 1988 edition, American Hospital Association, Chicago, 1988.
7. Knaus WA et al: An evaluation of outcomes from intensive care in major medical centers, Ann Intern Med, 104:410, 1986.
8. Department of Health and Human Services: The registered nurse population 1984, National Technical Information Service, Springfield, Va, 1986, (DHHS publication no [HRP] 0906938).
9. Secretary's Commission on Nursing: Interim Report, Department of Health and Human Services, Washington, DC, 1988.
10. Griffith H: Capital commentary, Nurs Econ 6(4):1988.
11. Weisman CS and Nathanson CA: Professional satisfaction and client outcomes: a comparative organizational analysis, Med Care 23(10):1179, 1985.
12. Survey by Hamilton/KSA (1989). Reported in Hospitals, p 32, Feb. 5, 1989.
13. McClure ML et al: Magnet hospitals: attraction and retention of professional nurses, American Academy of Nursing, Kansas City, MO, 1983.
14. Peters TJ and Waterman RH, Jr: In search of excellence, New York, 1982, Harper & Row Publishers, Inc.

IV

MANAGERIAL FUNCTIONS AND ISSUES

12

Other Health Professionals and Programs

The proliferation of health professions in recent decades has been one of the primary factors contributing to the increasing quality, cost, and complexity of health services and, consequently, complexity of its management. As in nursing and medicine, this has created role changes, ambiguities, and conflicts, as well as specialized expertise.

Table 12-1 lists employed persons in selected health occupations in 1985 (the last year for which such data were available). The census bureau categorized health occupations according to those who diagnose, those who can assess and treat, managers, technologists and technicians, and those in service occupations. It shows nursing to be the largest employment group in health services. It also shows there to be more than 100,000 managers; however, many professionals in other categories also have managerial responsibilities. The table confirms that the health occupations are female-dominated, with 77% being women. On the other hand, only 6% of dentists and 17% of physicians but 59% of managers are women. African Americans are under-represented in all professions except dietetics. Only 3% of physicians, less than 3% of dentists, and 8% of managers are black.

In Table 12-2, listed are 12 of the more common health professions other than nursing and medicine, and their educational characteristics and skills. We find that with each edition of this book, we must extend the training of at least some occupations, confirming the increasing skills of health professionals. One of the basic issues in the management of health services is the question of whether increasing skills and credential requirements serve the patient as much as the profession.

OTHER HEALTH PROFESSIONALS

On the following pages we discuss pharmacists, physician assistants, and nurse practitioners and very briefly discuss medical technologists and physical and occupational therapists. We focus on pharmacists because pharmacy represents one of the major treatment and expense categories in health services. Physician assistants and

Table 12-1   Employed persons in selected health occupations: 1985*

Occupation	Number (thousands)	Percentage Female	Percentage Black
TOTAL	5715	77.0	13.2
Health diagnosing occupa-tions†	728	14.8	3.2
Physicians‡	492	17.2	3.2
Dentists	131	6.5	2.6
Health assessment and treat-ing occupations	2006	85.6	7.0
Registered nurses	1447	95.1	6.8
Pharmacists	172	29.8	3.2
Dietitians	81	93.9	19.3
Therapists	257	76.2	7.2
Physician assistants	51	36.3	7.7
Managers, medicine, and health	106	59.2	8.1
Health technologists and technicians†	1115	83.4	13.6
Clinical laboratory	295	75.5	11.0
Dental hygienists	56	99.5	2.0
Radiology	121	73.8	7.5
Licensed practical nurses	402	96.9	19.6
Health service occupations	1760	89.9	24.5
Dental assistants	168	99.0	3.6
Health aides, except nursing	350	85.6	17.8
Nursing aides, orderlies, and attendants	1242	89.9	29.2

From US Bureau of the Census: Statistical abstract of the United States, 1985, Table 156 (Appendix 1, A1) Washington, DC, 1987, US Government Printing Office.
*Covers civilians 16 years old and older. Annual average is based on data collected by Bureau of the Census as part of Current Population Survey.
†Includes other occupations not shown separately.
‡Medical and osteopathic.

nurse practitioners are discussed because they are relatively new professions and they have unique relationships to physicians and each other. The other professions that are presented represent large numbers of health professionals and health service cost centers. Other health fields are omitted not because they are unimportant, but because this book is an overview and it was therefore necessary to limit its scope.

Pharmacists

Many will attribute the real advances in medical treatment since the 1930s to spectacular progress in drug therapy. The number of new, sophisticated, and therapeutically specific agents has increased dramatically during the past decade. The development of almost every therapeutic enhancement has occurred as a result, either directly or indirectly, of new drugs and drug delivery systems.[1]

The mission of pharmacy is (1) to promote and execute accurate and cost-effective drug therapy and delivery systems and (2) to systematically analyze and disseminate information on drugs.[2] It is estimated that in 1988, $36 billion was spent on drugs in the United States. The average expense for drug products in hospitals is approximately 6% of the average hospital's budget.[3] Management of drug procurement and dispensing is an increasing challenge with the introduction of more costly drugs within constraints on hospital revenues.

The role of pharmacies and pharmacists changed substantially in the 1980s. The independent neighborhood pharmacists are responsible for a decreasing portion of the total drug distribution volume. In the past they were responsible for compounding and dispensing drugs and acting as a primary source of health service support by advising customers on therapy for minor ailments and telling them where, when, and how to seek proper medical service. Currently, however, most drugstores are retail centers owned by large chains that employ pharmacists to count medications, insert them in a bottle, and type labels. Alternative approaches to drug dispensing include hospitals, mail-order prescription services, HMOs, and physicians' offices. The latter raises issues about disincentives to conservative therapy practices and is controversial within government and professional circles.

In hospitals, pharmacists have an increasingly important role. For example, with the shortage of nurses and increased sophistication of pharmacy services, a number of medication activities formerly performed by nurses are now being assumed by the pharmacists to improve accuracy and to relieve nursing workloads. In the past, 25% to 35% of a nurse's time was spent in various medication activities. In some hospitals it has dropped to as low as 10% with the transfer of more responsibility to the pharmacy department. It is now common to see advanced clinical pharmacy services provided with active involvement of the pharmacist working with physicians and nurses in providing direct patient care on inpatient units. For example, pharmacists participate in cardiac arrest calls, take patient drug-abuse histories, monitor medication effectiveness, and provide direct patient education and training.[4] Pharmacists have an important role in health service efficiency by working with the medical staff to have an efficient and effective drug formulary system, whereby drugs are purchased and dispensed generically. Expanded roles, more pharmacists, and multimillion dollar drug budgets have increased pharmacy department managerial responsibilities. In some hospitals the pharmacy has assumed broader functions of materials management for clinical departments.

With expanded roles for pharmacists, the supply of pharmacists has fallen behind the demand. The minimum time required for pharmacists to complete their training is 5 years. However, an increasing number have 6 to 7 years of training, resulting in a Pharmacy Doctor (Pharm. D.) degree. Also, master's degrees in hospital pharmacy are offered at several universities. With advancing knowledge in drugs, pharmacy specialties of radiopharmacists, parenteral nutritionists, and pharmacotherapists are recognized within the National Board of Pharmaceutical Specialties.

Table 12-2   Selected characteristics of representative members of health care team

Profession	Total length of professional training beyond H.S.	Basic curriculum structure	Indicator of academic achievement	Certifying bodies	Geographical location of training	Basic skills
Dietitian	5 yr	4 yr academic training 1 yr dietetic internship	B.S.—Foods and nutrition certificate for internship completion	American Dietetic Assn. (ADA)—registry exam (trend toward state licensure)	University setting Hospital, nursing homes, etc.	1 Determination of appropriate diet content for treatment of specific diseases 2 Source of information and advice to physicians
Respiratory therapy	Usually 2 yr, one summer	1st yr: 70%-80% didactic training; 20%-30% clinical training 2nd yr: 70%-80% clinical training; 20%-30% didactic training	Associate degree, inhalation therapy	American Assn., of Inhalation Therapists (AAIT)—registry board AMA-AAIT—review and approval of schools, state and local educational rules and regulations	Vocational technical school Hospital	1 Performs selected tests used in diagnosis of pulmonary diseases 2 Performs selected treatments for patients having pulmonary diseases 3 Maintain ventilatory control of acutely ill patients
Medical laboratory technician	24 mo	50% didactic training 50% clinical experience in affiliated lab	Diploma and certification	Amer. Medical Technologists (AMT) Amer. Society of Clinical Pathologists (ASCP) State and local educational rules and regulations National certifying agency	Vocational technical school	1 Hematology 2 Urinalysis 3 Bacteriology 4 Serology 5 Chemistry

	Length	Education/Training	Degree/Certificate	Accrediting Bodies	Setting	Duties
Medical technologist	4 yr	3 yr (90 credits) (basic sciences, liberal arts, etc.) 1 yr: 60% didactic training, 40% clinical experience in lab	B.S. in med. technology Certificate upon completion of internship	AMT AMA ASCP University approval NCA	University setting Hospital affiliated lab	Laboratory practice and theory: Chemistry Immunology Bacteriology Hematology
Occupational therapy	4 yr, 6 mo	4 yr academic (liberal arts and professional subjects—some "pre-clinical" experience, 6 mo. clinical experience	B.S. occupational therapy Certificate for completion of clinical experience (trend toward master's degree in O.T.)	Amer. Occ. Therapy Assn AMA—university approval	University setting Hospital	Practice in functional prevocational and home-making skills and activities of daily living. Sensorimotor, educational, recreational and social activities for patients Guidance in the selection and use of adaptive equipment Consultation and training concerning adaptation of physical environments for the handicapped
Pharmacy technician	1-9 mo	On-the-job training under supervision of trained technician and pharmacist or technical school	None	None	Hospital	1 Drug dispensation 2 Preparation of selected drugs 3 Maintenance of records

Continued.

Table 12-2   Selected characteristics of representative members of health care team—cont'd

Profession	Total length of professional training beyond H.S.	Basic curriculum structure	Indicator of academic achievement	Certifying bodies	Geographical location of training	Basic skills
Pharmacist-B.S.	5 yr plus usually 1 yr internship	1st & 2nd yr: liberal arts: 3rd-5th yr: professional courses & basic sciences	B.S. pharmacy	University standards & state licensure	University setting	1 Knowledge of drug action & human physiology 2 Responsibility for drug dispensing 3 Patient drug education 4 Source of information to physician, nurse, patient
Doctor of Pharmacy (Referred to as Pharm D.)	6 yr plus 1 yr internship	3rd thru 6th yr: professional courses	Doctor of Pharmacy	University standards and state licensure	University setting	Same as B.S. but more depth
Pharmacist—M.S. hospital pharmacy or Pharm D.	2-3 yr beyond B.S.	1 yr academic 1 yr residency or combination of the above in 2-3 yrs.	M.S. hospital pharmacy or Doctor of Pharmacy	University standards and state licensure	University setting Hospital	1 More highly developed understanding of clinical implication of drug use or 2 Improved development of management skills in hospital pharmacy
Physical therapist	4-6 yr; 4 mo. internship	4 yr academic 4 mo clinical experience	B.S., physical therapy	University standards Amer. Registry of Physical Therapists (certification) AMA	University setting Certificate for completion of clinical experience	Assess physical abilities and design therapy programs for patients involving physical means, e.g., exercise, heat, massage

	Duration	Curriculum	Degree	Accreditation	Setting	Functions
Radiographer (x-ray technician)	24 concurrent months to 4 yr programs leading to B.S. in radiological technology	Combinations of didactic training (physics, electronics, etc.) and clinical experience	Certificate	Amer. Society of Radiological Technologists (ASRT) AMA Amer. College of Radiologists (ACR)	Hospital	Performance of radiographic examination
Radiation therapy technologist	1-4 yrs depending on the program (1 yr must be graduate of radiographic program)	Anatomy, oncology, radiation physics, etc., and clinical experience	Certificate	ASRT, ACR, AMA	Hospital	Administration of prescribed course of radiation therapy
Social worker	4 yr	3 ½ yr didactic training ½ yr clinical experience	B.S.W. social work or B.A. social work	Council on social work education	University & selected agencies	1 Knowledge of human behavior & social environment 2 Structure and function of community agencies 3 Understanding of development of social welfare policy and services 4 Planning and evaluation of treatment using above knowledge (casework, group work, and community organizations)
Social worker, M.S.	1 to 2 yr beyond B.S.W.	Didactic training—50% clinical experience—50%	M.S. social work (M.S.W.)	Council on social work education	University & hospital or health agency	Advanced practice

Changes within the pharmacy profession are good examples of increased professionalism raising challenges to health services management. Knowledge has advanced dramatically, enhancing opportunities for better patient treatment. By the same token, drug dispensing requires education, surveillance, and controls to assure quality and efficiency.

Physician Assistants (PAs) and Nurse Practitioners (NPs)

Among the health professions to develop in the mid-1960s through the 1970s were physician assistants and nurse practitioners. Nurse practitioners were described in the previous chapter. Figure 12-1, developed by Barbara Bates, M.D., a former nurse, figuratively represents the relationships between nursing, medicine, and physician assistants. It shows some overlap among these three groups in meeting psychological needs and tasks instrumental to diagnosis and treatment. The physician assistant usually functions within the sphere of medicine, overlapping to some extent with nursing with regard to tasks instrumental to diagnosis and treatment and to a more limited extent in meeting psychological needs.

The first formal training program was developed at Duke University in 1965. By 1977 there were 56 accredited training programs across the country but this declined to 51 accredited programs by 1989. Titles and type of training vary considerably. Most PAs are in primary care.

At the insistence of organized medicine, physician assistants function under the supervision of, and in almost all cases are employed by, physicians. Such relationships have been written into statutes in a number of states. In certain rural areas, for example, in Alaska and Wyoming, physician assistants may work more than 100 miles from their supervising physicians, maintaining communication via telephone or other communication devices.

What impact have physician assistants and nurses practitioners had on the delivery of health services, that is, access to care, cost, and quality? PAs and NPs appear to increase access by distributing themselves in a different way from physicians. More go into rural areas and innercities, and larger proportions function in primary care—ambulatory settings. They also seem to increase the availability of service by increasing the productivity of physicians, enabling them to serve more patients. However, services added when PAs and NPs are introduced vary, and their impact on community access has had little study. Consumers and physicians seem to accept PAs and NPs, particularly after having received care from them or having employed them. Interestingly, physicians seem to prefer physician assistants to nurse practitioners,[5] but the public seems to accept nurse practitioners more readily than PAs.[6]

Studies suggest that PAs and NPs at least generate sufficient revenue to offset the costs to employ them in fee-for-service settings and they may indeed be quite profitable for the employing physicians. In controlled settings, such as HMOs, they may even result in reducing the cost of medical services if they serve as true substitutes for physicians. However, in terms of their impact on the cost of health care, it is likely that PAs and NPs have contributed to rising costs. They add to services provided to people. Moreover, millions of federal, state, and personal dollars have been expended in training such persons.

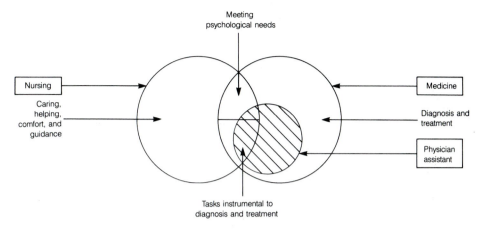

Fig. 12-1   Role of physician assistant who has military service corps background in relation to nursing and medicine. (From Barbara Bates as presented by Andrus LH and Gayman JP. In Conn HF, Rakel RE and Johnson TW, editors: Family practice, Philadelphia, 1973, WB Saunders Co.

All studies seem to conclude that the introduction of PAs and NPs into the health team in no way reduces quality in terms of process or outcome measures and in some instances is associated with marked improvement in access to care, patient satisfaction, and outcome measures of quality.

Although there has been some conflict between PAs and nurses at the national and institutional management levels, anecdotal evidence suggests that PAs and nurses generally have harmonious relationships at the work level because they recognize each others strengths. Both NPs and PAs can prescribe medications in some states, but training and roles differ. In HMOs, NPs and PAs work in a team with physicians. PAs trained in a university setting have an educational emphasis on science, differential diagnosis, counseling, and patient education. Nurse practitioners have more behavioral training and more emphasis on nutrition and long-term counseling and family relationships. NPs are independent practitioners in many states; PAs depend on physicians and must, for example, be within 15 minutes of at least telephone communication with a physician. Although PAs were initially men, representing corpsmen returning from Vietnam, today about half of the students in training are women.

With the impending surplus of physicians, questions are raised regarding PAs exacerbating the problem. Although a PA performs 80% of the tasks of primary care physicians, the number of PAs is small compared with physician numbers, and many PAs are located in rural and inner-city areas where physician shortages continue. Moreover, PAs are filling roles formerly held by interns and residents and foreign medical graduates. Starting salaries for PAs in 1989 was $26,500, yet they generate more than $100,000 annually because their time is usually billed at a physician's rate in fee-for-service practice. Although PAs contribute to physician profits as well as productivity, staff model HMOs tend to use PAs as substitutes for major portions of physician services to help contain costs.

Rehabilitation Therapists and Other Professionals

Services to rehabilitate persons with acute or chronic conditions have exploded in recent decades. In the past, people with disabilities had to depend on others for normal daily routines. One of the more remarkable successes of our health system is the transformation of lives of many disabled to independence and productivity. Intensive services from a broad scope of professionals make vast differences in the lives of disabled persons and their loved ones. Examples of the many professional skills serving such persons are physical and occupational therapists, audiologists, vocational therapists, speech pathologists, recreation therapists, music therapists, art therapists, social workers, dietitians, exercise physiologists, respiratory therapists, physiatrists (physicians specializing in rehabilitation), and others. As the reader will recognize, many of these people provide health promotion, preventive, diagnostic, and treatment services, as well as rehabilitation therapy.

Physical therapy (PT) is one of the better-known professions and a good example of dramatic advances and changes in health professions. As physical fitness, sports medicine, industrial medicine, and cardiac, burn, and other rehabilitation services have developed and advanced, the demand for physical therapists has soared. In 21 states there is legislation allowing physical therapists to practice independently, that is, without physician referral. A large proportion of physical therapists practice in physical therapy groups, contracting their services, for example, to hospitals, physician clinics, industrial plants, and schools. Starting salaries for PTs in 1989 was $25,000 to $38,000, and potential earnings are comparable with that of physicians. Graduates have averaged at least two job offers. Entry level training is 4 years of didactic training at the baccalaureate level plus an 18-week internship. A master's degree is another 1½ to 2 years in which the therapist would specialize in fields such as pediatrics or developmental disabilities. There have been attempts by some physical therapist spokespersons to lengthen entering requirements to the master's level. Such attempts have been resisted because there is no evidence that current training is inadequate. Moreover, although extension of training may enhance professional status, it exacerbates shortages of PTs and adds to costs.

Occupational therapy (OT) has also experienced a great demand for its services. It is one of the five fastest growing health professions in the United States. The field has moved from a focus on arts and crafts to emphasis on physical disabilities and psychosocial services. OTs are especially valuable for services to an aging population, and they have recently moved into the elementary schools for early identification of problems among youngsters. The expansion of home, mental, and industrial health services have increased demands for OTs. Although length and rigor of training is similar to that of PTs, starting salaries for OTs ($23,000 to $30,000) has lagged behind that of PTs.

Social workers can trace their roots in health services to 1893 when Jane Addams established a medical dispensary at Hull House in Chicago. Social workers can be found in all types of health services, especially mental health services where they serve as case managers, counselors, and directors of community mental health centers. Hospitals, nursing homes, HMOs, clinics, and rehabilitation services are also major employers of social workers. Social workers enhance the problem-solving capacities of people by assisting patients and families with the social aspects of illness, disability, and recovery. They serve as linkages for entry into the coordination through the health system. They promote effective and humane operation of health systems, and in their advocacy role, they contribute to the analysis and improvement of social policy and program development. Bracht summarizes basic premises that underlie social work as follows:

1. Social, cultural, and economic conditions have a significant and measurable effect on both health status and illness prevention and recovery.
2. Illness-related behaviors, whether perceived or actual, frequently disrupt personal or family equilibrium and coping abilities.
3. Medical treatment alone is often incomplete and occasionally impossible to render, without accompanying social support and counseling services.
4. Problems in access to and appropriate utilization of health services require community action and institutional innovation.
5. Multiprofessional health team collaboration on selected individuals and community health problems is an effective approach to solving complex medical problems.

Because patients increasingly are treated in the community (outside hospitals) and because they are discharged from hospitals sicker and sooner, linkages provided by social workers become ever more important.

Because nursing has moved into psychosocial roles, there has been some tension between roles of social workers and nurses in discharge planning in general hospitals. Management needs to facilitate the application of unique skills of both and enable them to focus on common goals for patient services and not on turf issues.

Medical technologists who work in hospital clinical laboratories are currently experiencing an increased demand for their services. This is a reversal from several years ago when there were reductions in laboratory tests because of Medicare PPS utilization disincentives. Because of some reductions in employment opportunities, enrollment in medical technology training also declined. However, demand for medical technologists has increased dramatically because of recent advances in laboratory diagnostic technologies and increasing demand for testing, such as for AIDS.

Cytotechnology, x-ray technology, respiratory therapy, and others have experienced increased demand for their services as medical knowledge and technology have advanced. There is increasing evidence that diet has an important relationship to health promotion and is a contributing factor to illness and even to cure, such as cholesterol problems. Dietitians, consequently, have an increasingly important health team membership role.

MANAGEMENT OF PROFESSIONAL SERVICES TO PATIENTS

In this section we take a microview of management, focusing on how to coordinate the broad scope of health professional services available to patients. The objective is to deliver the most appropriate skills and technologies at least cost. Using a mentally ill patient as an example, the various beneficial services will be listed, beginning with a psychiatrist. Within the field of psychiatry there are a large number of psychiatric interventions that might be applied, and each psychiatrist will likely have his or her preferences as to what is best for a particular patient. They might include medication therapy, shock therapy, psychoanalysis, social-milieu therapy, hospitalization, half-way house services, and a variety of community support services. There are also numerous combinations of interventions. In addition to these services, special skills of a variety of health professions can facilitate patient care. For example, there are clinical psychologists, social workers, nurses, OTs, recreation therapists, art and music therapists, vocational rehabilitation counselors, and other professionally trained persons available to help meet patient needs.

The first task is to diagnose the patient's problem and determine which therapies and services would be most helpful to the patient. Who should make such decisions? Should the psychiatrist make it unilaterally, in consultation with others, or should it be a group decision by a team? What is the role of the patient, family, employer, and legal system in such decisions and in the therapy and support services themselves?

The next step is to coordinate services to ensure proper timing for a broad scope of services in relation to patient needs and progress and for efficient use of time by the professionals. Coordination also includes the essential element of obtaining evaluations from the different disciplines and making decisions for alterations in the patient's care plan. There are a number of barriers to coordination of a broad scope of professional skills, be they in an acute medical or surgical facility or in a psychiatric inpatient or outpatient service. Each discipline brings its own values and cognitive mapping of patient problems and recommended interventions. Although this is a strength in terms of bringing a broad scope of knowledge to patient needs, it also complicates communication among the disciplines. Each discipline desires autonomy to practice its own skills, yet independence is limited in group settings. Status and respect are important to every individual, but these will be perceived as being compromised at times, particularly in interdisciplinary settings. Differing professional languages also contribute to misunderstandings. Role conflict and ambiguity, described in Chapter 17, are also more prevalent in interdisciplinary settings. Ways to mitigate conflict are also presented in Chapter 17. Here organization structural considerations in the coordination of health professions at the patient level are discussed.

Figure 12-2 summarizes different organizational patterns within three models. It presents them in a mental health context, either in an inpatient or outpatient setting. The models show only a few of the different professions that might be used in patient care. The reader should also remember that the variety of community services that require coordination are not shown. Although these are presented in a mental health setting, the models are relevant to medical, surgical, and other somatic services.

In the traditional medical model, the physician makes patient diagnostic and treatment decisions unilaterally or in consultation with others. Even though the physician might consult with others, he or she is clearly in charge and orders services from other disciplines. In a hospital setting, the physician will usually have standing orders and make exceptions as appropriate for the individual patient. The head nurse is usually in charge of the unit and responsible for coordinating other services. Within nursing, a team or primary nursing structure might be used. Coordination of patient evaluation and changing needs is facilitated by daily unit reporting on each patient. The medical

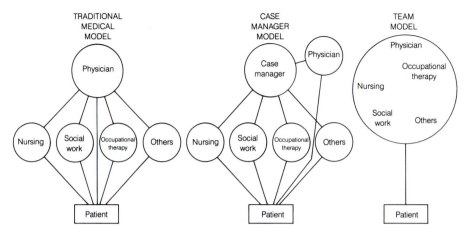

Fig. 12-2   Models for professional relationships.

record is also an important vehicle for communication among disciplines and with the attending physician. Physicians also have discussions with the various professionals, at times in a team setting.

The traditional medical model worked quite well before the proliferation of health professions. Physicians had close working relationships with nurses, who provided most of the services to patients. It is still the prevalent model for inpatient and outpatient somatic services. In complicated cases there may be a team of doctors, who then must come to consensus on treatment. However, with the broader scope of professional services to patients, with more intensive services per patient, and with staff shortages and cost pressures, it is an increasingly burdensome structure. It must rely on informal communications among disciplines and tends to give rise to conflicts and to compromise perceptions of status and autonomy.

The case manager model shown in Fig. 12-2 is widely used in ambulatory psychiatric services. More recently it is applied in general hospital nursing services. In ambulatory psychiatric services for the chronically mentally ill (CMI), the case manager has primary responsibility for the patient and coordination of all other services. The psychiatrist in this model serves as a consultant to the case manager, primarily for medication. It is an intensive service model with the manager having a case load of, for instance, 20 patients for whom he or she is responsible 24 hours a day. The case manager may be a clinical psychologist, social worker, or nurse. The legitimate authority of the case manager clarifies roles and responsibilities to facilitate coordination. The case manager system in a hospital medical or surgical unit works the same way except that the patient's physician has primary responsibility and takes an active role in the patient's treatment but delegates responsibility for executing services for the specific patient to the case manager. Where it has been applied to nursing units, patients, their families, nurses, and physicians are reportedly more satisfied. Moreover, there is evidence of some savings through reductions in length of stay and patient acuity levels.[8]

The team model is also widely used in both inpatient and outpatient mental health services. It is also used in staff model HMOs and community health centers. In somatic services the team might include the primary care physician, PA, NP, nurses, and home health workers. Teams with group decisions have the advantage of potentially better decisions in as much as different perspectives and a broader scope of knowledge are brought to bear on patients' needs. Group decisions are recommended in situations where issues are more subjective and not easily answered by facts, where commitment to action is needed by the decision makers, and where time can be taken for group discussion.[9] Ambulatory psychiatric services lend themselves to such criteria, whereas surgery, where unilateral decisions must be made by the surgeon, would not. Heterogeneous teams can be more innovative, and there is more agreement and commitment to goals and more continuity of care.

The team model also has weaknesses. First, it takes time and effort to develop a smooth operating team. When the British National Health Service implemented team management for health districts, most reported that it took nearly 2 years to achieve an effective team.[10] Experiences in interdisciplinary teams in neighborhood health centers also found it took considerable time to overcome barriers to team effectiveness and member satisfaction. Team decisions are considerably more time consuming than unilateral decision processes. Personnel turnover can create serious problems to team continuity and effectiveness. However, ingredients for successful teams include the following[11]:

1. Clarity in team goals
2. An improvement plan to achieve goals
3. Clearly defined roles
4. Clear communication
5. Beneficial team behaviors
6. Well-defined decision procedures
7. Balanced participation
8. Established ground rules
9. Awareness of the group process
10. Use of the scientific approach

Whatever the structure for coordination of patient care professional and support services, ultimate effectiveness of such services and relationships among professionals rests with unit and organization managers. Such managerial functions are discussed in the balance of this book.

REFERENCES

1. Kwan JW: High technology I.V. infusion devices, Am J Hosp Pharm 42(2):320, 1989.
2. McLeod DC: The philosophy of pharmacy practice. In McLeod DC and Willer WA, editors: The practice of pharmacy, institutional and ambulatory pharmaceutical services, Cincinnati, 1981, Harvey Whitney Books.
3. Wagner M: Pharmacy heads fight battles on two fronts, Modern Healthcare, 19(9):35, 1989.
4. ASHP statement on the pharmacists' clinical role in organized health care settings: *Practice standards of the ASHP 1988-1989 American Society of Hospital Pharmacists,* Bethesda, MD, 1988.
5. Fottler M: Physicians' attitudes toward physician extenders: a comparison between nurse practitioners and physician assistants, Med Care 17(9):536, 1979.
6. Storms D and Fox J: The public's view of physician assistants and nurse practitioners, Med Care 17(9):526, 1979.

7. Bracht NF: Social work in health care, Haworth, New York, 1978, The Haworth Press, Inc.
8. Ethridge P: Professional nurse/case management reduces hospital costs, Ariz Nurse 41(5), 1988.
9. Schulz R and Filley AC: Participation in management: when it is and is not appropriate, Administrative Briefs of American College of Hospital Administration, pp 1-5, Summer 1979.
10. Schulz R and Harrison S: Teams and top management in the NHS, King Edward's Fund for London, 1983.
11. Scholtes PR: The team handbook, Madison, Wis, 1988, Joiner Assoc.

13

Functional Managers

In this chapter we will suggest ways to improve the utilization of the managerial specialties of functional managers, such as accountants, industrial engineers, and planners. We will not attempt to review the bodies of knowledge from these disciplines, which are beyond the scope of this text and are described in other publications. Moreover, further consideration is given to some of these issues in later chapters on management of quality, costs, and conflict. In addition to discussing functional managers concerned with quantitative methods, this chapter also briefly considers specialists in marketing, materials management, personnel, public relations, planning, risk management, and the employment of consultants.

The knowledge and skills of functional managers are becoming increasingly important in the management of hospitals for the following reasons:

- The increasing size and complexity of health care organization operations require more formal procedures than have been necessary in the past. Informal contacts between the medical staff, nursing, and other departments and the administration are no longer sufficient, and communication problems are increasing.
- It is difficult for the CEO to keep informed about internal operations, since he or she spends more time on external affairs important to the organization.
- Assuming that everything is satisfactory unless management hears complaints is no longer an acceptable approach, because the environment in which a hospital, in particular, operates is changing so rapidly. Moreover, complaints seem to be increasing, and continually putting out fires is not effective managerial control.
- Health care organizations are coming under increasing scrutiny. Managers need measures of effectiveness to have better control over institutional destiny.
- Resources with which to operate health care organizations are becoming increasingly scarce. In years past organizations could raise rates or increase volume almost at will to obtain additional resources. Today more mileage must be obtained from very limited resources.
- Management has less authority today. Employees, public agencies, and consumers often must be convinced to act in certain ways, and administrators and trustees must back up their requests with proof.
- Managerial knowledge and skills have advanced to a point where specialists are needed to cope with and apply them.

In other words, administrators, governing board members, and others involved in the management of health care organizations need both useful information and the skills of experts who are qualified to generate and help analyze it.

Table 13-1 summarizes the specialties of a number of functional managers, listing some of their tools and the university disciplines that supply their training. It is important to stress that these are only examples; there are many other titles, combinations of functions, and disciplines of training that may be found in larger health care organizations. Clearly there is a need for better definition of tools and their uses, in addition to more teamwork among functional managers.

Table 13-1 Examples of management specialties, tools, and training

Functional specialty	Tools	University discipline as a site of training
Financial management or controller, accountant, business office, etc.	Accounting reports, budgets, responsibility accounting, cost volume analysis, cost accounting, operations research (OR), tools, credit extension, management of cash, inventory and capital structure, etc.	Business (accounting and/or finance)
Systems engineering or industrial engineering, methods improvement, systems design, etc.	Design, implementation, control and evaluation techniques, time and motion, facility layouts, OR techniques, etc.	Industrial engineering (IE), production management
Data processing or computer services, information systems, etc.	Computers, OR techniques, etc.	Accounting, IE, computer sciences, economics, statistics, etc.
Planning or institutional research, R & D, etc.	Statistical analysis, computers, group process techniques, OR tools, marketing, etc.	Marketing or generalist background in health administration or planning
Personnel management	Job design, position descriptions and controls, training, etc.	Business (personnel management)
Public relations	Surveys, communications devices	Generalist or journalism, etc.
Materials management or purchasing agent, etc.	Inventory control techniques	Business, pharmacy, nursing, IE, etc.
Risk management	Statistical analyses, legal analyses, claims examination, site examination	Business (risk management), law

FUNCTIONAL MANAGERS

In this section the functions of financial management, systems engineering, computer applications, marketing, planning, human resources management, materiels management, risk management, public relations, and volunteer services will be considered.

Financial Management

One of the most dramatic changes in health care management, especially hospital management, in the past 15 years has been the development of financial management and the chief financial officer (CFO). Specialists in accounting functions have been in health care organizations for many years. However, theirs has been (and in some institutions still is) mainly bookkeeping and a financial accounting and collection function. The emphasis was on internal reporting of routine planning and control decisions, external reports to capital providers (such as banks, government agencies, and physicians) and reporting to third parties providing operating resources in some form of reimbursement. Beginning with the Medicare/Medicaid (Title XVIII and Title XIX of the Social Security Act) legislation of 1966, financial management has been increasingly concerned with cost accounting and total financial requirements.[1] This more comprehensive approach is emphasized in the American Hospital Association's statement in 1979, indicating the need for the accountability of the total financial requirements of health care providers:

> Financial requirements, as differentiated from accounting costs, are defined as those resources that are not only necessary to meet current operating needs, but also sufficient to permit replacement of the physical plan when appropriate and to allow for changing community health and patient needs, education and research needs, and all other needs necessary to the institutional provision of health care services that must be recognized and supported by all purchases of care.

What does it take to determine the total financial requirements of a health care organization? Newmann, Suver, and Zelman[1] suggest the following (p. 9):

1. Costs of doing business, such as salaries, supplies, utilities, bad debts, and taxes
2. Costs of staying in business, such as maintenance of working capital and maintenance of assets
3. Costs of changing business, to meet competitors and take advantage of new opportunities, such as additional assets and working capital
4. Costs of attracting and/or holding capital, or returns to capital sources, such as interest on debt, payment of debt, required returns to equity holders, and maintenance of the equity base

Generally, financial management personnel are increasingly involved in the strategic management process by providing information for planning purposes, often in the form of "what-if" questions, the implementation of plans via budget preparation, and acquisition of funds and control through internal monitoring of financial activity and providing the necessary reports.

Suver and Neumann[2] suggest a management control model for financial managers related to the establishment of objectives and subsequent program development via budget preparation and collecting and organizing accounting information relative to the operating activity of the health care organization. Two primary concerns of operating activity review are the evaluations of effectiveness and efficiency. These activities indicate the active and significant participation of financial officers in formulating, implementing, and controlling strategies in health care organizations.

Recently the fear of financial failure appears to be growing among top hospital executives. In a 1988 survey by Touche Ross & Co., Boston, 46% of hospital executives surveyed feared institutional failure, compared with 43% in 1986. "The new survey, a repeat of a 1986 study, reveals an apparent paradox: while fear of failure has grown, executives are falling back on traditional tactics—that is, cutting capital expenditures—while implementing newer strategies less often than they had planned"[3](p. 20). On the other hand, there was an optimistic note in terms of an expected increase in overall revenues beyond the inflation rate during the next 5 years. The problem is whether revenues will increase sufficiently to cover increased costs.

These concerns among top executives can lead to increasing responsibilities for CEOs. Health care organizations have, as we have pointed out a number of times, become more competitive. Kiser[4] suggests that "the health care business has evolved from a cost reimbursement environment where price had little impact to a highly competitive, risk-based industry. At the same time, the role and responsibility of the financial manager has also changed" (p. 72). She goes on to point out that the CFO must now understand the *total* business, including the clinical departments. Ross[5] suggests that "leadership in health care today must be a team effort; relationships must be built. CFOs must push key financial issues to the forefront, and to do this effectively, issues must be researched, strategies identified, recommendations made and defended, and new relationships developed" (p. 74).

Silver[6] concludes that there will be a "super CFO" by the year 2000, who will be surrounded by a group of specialists, including government relations analysts—financial control experts assisted by physicians and nurses trained in budgetary control. These specialists, according to Silver, will be organized in sections, such as for cost accounting, budgeting, cash investments, strategic financial planning, physicians contracts, and economic projections. Although some CFOs will move into CEO positions (as is frequently the case in other industries), others expect that CEOs will continue to come from more generalist training settings, such as Health Service Administration (HSA) programs.[7]

Although there have been dramatic improvements in hospital fiscal management, problems remain. For example:

- Participative accounting practices, such as responsibility accounting, still are not widely utilized.
- There is considerable evidence of communication difficulties between hospital financial managers and heads of professional departments because of language barriers caused by technical terminology and mistaken perception of motives. For example, many professionals believe financial managers are not interested in patient care—only in money. And financial managers believe professionals have no interest in costs.

- Incentives for financial management are lacking because of the ease of obtaining higher income until recently by raising rates and increasing volume of service. There have been more incentives for income maximization and larger facilities than for cost containment.
- The personal characteristics of some financial managers—their attitudes and behavior—limit their effectiveness.
- Financial managers need to be particularly skillful in communicating with nurses, physicians, and other health professionals who lack the knowledge of and motives for financial control (unlike managers in industry with whom financial managers work).
- Many financial managers have been hired from commercial enterprises and are unfamiliar with such matters as hospital objectives, dealing with professionals, and patient care programs.

Hospital Systems Engineering

Hospital systems engineering, or management engineering, has its basis primarily in the discipline of industrial engineering. This discipline had its origins with Frederick W. Taylor and Frank Gilbreth around the turn of the century and used tools of time-and-motion studies and related work-measurement approaches.

This traditional "efficiency expert" approach is not evident today in most hospital programs. The role of the hospital systems engineer now focuses on larger systems of labor productivity, resource utilization, and operational planning and improvement rather than the time-and-motion study emphasis of earlier industrial engineers.

The following list includes several specific functions for management engineers in hospitals:

Hospital-wide productivity reporting systems
Standard setting in hospital departments
Work simplification and systems improvements in departments
Functional space utilization and layout
Staff scheduling
Capital budget decisions
Purchase versus lease decisions
Quality definition and evaluation
Internal consultants
Cost accounting systems
Position control systems
Information systems and computer evaluation and development
Long-range planning
Contract versus in-house service decisions
Management education
Inventory control
Consultants to other health institutions

The American Institute of Industrial Engineering (AIIE) has adopted the following definition, which indicates a broadened role for industrial engineering[8] (p. 4):

Industrial engineering is concerned with the design, improvement and installation of integrated systems of people, materials and equipment. It draws upon specialized knowledge and skill in mathematical, physical and social sciences together with the principles and methods of engineering analysis and design to specify, predict and evaluate the results to be obtained from such systems.

This definition has been adopted also by the Hospital Management Systems Society.

A unique aspect of systems engineering is its emphasis on improvements; in contrast, administrators, physicians, and others are sometimes more concerned with maintenance. It is apparent that improvements, like maintenance, require teamwork. Good relationships between the engineer and administrators, physicians, nurses, and other professionals are crucial to success.

Gustafson et al.[9] suggest that systems engineers can have an important role in accomplishing the following in hospitals:

- Facilitating and obtaining agreement on goals, and plans to achieve goals
- Organizing and coordinating services to reduce costs and improve accessibility of care
- Setting up more effective ways of evaluating and improving the quality of care provided
- Improving personnel utilization
- Improving work methods

They suggest that, to accomplish these, the engineer would work in a multidisciplinary team as a specialist in technical facilitation, designing and changing strategies during the design, implementation, and evaluation phases of a hospital project. The engineer should be able to set up, obtain, and analyze measurements for achieving the above with help from others in the hospital team and build conceptual design and mathematical models for decision making with assistance from content experts, such as administrators and physicians. Some variation in training is needed, depending on which of the problems the engineer is going to handle.

As was true of other functional specialists, Gustafson et al.[9] found that in only a few instances were systems engineers fulfilling the theoretical roles described here, or having a major impact on hospital problems. This is interesting when the AHA[10] reports that 55% of 6079 hospitals responding to their survey report that they employ industrial engineers on a full-time, shared, or consulting basis.

In personal experience we have found that until the late 1970s management mainly gave lip service to systems engineering, apparently believing that as long as they had appointed someone to improve productivity and control costs, they were meeting responsibilities to their community for this function. Today, however, with more concerns for cost containment, management places more importance on systems engineering, and demand for such managers is increasing. Gustafson et al.[9] found problems in the effectiveness of some engineers, with social and political failures more prevalent than inadequacy of engineering technical skills. Conflict among the overlapping functional specialties of financial management, data processing, engineering, and others was not uncommon. An appropriate team approach among these closely related functions was lacking in a number of cases, to the detriment of the potential of each. Chapter 17 presents some suggestions for ways to reduce such conflict.

Although many hospital engineering programs seemed to have little impact, in others significant results were found. In one large hospital that one of the authors surveyed, the administrator documented real savings of more than $1 million annually, primarily as a result of the efforts of a systems engineering program. Five major characteristics of this program that were lacking in those not as effective were the following:

Top management was committed to cost reduction, was knowledgeable about industrial engineering practices, and was very supportive of engineers.

Engineers were knowledgeable about hospital objectives, operations, and problems.

Engineers were not only competent in their field, but also had personal stature and élan. They communicated well with professionals and would be found at coffee or lunch with nurses, physicians, and others, rather than clustering as a group by themselves, as was evident in other hospitals.

The hospital appeared to fit into a type D model (see Chapter 6). It was not hierarchically organized; that is, communication was generally across the organization between individuals rather than vertical, as in traditional lines of authority. Physicians, nurses, and others would contact or be contacted directly by the engineers rather than go through formal lines of authority. There were good relations and respect among various functional specialists, all of whom appeared to be very strong.

Engineers were technical facilitators in designing, implementing, and evaluating, rather than traditional work measurement engineers.

In addition to productivity/savings issues, health systems engineers have directed their attention to quality improvement programs. Their contributions include the following:

- Decision models that can measure quality
- Information systems that allow quality changes to be tracked
- Human factors approaches that allow engineers to suggest methods for the reduction of stress so that employees can perform their jobs better
- Statistical approaches (experimental design and analysis) that allow health systems engineers to track experiments aimed at improving quality

We suggest that many of these findings, models, and complementing approaches by health systems engineers regarding important ingredients for success might apply equally to other functional areas of specialization.

COMPUTER SYSTEMS—MEDICAL AND MANAGEMENT INFORMATION SYSTEMS—DECISION SUPPORT SYSTEMS

In the late 1960s and 1970s computerization and automation were hailed as the solution to the rising costs of a labor-intensive industry and to the problems of coordinating increasingly complex health care services. Many hospitals were eager to install computer systems. A few hospitals as small as 100 beds have rather elaborate computers. Trustees, administrators, and physicians have been proud of their computers, seeing them as an indication of their hospital's sophistication and progress.

Management information systems is a commonly used term to describe the total data gathering and analysis system of the hospital. Gillette et al.[11] suggest that there are eight information subsystems in a hospital:

1. *Patient diagnosis and treatment system,* which would include information derived from such hospital departments as clinical laboratories, pathology, electrocardiology, diagnostic radiology, pharmacy, rehabilitation services, and nursing services
2. *Patient record system,* which would involve departments such as medical records, admissions, and insurance, in addition to the above departments
3. *Patient scheduling and order system,* which would include all patient care departments and support services, such as dietary and housekeeping
4. *Patient accounting system,* which involves most of the above plus, for example, accounting, and credit and collection offices
5. *Expenditure and general accounting system,* which includes budgeting, payroll, materials, and plant systems, in addition to patient service departments
6. *Personnel system* of employee and position information
7. *General supportive services system,* which includes such departments as industrial engineering, data processing, and plant management
8. *Management control system,* which runs through all systems for effective and efficient management

Most computer applications in health care organizations are in routine accounting functions, such as payroll and patient billing. The clinical laboratory and hospital pharmacy have also been areas of computer application in a number of hospitals. Automated history taking, diagnosis, and patient records have been subjects of considerable research, as have menu planning, employee staffing, patient scheduling, and so forth. A number of companies, for example, aerospace companies and computer manufacturers, are currently marketing total hospital information systems.

Computer applications have increased substantially during the 1980s. Moreover, medical information systems are being developed rapidly and are being linked with management information systems. For example, a total hospital information system (HIS), a real-time computer-based system that nurses, physicians, and other health care professionals and management interact with in the delivery of care to patients, was developed at El Camino Hospital in Mountain View, California. It automates substantially all clinical and administrative information handling and interfaces with the nurse, physician, laboratory, radiology, other medical services with administrative functions, such as admissions, business office, and medical records. Evaluation of this system documented improved quality of care and increased productivity of the nursing staff. With continued advances in information gathering, storage, analysis, and retrieval, it is likely that HIS and similar programs will have a major impact on hospital operations in the decade ahead.

With the development of information systems, there has been increasing concern about collecting and aggregating data for its own sake. More recently it has been recognized that information is only a means to an end. That is, decision requirements should be established first, then information support systems designed to meet decision requirements. Consequently, decision support systems (DSS) are a current field of study. Such systems will be of increasing importance for the health care manager in the future.

Organizationally, computer information systems may be found in the fiscal management area (especially if computer applications are primarily in accounting systems) or they may be in a separate unit, in systems engineering, or in another location. The head of the unit may have received his training in any one of a number of disciplines or received on-the-job training from a computer manufacturer or a software consulting service.

With increasing numbers of interorganizational and interdepartmental arrangements, health care organizations need to think more and more about electronic data exchange. Electronic data exchange involves computer-to-computer exchange of documents in standard formats. Savings include direct monetary savings, increased accuracy, and speed. In many cases there may be better documentation, especially in data or document exchange systems.

In site visits to a number of institutions, we found the same sort of problems with computer services as we did with other functional specialties, for example, poor communications, jurisdictional disputes, and inability to evaluate current operations or potential for computers among top administrators. In the institutions we visited, computer services did appear to be a more aggressive operation than some other staff services and also appeared to have more organizational support.

MARKETING

Although we devote an entire chapter to the marketing function, it is appropriate to summarize key elements involved here so that this specialization can be viewed in juxtaposition with the other functional managers making up the managerial team. Marketing has received tremendous impetus during the last decade, but this emphasis has also resulted in considerable confusion. Smith and Reid[12] describe it as follows (p. 185):

> If the sum total of all available written material on hospital marketing were placed before a chief executive officer and if that executive were required to read it, the result would be a very confused executive. For years hospitals carefully maintained a low profile in advertising–much less marketing. In the early 1980s, there was a virtual explosion of ideas. When one read the professional journals in the hospital field, the conclusion to be drawn is that hospitals could not exist without well-conceived marketing plans. How did hospitals ever survive without marketing? A better question is whether hosptials can survive with marketing.

Why has this situation developed? We cannot present a completely definitive explanation, but we can make some suggestions. Consider the following:

- Marketing concepts have their foundation in for-profit organizations. In some situations these philosophies and processes were not necessarily adapted to health care organizations. For example, Certo and Peter [13] make this comment when discussing the nature of marketing relative to for-profit organizations (p. 278):

> Although there is no clear distinction between some aspects of strategic management and strategic marketing, the major focus of strategic marketing is on knowing, adapting to, and influencing consumers in an effort to achieve organizational objectives. Marketing strategies are usually designed to increase sales and market share in order to increase long-run profits.

- Health care organizations have broader objectives than increase in sales in market share relevant to profits.
- There has been in many organizations an over-emphasis on promotion of health care as opposed to determining needs of consumers. There are probably several reasons for this. Promotion no doubt brings immediate short-run advantages but may result in misconceptions by the public as to the nature of the health care organization. Also, many health care chief executives looked only at the tip of marketing because they utilized their own life experiences with advertising without study of the true nature of marketing. After all, their formal educational experiences probably did not include a marketing course.
- Deregulation of the health care industry removed many governmental constraints so that CEOs were able to make changes that often were experimental in nature without any firm base of data development and analysis.
- The advent of DRGs provided a base for segmentation of services and in turn focused on those that were cost effective.
- Increased competition no doubt made many executives more fearful of failure as opposed to the earlier cost-plus periods, and marketing appeared to provide an approach to avoiding failure but often ignored the service aspects of marketing.
- Marketing departments were established, and too often these were staffed by people who did not understand health care organizations but still were expected to be successful.

Given these and other developments, one might ask how such misunderstandings can be prevented or at least mitigated. We suggest some ideas.

First, as Folland, Ziegenfuss, and Chao[14] point out (p. 29):

> A comprehensive accounting of the marketing implications of DRGs requires a broad concept of marketing. As often noted, hospital marketing in practice is too narrowly construed and becomes synonymous with promotion.

They suggest a broader concept of marketing such as proposed by Kotler and Levy[15] (p. 15):

> The concept of *sensitively serving and satisfying human needs* . . . Perhaps the short-run problem of business firms is to sell people on buying the existing products, but the long-run problem is clearly to create products that people need. By this recognition that effective marketing requires a consumer orientation instead of a product orientation, marketing has taken a new lease on life and tied its economic activity to a higher social purpose.

In other words, chief executives must stress community health needs and purpose, as well as organizational purpose, in developing and approving marketing strategies.

Second, top executives need to recognize and take advantage of the marketing specialists' expertise in the analysis of the environment and the health needs of all community members. Recall that this is one of the tenants of strategic management relative to strategy formulation. All marketing specialists should have this ability and should be encouraged to use their skills. This approach assumes the determination and satisfaction of human health needs as a goal of market research.

Third, the CEO and his or her staff need to understand the general nature of the marketing process and the fundamental concepts and tools. Among these are the following:

- *Marketing segmentation* The idea behind market segmentation is to divide the total market into targets or segments and then serve only those segments the organization can best service. The idea is that not all patients have the same needs. Carried to its ultimate conclusions in for-profits terms, this approach would call for serving only those segments where the resulting provision of service would result in a cost-effective or profitable position. Of course, the key question is what happens to the nonserved, such as the poor and/or disabled. Obviously they must be served, and if the present system does not make such provisions, alternatives must be developed.

- *Differentiation of products and services* This is often referred to as marketing mix. The health care organization seeks to distinguish its products from competitive organizations. Some of the practices include executive suites, family birthing rooms, and highly specialized services. However, the differentiation should be on service and quality rather than superficial activities.

- *Product pricing* The services of the hospital may be set to increase market share (usually by lowering price) to attract certain patients (a two-tier pricing approach) or to increase quality (often a higher price based on superior delivery practices). How will pricing affect the needs of patients? This should be the guiding principle in pricing.

- *Promotion* This generally includes advertising and the lay person usually associates advertising with mass media utilization. However, promotion may also involve physicians, nurses, and all other people who have contact with patients. These clinicians have greater impact on patients than does mass media.

- *Organizational structure for the marketing function* This involves ascertaining the training and experience of marketing personnel, including the chief marketing officer (CMO) and his or her relationship to the CEO and his or her staff. It may well be that some form of matrix organization will evolve that includes organizational relationships on a professional basis with physicians, nurses, and other clinical personnel.

- *Policies* These need to be established to guide the marketing function and its relationships, both externally and internally. Policies might include subjects such as morality and public service, quality issues, community service, behavior of personnel, relations with patients, including grievances, and promotion/advertising (what is in good taste).

In conclusion we include a summary statement from the report of the Amherst Study of Hospital Marketing Practices [16] (p. 87):

> The study findings identify two major areas of concern related to marketing and the direction the field is taking. First, health care marketing—though much discussed and expensive—is still in a stage of immaturity. As practiced in hospitals today, marketing is frequently synonymous with advertising. Second, marketing in health care will not ultimately be a "clone" of marketing practices in industry and retailing. Though hospitals are looking to those areas for knowledge and expertise, the unique character of the product will cause health care marketing to evolve into a practice uniquely different from that in other industries.

PLANNING

Health care planning is generally considered to be one of the most important functions of management. The dynamics of health care, the need to improve the delivery of health services, and the increasing pressures on organizations all argue for long-range planning. Some may say that things are changing so fast that it is fruitless to plan, yet rapid change and the organization's increasing difficulty in controlling their own destiny are precisely why planning is so important. Long-range plans are a blueprint for health care decisions and are preferable to making decisons in a vacuum or not making them at all, which usually results in the worst kinds of outcomes. Plans provide an opportunity for the health care organization to be proactive and a leader, rather than reactive, and if they are developed and understood by the health care community, they can help unify diverse interests and goals.

There are a number of important criteria for effective long-range planning:

- Plans should be based on a thorough study of the needs the organization is established to serve. This is not an easy task. It requires study of community needs and advice from consumer representatives and scholars of community needs.
- Broad participation is important to effective planning and implementation of plans. In addition to consumers (whose participation can be accomplished through group process techniques, such as nominal groups, the medical staff and other members of the hospital family should be included.
- Plans should be comprehensive and developed in a continuum from the following:
  Definition of community needs
  Definition of objectives
  Programs to achieve objectives
  Organizational arrangement for fulfilling programs
  Staffing required
  Facilities needed
  Financial requirements (this is likely to result in revisions of objectives pro-grams, staffing, etc.)
  Relationships with others
- Plans should be flexible, action-oriented, and continually updated consistent with other changes.

- Plans should strive for higher levels of achievement.
- Plans should be realistic within constraints of resources.
- Plans should be time-phased from long-range back to the forthcoming year.
- Plans should be a basis for hospital operation, for example, decisions, budget systems, and evaluations

Despite the federal requirement for planning, but possibly because of its magnitude, few hospitals have plans that meet the above criteria. Many organizations have long-range program and facility plans, but these are only means to ends. Some organizations plan facilities and then must attempt to fit programs into facilities rather than designing facilities to meet the programs.

Many hospitals have planning committees as a part of their governing board, and occasionally they include operating personnel as well. Staff services so essential to the planning process are usually left to the administrator or someone else who is committed to many other tasks. Consultants frequently provide planning services but usually on a one-shot basis, so plans become outdated rapidly.

Institutional research and development (R&D) aimed at improving organization services is another function usually neglected by all but the largest hospitals. Anyone with the title of head of hospital development is usually a fund raiser. Research and development are important functions of the more progressive industrial corporations, but it is more difficult for organizations than for industries to demonstrate tangible returns on R&D investments. Most organizations depend on universities for research in the delivery of health services, but they could do a great deal of R&D either in association with universities or on their own.

Funding for R&D can be obtained from both federal and private sources. Local industries may be willing to support a hospital research and demonstration project even when they would not support other hospital activities.

HUMAN RESOURCES MANAGEMENT

Human resources management is an increasingly important specialized function in the modern hospital. The principal objective of human resources management is to enable administrators and department heads to integrate organizational and employee needs. In a labor-intensive organization, such as a hospital, this indeed is a significant function.

Of the many activities performed by the human resources department, the procurement of employees is the most basic. The responsibilities range from the recruiting and initial screening of employees to the actual hiring of some employees. The basic human resources management philosophy is for the department to perform actual recruiting and initial screening but for the managers to make the final decision to hire. In practice, it appears that the human resources department often does the hiring because department heads have confidence in the ability of the human resources staff and accept their recommendations regarding potential employees.

In the procurement activity, the members of the human resources department should be proficient in developing labor market information, carrying out recruitment campaigns, developing job descriptions, evaluating and validating selection instruments, such as tests, administering selection tools, such as application blanks, maintaining files of accepted, as well as rejected, applicants, and aiding in the orientation of new employees to the health care organization.

A second activity or function performed by the human resources department is assisting managers in the evaluation of employee performance. This may involve developing evaluation instruments, training management personnel to evaluate employees, and discussing results with them, as well as auditing promotions, transfers, salary increases, dismissals, and resignations.

Wage and salary administration is a third function assigned to human resource specialists. The purpose is to develop and maintain equity in wage and salary payments, as well as to evaluate the overall labor budget.

Because of the increasing importance attached to training and development, human resource specialists have been appointed as training directors. The general objective is to enable department heads and administrators to meet their employee development responsibilities by using training techniques and general educational programs. In larger organizations, the training function may be established as a separate unit or department.

As health care employees become unionized, specialists in labor relations to aid in contract negotiation and administration are hired and are often affiliated with the human resources department.

With the passage of the federal Occupational Safety and Health Act and the development of standards for hospitals, the safety function is frequently made a part of the human resources department's responsibility.

Personnel records may or may not be the responsibility of the human resources department, but auditing the personnel function and assisting in developing effective personnel policies should be. The auditing function includes examining such indicators as turnover records and grievances. Policy recommendations are concerned with equity concepts and changing employee needs and expectations, as well as organizational needs. Thus the personnel specialist usually has direct access to the chief executive officer, even if he or she does not report directly to the CEO.

MATERIALS MANAGEMENT

It has been suggested that "up to 46% of the hospital expense budget centers around materials management"[12] (p. 4). Other situations suggest about 30% of total costs relate to materials, depending on how capital costs are allocated. Regardless of the percent of total expenditure, the amount of money involved is significant and a small deviation in percent of total expenditures can result in sizeable dollar savings.

One of the interesting changes in health care management during the last two decades has been the increasing importance of materials management. This function is concerned with the following:

- Negotiation and purchasing material
- Receiving and expediting
- Supply and inventory control
- Processing
- Distribution

■ Product/materials standardization

If indeed health care organizations do compete in quality, price, and availability of services, increased emphasis can be expected to be directed to materials management in terms of how the organization can achieve a more competitive position using the activities of materials management.

Recognizing the major effect that procurement and materials management has on costs, the management role for this function has broadened and increased substantially in many hospitals, particularly in larger institutions. In the recent past, a purchasing director's responsibilities were usually limited to supply procurement and inventory control in most hospitals, but a new materials manager role has evolved in the past few years. Biomedical engineering to maintain equipment and perform other procurement functions, such as professional service contracts, might also be included in a broadened definition of procurement and management.

The following are ways to contain procurement and materials costs through management practices:

■ Standardization of supplies and equipment
■ Value analysis studies
■ Inventory control
■ Group purchasing
■ Educational programs for more efficient materials management by professionals
■ Consignment arrangements
■ More efficient distribution systems
■ Extending equipment life and efficiency

Although quantitative techniques are important tools, the real key to being an effective manager is relating well to health professionals and other key managers to bring about standardization, control techniques, and other practices.

RISK MANAGEMENT

Risk management is a relatively new health care management functional specialty. It grew out of the dramatic changes in medical malpractice during the 1970s. Its initial purpose was liability control by (1) reducing incidents of patient injury, (2) identifying potentially injurious events, (3) increasing patient satisfaction, (4) documenting procedures that deviate from the norm, and (5) standardizing procedures for disaster calls. At the time of Bryant and Korsak's survey,[18] most risk managers had been hospital employees with training in hospital administration, insurance, or safety engineering. The field has expanded dramatically in a very short period—yet another example of the dramatic changes in the management of health care organizations during recent years. The American Hospital Association formed a national group dedicated to hospital risk management in 1980—the American Society for Hospital Risk Management (ASHRM). This association has well over 1000 members.

The three major aspects of risk management are identification, measurement, and resolution or treatment. Subject components include insurance (product, property, malpractice), safety (workers' compensation, patient/employee complaints, counseling), and risk audits. Kraus[19] defines risk management as "a series of tasks and functions the purpose of which is to reduce unplanned or unexpected financial loss to an organization." (p. 1).

Risk identification involves determining where exposure areas exist (such as technology; medical, nursing, and other professional malpractice; drugs; and employee practices.) Such a list of potential exposure areas can be lengthy indeed. However, the extent of the risk associated with each must be evaluated. This involves the measurement of potential losses. Kraus[19] states that the "risk management process requires the risk manager to measure, analyze, and evaluate data in order to make an intelligent and appropriate decision regarding how to deal with the risks and potential financial losses to which the organization is exposed" (p. 7). The intention is to determine the probable severity and possible dollar loss. This is the resolution or treatment aspect.

The resolution or treatment process can be thought of in two broad categories. One category is the financing process and involves the purchase of insurance. In other situations, the health care organization may decide that the risk is low enough and funds would be available from operations to cover the loss. In still other situations, the health care organization may use self-financing but would include the establishment of a fund to cover prospective losses.

Ideally, risk managers would like to be able to control the internal environment sufficiently so that risk is avoided. This is impossible, in some situations at least, because people do make mistakes, some of which can be very costly. Training programs often can reduce the risk by calling attention to the possible problems and developing the attitudes and skills necessary to reduce unsafe acts.

In 1983 ASHRM conducted a survey of risk managers. The results were published in the 1983 survey of Hospital Risk Management Responsibilities and Salaries. One of the results of that survey was an examination of the tasks performed by the managers together with time allocated to the tasks or program components. This information is shown in Table 13-2. The program components that 50% or more of the respondents identified as performing were the following:

- Risk identification/evaluation
- Loss prevention
- Safety administration
- Handling patient complaints
- Property/casualty claims
- Product liability claims

No doubt there will be considerable variance among different types of health care organizations, but the table does identify major components of the risk manager's task responsibilities.

Another function that may or may not be directly associated with risk management is quality assurance; that is, the two functions of risk management and quality assurance may or may not be in the same department. Emphasis on quality assurance has been given through the Joint Commission on Accreditation of Healthcare Organizations (JCAHO) self-assessment activities. The JCAHO requires quality assurance programs

Table 13-2 Comprehensive risk management program responsibilities: percentage of respondents with responsibility for handling individual components of a comprehensive risk management program

Program component	Percentage of respondents with responsibility (number)		Percentage of individuals whose authority is:			Average percentage of respondent's time spent
			Complete	Shared	Consulting	
Risk identification/evaluation	94.3	(2864)	39.5	55.9	4.6	12.6
Loss prevention	87.8	(2665)	33.2	61.0	5.8	7.9
Safety administration	73.7	(2239)	34.4	53.5	12.1	6.1
Handling patient complaints	65.9	(2001)	24.3	66.1	9.6	4.3
Property/casualty claims	65.5	(1989)	40.6	52.2	7.2	4.8
Product liability claims	52.9	(1607)	38.1	51.3	10.6	1.8
Security	51.2	(1554)	39.8	43.5	16.7	3.2
Workers' compensation claims	45.2	(1373)	40.7	45.0	14.3	2.7
Conducting patient satisfaction surveys	40.6	(1234)	27.3	58.2	14.5	1.6
Other employee benefits: design/administration	31.2	(949)	29.5	54.4	16.1	1.3
Premium forecasting/budgeting	30.2	(916)	35.8	49.2	15.0	.9
Group insurance plan: design/administration	29.2	(888)	31.0	53.0	16.0	1.3
Group insurance benefit claims	28.6	(868)	39.5	46.7	13.8	.1
Insurance accounting	27.0	(821)	33.4	52.1	14.5	1.0
Management of department personnel (2+)	25.6	(778)	66.6	28.4	5.0	3.4
Pension/retirement income payments	21.8	(663)	39.5	45.0	15.5	.6
Family counseling	20.3	(616)	22.9	55.3	21.8	.9

From Summary Report, Survey of Hospital Risk Management Responsibilities and Salaries—1983. Published by the American Hospital Association, 1984. Reprinted by permission.

for hospitals, as does the federal government through Medicare. Richards and Rathbun[20] identify the following "essential components of a sound quality assurance program-in-the-aggregate" (p. 53):

- Identification of important or potential problems or related concerns in the care of patients
- Objective assessment of the cause and scope of problems or concerns, including the determination of priorities for both investigating and resolving problems; ordinarily, priorities shall be related to the degree of impact on patient care that can be expected if the problem remains unresolved
- Implementation by appropriate individuals or through designated mechanisms, of decisions or actions that are designed to eliminate, insofar as possible, identified problems
- Monitoring activities designed to assure that the desired result has been achieved and sustained
- Documentation that reasonably substantiates the effectiveness of the overall program to enhance patient care and to assure sound clinical performance

Whether to coordinate risk management and quality assurance in the same department or unit is not the basic question. The CEOs basic concern is to make the necessary arrangements so that both functions are performed. As Brown[21] concludes (p. 7):

> But risk management is only a term for a very serious subject. It sounds like a business term, drawn from the realm of pure financial management with minimal human involvement. Placed in a hospital setting, the reverse is true. Here, risk management is dominated by the human element.

Related to the overall risk mangement emphasis is the relationship to the legal profession. Often lawyers are employed (1) on an ad hoc approach as needed, (2) contracted for via a contingency arrangement, or (3) in larger organizations employed in a legal department that is directly associated with the risk management department. As legal contingencies increase, there will be increasing demand for the services of lawyers for interpretation, advice, and representation.

PUBLIC RELATIONS AND VOLUNTEER SERVICES

The public relations function was usually conceived of as a publicity or fundraising function in hospitals. We suggest that its functions could be considerably broader, particularly in this era of consumer activism. Market analysis, use of ombudsmen, and evaluation of patient and community needs and satisfactions are functions that are often neglected by health care organizations even though they are critical to the two-way communications so important to effective relations. Most health care organization public relations programs, recognizing the importance of employee relationships with the public and patients, consider this an important part of their responsibility.

Volunteer service (relationships with the auxiliary) is a common staff service in health care organizations. It is usually a separate department run by a paid employee who has good rapport with the volunteers. Hospital volunteers provide important services in the hospital, such as transporting patients and providing recreational and social services. They can be effective spokespersons for both the hospital and a large segment of the public and aid in raising funds.

CONSULTANTS

The need for staff expertise varies: consequently, health care organizations have increasingly turned to consultants. In many health care organizations, functional activities are performed in whole or in part by consulting agencies. There are a number of different types of consultants. For example, there are diversified and large general management consultant firms that have different specialists and serve a variety of industries, including health services. Their professional organization is the Association of Consulting Management Engineers (ACME), and a listing of such firms can be obtained from ACME. There are the large accounting firms that are providing consultation services well beyond fiscal management. There are firms and individuals that specialize only in hospitals, and their professional organization is the American Association of Hospital Consultants (AAHC). Architects are consultants, and there are consultants that specialize, for example, in systems engineering, finance, and laundries. Consulting psychologists are used for conflict resolution, screening candidates for top management postitions, and other services. University professors will frequently serve as consultants to health institutions, providing scholarly expertise or possibly group process assistance to help the institution use its expertise more effectively. Well-known practitioners, for example, CEOs, directors of nursing, and medical record librarians, will also serve as consultants to other organizations. All have certain advantages and disadvantages.

Consultants can be helpful to health care organizations by providing the following:

Time that personnel may not have to work quickly and without interruption, for example, to solve a problem or plan

Knowledge and experience from other settings

Objectivity and understanding to approach a problem from an independent perspective

Analytical skills from experience

Perspective to see facets that an organization may not see

They are useful when an institution needs one or more of the following:

One-time assistance

Help with internal communications

Outside appraisal

Reasons (for example, tension) for change to take the onus off people within the organization

Help with conflict resolution

Long-range plans

Expert advice or time

In selecting consultants it is important to carefully define the problem and scope of work required. It is also important to interview several firms when a large assignment is involved, to check on work they have done and to determine who will actually do the work. To ensure that results will be accepted, it is essential that all who will be concerned with recommendations approve of the consultant selected.

A number of factors can be helpful in using consultants most effectively. For example, for a major consulting assignment, it is important that the consultants develop a work plan and schedule, and specify expectations for the assignment at various stages of the project. All concerned with the project should agree on expectations in advance to avoid misunderstanding of the expected results in relation to costs of the project. Financial arrangements on a time and expense basis with a definite ceiling hold a consultant accountable for the time invested in the assignment, as well as for results.

The consultant and client should work as a team during the project, for example agreeing on objectives, alternative solutions, criteria for evaluating alternatives, and recommendations. When possible, implementation of recommendations should be initiated while consultants are still working. A plan of action with identified responsibilities and a mechanism for continual updating should also be developed. Evaluation is essential and should be based on expectations agreed on at the outset.

Because of the increasing complexities, challenges, and opportunities facing health services, the use of consultants should continue to increase. It is surprising, however, that when harder times fall on organizations, they frequently drop the use of consultants first, much as corporations with falling sales may cut their advertising budgets first in order to cut costs. We have found that it is usually the stronger and leading organizations that use consultants; for example, most of the 500 largest corporations in the United States use consultants, whereas many smaller companies who need them most will not seek outside help. Using consultants can be a good investment and should not be considered a sign of weakness.

MANAGEMENT CONTRACTS

Still another area of health care management that has changed dramatically over the past decade is the use of private firms or other larger hospitals to manage organizations. Such a practice might be considered an extension of consulting services, and it is consistent with trends of multihospital systems. Extrahospital management allows a local community to retain control of the community needs it wants to serve and, through contractual arrangements, to hold the firm or contracting hospital accountable for agreed-upon results.

FACTORS THAT MIGHT IMPROVE EFFECTIVENESS OF FUNCTIONAL SPECIALISTS

In previous sections we discussed problems associated with functional specialties and managers. Because of increased knowledge and the need for more effective management of costs and quality of service, there will be increasing emphasis on most of these specialties. We suggest a number of conditions that might improve the effectiveness of functional specialists:

Executive officers, trustees, medical staff, and heads of professional departments should be more knowledgeable about the contributions functional managers could offer for improved patient care and hospital efficiency.

Functional managers should be able to relate more effectively with providers of care and administrators.

Executives should be oriented toward more participative management. Line department heads, such as nurses and chiefs of professional services, should have responsibility and accountability for management of their departments and seek help and information directly from functional specialists.

Functional managers should have the capability and opportunity to move up on the administrative ladder. Without more general administrative and health care knowledge—a calling card of masters in health administration and communication skills—most functional specialists will be locked into their jobs. In industry, functional managers have the opportunity to move up to the chief executive position.

A type D administrative organization with a matrix rather than a hierarchical organization would foster communications between functional specialists and health providers and increase managerial responsibility among specialists.

Programs in health administration might consider giving students training as specialists, to qualify them for first-job opportunities as functional specialists, in addition to training for the chief executive role. Many business schools have moved away from generalist training (that is, training students to be presidents of corporations) and toward giving them first-job skills in such areas as marketing and production management. Ansoff[22] suggests that the differentiated specialist will be the manager of the future. Such an approach would seem to be particularly relevant for hospitals, because few hospitals can offer management training comparable to that provided by large corporations for MBA or baccalaureate graduates. This is not to suggest that functional specialists should not have "star" status in their own right. On the contrary, in the type D organization we suggest that the functional manager could have a status similar to that of the CEO. As we have noted, status is related to expertise in professional organizations. Indeed, a number of studies suggest that administrative line authority does not have much status among physician and nursing professionals.

Making changes through educational programs in health services administration is, however, a slow way of solving problems. Some more immediate ways are through continuing and in-service education programs, and changing administrative roles toward Type C and, more ideally, type D. External planning and regulatory pressures are making the role of the functional managers more influential. It is important to note that specialists have a major influence on quality improvements and control, as well as on costs.

We believe that more effective application of specialty skills is one of the best ways of improving the management of health care organizations. It deserves concern and effort from trustees, CEOs, and providers and from their training programs. Some of the more exciting opportunities for hospital administration are likely to be related to these management specialties. This is discussed further in later chapters on management of quality, costs, and conflict.

CONCLUSIONS

Since World War II, health care organizations have experienced a revolution in medical technology. In the 1980s a managerial technological revolution took place. Health care organizations are now seeking to apply advances in managerial techniques to the increasing challenges of hospital management. The employment of well-trained managerial functional specialists has helped to introduce some of these advanced techniques. However, the application of such knowledge to improve the effectiveness and efficiency of health services depends on the ability of the functional specialists to relate to health professionals, and vice versa, and of the functional specialists to relate to each other. The other great challenge is to ensure that the application of advanced managerial techniques is used to improve the health of the community and not only the health of the health care organizations.

As a conclusion to this chapter, we believe this quotation from Peter Drucker[23] puts this chapter in proper perspective relative to the mission of a health care organization (p. 76):

> Finally, the single most important thing to remember about any enterprise is that there are no results inside its walls. The result of a business is a satisfied customer. The result of a hospital is a healed patient. The result of a school is a student who has learned something and puts it to work 10 years later. Inside an enterprise, there are only cost centers. Results exist only on the outside.

REFERENCES

1. Neumann BR, Suver JD, and Zelman WN: Financial management: concepts and applications for health care providers, ed 2, Owings Mills, Md, 1988, National Health Publishing.
2. Suver JD and Neuman BR: Management accounting for healthcare organizations, ed 2, Oakbrook, Ill, Health Care Financial Mangement Association, Chicago, Ill, 1985, Pluribus Press, Inc, Divison of Teach em, Inc.
3. Traska MR: Fear of failure and what hospitals did about it, Hospitals, 62(13):20, 1988.
4. Kiser JJ: The role of the financial manager: how much has it changed? Hosp Finan Manage 42(8), Aug 1988.
5. Ross JD: Developing and maintaining new relationships, Hosp Finan Manage 42(8),Aug 1988.
6. Silver AP: 2000—The year of the "super CFO," Topics Health Care Finan 7(1):47, 1980.
7. Dolan RC: Key questions about careers in health care management, Topics Health Care Finan 7(1):57, 1980.
8. AHA: Management engineering for hospitals, American Hospital Association, 1970.
9. Gustafson D, Rowse G, and Howes N: Roles and training for future health systems engineering. In Education for health administration, vol 11, Ann Arbor, Mich, 1975, Health Administration Press.
10. AHA: Research capsule no. 15: hospital use of industrial engineers, Hospitals 49(3):186, 1975.
11. Gillette PJ, Rathbun PW, and Wolfe HB: Hospital information systems—part 2, Hospitals 44:45, 1970.
12. Smith HL and Reid RA: Competitive hospitals: management strategies, Rockville, Md, 1986, Aspen Publishers, Inc.
13. Certo SC and Peter JP: Strategic management: concepts and applications, New York, 1988, Random House, Inc.
14. Folland S, Ziegenfuss JT, Jr, and Chao P: Implications of prospective payment under DRGs for hospital marketing, Health Care Marketing 8(4):29, 1988.
15. Kotler P and Levy SJ: Broadening the concept of marketing, J Marketing 33:10, 1969.
16. Robbins SA, Kane CM, and Sullivan DJ: J Health care marketing: minicase, J Health Care Marketing 8(1):86, 1988.

17. Housley CE: Hospital material management, Rockville, Md, 1978, Aspen Publishers, Inc.
18. Bryant Y and Korsak A: Who is the risk manager and what does he do? Hospitals 52(16):42, 1978.
19. Kraus GP: Health care risk management: organization and claims administration, Owings Mills, Md, 1986, National Health Publishing, A Division of Rynd Communications.
20. Richards EP III and Rathbun KC: Medical risk management preventive legal strategies for health care providers, Rockville, Md, 1987, Aspen Publishers, Inc.
21. Brown BL: Risk management for hospitals: a practical approach, Rockville, Md, 1979, Aspen Publishers, Inc.
22. Ansoff JI: The next twenty years in management education, 43(4):293, 1973.
23. Drucker PF: Management and the world's work, Harvard Bus Rev 66(5):65, 1988.

14

Management of Access: an Epidemiological Approach to Marketing

Health services are no longer service driven—they are market-driven organizations.

This often heard statement describes the changes that have taken place in health services management in the 1980s. Service-driven care focuses on the product or service and delivering it to those who need the service. A market orientation means focusing on the needs and demands of the target markets and providing the products they need. However, some health service organizations are neither primarily service nor market, but marketing driven. The marketing driven are sales-oriented organizations that focus on stimulating interest of a target group (that is, paying patients) in buying the organization's services.

Most health services were originally established by a religious or community group or by philanthropists or physicians to serve unmet needs of the sick and injured. Such a service approach was supported by post–World War II reimbursement incentives that rewarded health services by paying higher costs for more services to more people, which in turn increased provider income, size of facilities, and quality of service. In the civil rights era of the 1960s and 1970s, health care was considered a right of all people and programs were launched to increase access to care. However, in the 1980s cost-containment incentives described in Chapter 2 rewarded providers to serve full-pay private patients and penalized them to serve the elderly and poor, who were partial-pay or nonpay patients. Marketing became the key to success of health services: that is, market to those who can pay, but if the organization is to prosper or even survive, neglect and perhaps demarket to those who cannot.

Can a health services organization serve both the health of the community for access to care and at the same time its own organizational health and survival? Health services need to serve both the community and themselves. If the institution is not healthy, it cannot serve the community. Patients are necessary for a healthy institution; however, a health service must guard against inverting ends and means. Patients are ends, not just means to health of an institution. In this chapter we propose a market-driven epidemiological approach to serve community needs for access to health while also meeting organizational needs.

From the patient's perspective, it is important to have access to care that will improve or maintain health. Access to care includes the five "A"s of availability, accessibility, accommodation, affordability, and acceptability, as discussed in Chapter 2. Providing access to care for people who are in need should be an objective of health services organizations. Achieving access and the five "A"s translates into marketing from the institution's perspective.

MARKETING AND DEMARKETING HEALTH SERVICES

Marketing has become one of the most important managerial functions in a health service. Patients are the primary, if not only, source of income, and in a very competitive environment health service facilities feel they must sell their services directly to patients, as well as to physicians, just as any other consumer product industry. Marketing has become a goal of some hospitals, not simply a means to community service. As stated by one author, "hospitals must build powerful marketing organizations, not just powerful marketing departments."[1] Emphasis on market management in the 1980s resulted in the rapid application of "product line management," that is, treating services as separate profit centers organized around marketing plans. Women's and children's health, cardiology, and oncology are examples of product lines. However, product line management has faded in a number of hospitals because of problems implementing the matrix organizational structure in which product line management usually falls.

In 1986 hospitals in the United States spent more than $1.1 billion on marketing.[2] This represented a 56% increase in just 1 year. This estimate is probably an understatement, since marketing is frequently defined narrowly, including mostly promotional and direct marketing costs. If one adds to this $1.1 billion the much larger amounts expended on marketing health insurance, pharmaceuticals, and other health products, he or she can see that a portion of the increase in health care costs can be attributed to marketing the services.

At the same time that billions are spent on marketing health services, in 1987, 37 million Americans had no (or insufficient) means to seek health care. The dilemma for health providers is they must attract paying patients to survive. It also means that if they serve mainly the poor and underserved who are usually most in need of care, the hospital may go broke. Indeed, most of the hospitals that have had to close are those that served large numbers of the urban and rural poor. Consequently, while health care providers aggressively market to those who can pay, some demarket to those who cannot. In an earlier chapter we described some of the more subtle means of rationing health service. An American Hospital Association work group was more explicit in describing alternative ways a hospital might demarket its services to those who cannot pay hospital costs.[3] They included the following:

Allow lengthy waiting time for nonurgent patients in the emergency room

Require cash payment or proof of insurance before rendering service to nonurgent patients

Provide little or no parking for emergency department patients

Screen all nonurgent patients and refer poor ones to other providers

Transport poor, trauma, or critical care patients to other providers after initial stabilization

Provide an unlisted number for the emergency department

Segregate waiting areas for paying and nonpaying patients; in the area for nonpaying patients provide few seats, poor lighting, few signs, and no food or drink

Segregate treatment areas, providing fewer staff and less equipment in areas for nonpaying patients; in other words, develop and offer a two-class system of care based on patients' ability to pay

It is important to note that the above is not a recommended policy proposal of the AHA. Indeed, such a statement conflicts with AHA ethical standards for hospitals presented in Chapter 18. Nevertheless, some believe such demarketing practices have become necessary for some hospitals to survive.

Providing access to care is a mission of a health care system. Although access to care is primarily a policy issue at the national level, it is implemented at the service level. We propose that a broadly based market-driven strategy using an epidemiological approach may help health services manage access between counterforces of serving needs and marketing for resources.

AN EPIDEMIOLOGICAL APPROACH TO MARKETING

We noted in Chapter 5 that marketing is an integral part of the strategic planning process. Indeed, in our broad approach to marketing, strategic planning and marketing are nearly synonymous. In common usage, marketing means promotion and selling activities. To professional managers, however, marketing incorporates all of what we described as strategic planning. In the first part of this Chapter we discuss marketing. We next describe epidemiology, and finally an epidemiological approach to marketing is proposed.

MARKETING

During the past decade, health services administrators have attached increasing importance to the marketing function. However, there has been considerable confusion as to what marketing really is. It is the purpose of this section to examine the marketing process.

The Marketing Philosophy

It is important to realize that the marketing concept, which places primary emphasis on the consumer, arose as part of the evolutionary growth stage of business. Although Adam Smith in his *Wealth of Nations* placed the consumer as the central actor in his concept of business and commerce, the customer has not always occupied this preeminent position. In fact, businesses have passed through a production orientation, to a sales orientation, and finally to the marketing orientation.

A production orientation is found in those economies where scarcity exists. Attention is directed primarily to providing for the basic physical needs of food, clothing, and shelter. This was the situation in the United States during most of the nineteenth century and even into the early twentieth century in some areas. It is the situation found in most developing countries. Kotler[4] suggests that this philosophy is also representative of many nonprofit organizations.

When citizens become more affluent, their demands shift from meeting physical needs to spending discretionary income. This income is allocated to personal tastes or demands. Under a sales orientation, it is assumed that these personal tastes or demands can be influenced or induced so that individuals will purchase given products or services. An organization that has products or services to sell or to provide takes steps to induce the potential buyer to purchase said products or services. By means of various sales techniques including advertising, the potential customer is "convinced" or "sold" on the product or service. In other words, a need for the product or service is aroused. The problem of course is that if the purchasers are oversold, distrust will set in and the customers will withhold purchases or demand that controls be established by governmental agencies.

Many health services managers today have this "sales" orientation of marketing. If larger and better appointed buildings are erected, physicians and hence patients will more likely make use of the facility when faced with a medical use decision— the "bigger is better" philosophy. A similar situation exists with the duplication of services in order to offer a "full range" of services or to "keep up with the Joneses." Moreover, many hospitals seem to be taking a sales approach to hospital survival; that is, what new products can they sell or how can they repackage services to increase patient volume in competition with other hospitals. They do not focus on community needs and the possibility that the community's health may be better without them.

During the 1950s the business segment of the U.S. economy began to recognize limitations of the sales orientation and realized the necessity of meeting needs rather than selling a product by creating needs. Levitt[5] suggested that an industry should be viewed as a customer—satisfying activity rather than a goods-producing process.

Although there are those organizations that do not understand the marketing concept, what the typical citizen really sees is the tip of the iceberg. The research activities involved in determining customer needs are not usually visible. Then what is marketing? Kotler suggests a definition of marketing.

> Marketing is the analysis, planning, implementation and control of carefully formulated programs designed to bring about voluntary exchanges of values with target markets for the purpose of achieving organizational objectives. It relies heavily on designing the organization's offering in terms of the target markets' needs and desires, and on using effective pricing, communication, and distribution to inform, motivate, and service the markets.

In the following paragraphs these aspects of marketing will be reviewed: identification of customers (publics), determination of needs, satisfaction of needs, and evaluation of results.

Identification of Publics

Although often used, the word *customer* does not seem to be the appropriate term to identify those groups of people or organizations that have an actual or potential interest or impact on the hospital. The term *publics*, employed by Kotler, is more appropriate and will be used in this discussion.

Simon[6] identifies five groups and organizations as publics of the hospital: (1) patients; (2) physicians; (3) employer or union groups; (4) government and regulatory agencies; and (5) employees. During the past 10 years, each of these publics has become more concerned about the efficiency and effectiveness of hospitals, at least so far as the government is concerned. There is no question about the key role played by physicians and patients. These publics have been discussed at some length in earlier chapters. With the inclusion of hospitals in collective bargaining regulations through extension of the Taft-Hartley Act to cover hospitals, unions have become interested in organizing hospital employees and have therefore become a public of the hospital. Employers in other organizations are becoming more concerned about the costs of their health insurance programs and, in turn, concerned about hospital operations. We are constantly reminded of the increasing influence of governmental and regulatory agencies on hospitals. These publics present a challenge to hospital managers to develop innovative administrative and operational procedures. Employees constitute a significant public of hospitals. Every practicing CEO has either personally experienced or knows of situations where the quantity and/or quality of service has been disrupted because of either actual or perceived lack of understanding of employee attitudes and needs.

Other publics that should be identified include the community where the hospital is located. Relatives and friends of patients constitute another public of hospitals. In many communities, other hospitals constitute an important public of hospitals. This public is particularly significant in light of evaluations by health services agencies under health-planning legislation.

Because each of the publics serves a different function, it is important to identify the normal or usual function of the public and how the hospital can better serve the needs of the public. Some publics are more directly involved in hospital operations than others. For example, physicians, patients, and employees are directly involved, whereas the other publics, such as the government, have a more intermittent though powerful involvement.

Determination of Needs

Determination of the needs of the publics is one of the basic research efforts of marketing. Needs assessments that identify the strengths and weaknesses of present programs and services relative to the various publics are a requirement of successful marketing. Such activities also examine the changing environment within which the hospital exists.

Fink[7] suggests that the hospital should begin with an analysis of utilization records over the past several years and tie this information to financial data. This will give input regarding services and programs used by patients and physicians over the period of study. He says, "The hospital should also try to determine the needs, wants, and attitudes of its major market segments" (p. 52).

MacStravic[8] points out that marketing professionals in business settings have defined "need" in terms of what products or services consumers want to buy. He also suggests that marketing research involves determining motives of customers or publics and the subconsious factors that influence buying. However, health care planning and delivery have defined "need" in a different context. Need is defined in terms of "what persons should be provided in order to protect, promote, or restore health" (p. 60). He goes on to say that health-related needs are determined by the identification of the incidence of a given disease or injury and the risk factors associated with it.

It is the health care professional's decision-making function to relate these determined-by-assessment techniques, such as surveys or population studies, to the ability of the hospital to meet such demands and expectations. No service or program can be completely controlled by a hospital in today's environment of competing organizations, planning agencies, rate review boards, and third-party reimbursement policies and practices. In addition, MacStravic indicates four errors hospitals and related health care organizations often make concerning needs (p. 62):

1. It may ignore unmet needs and satisfy itself that as long as it serves all who enter its doors, it has fulfilled its obligation.
2. It may provide services in excess of need, perhaps excusing itself on the grounds that it is providing what the consumer wants.
3. It fully accepts its obligation to serve the community, but fails to ration the community's scarce resources; it insists on developing capacity in response to need but ignores the extent of demand, producing overblown capacity and underutilization.
4. The biggest danger in health care services facilities' need-oriented approach is that obligation, not cost, is usually placed first.

Satisfaction of Needs

One area of increasing interest among consumers is that of health promotion or "wellness" programs. The Surgeon General's Report *Healthy People*[9] states that Americans are healthier than ever but that we as a nation can do better. In fact, the report points out that Americans are now very interested in improving their health (p. 7):

> Prevention is an idea whose time has come. We have the scientific knowledge to begin to formulate recommendations for improved health. And, although the degenerative diseases differ from their infectious disease predecessors in having more and more complex causes, it is now clear that many are preventable.

Of course, consumer health programs are not the only approach health services has available to implement their marketing activity. However, these programs are illustrative of how they could meet the identified needs of consumers. Obviously, if our need pattern as we define it is not in keeping with good health, it should be changed through encouragement from the health services staff if this approach is appropriate. However, we should not be expected to change our need pattern for the sole purpose of cost containment. Cost containment is important, but it must take a back seat to the maintenance of health in the community.

Evaluation of Results

In this section we are concerned with how well the health service develops and carries out its marketing activity. Assessment of marketing activity in the business organization is easier than in a health service because the business measurement is discrete, such as the number of units sold or the profit attained after the marketing program was implemented. Remarking about the activities of 25 hospitals involved in community health programming, Longe stated[10] (p. 172):

> Only a few of the participants have begun to incorporate evaluative research into the evaluation designs, control groups, precourse and postcourse testing, standardized instruments, random assignment of participants to experimental and control groups, and a representative sample of participants. Some of these hospitals are just beginning to show results from the evaluative research. Many of the participants said it was necessary to do program evaluation in order to justify their existence to the hospital administration and governing board. However, the evaluation process is considered one of the most confusing and difficult tasks to do.

The marketing function in the hospital should be properly viewed as a series of programs, each subject to evaluation in terms of its goals or objectives. Green[11] believes that there are three levels of evaluation: process, impact, and outcome. Process evaluation revolves around professional practice, and assessment is made of professional conduct or practice in terms of professional standards. Impact evaluation involves the measurement or determination of the impact of the program on health, knowledge, attitudes, needs, environment, or behavior. Outcome evaluation concerns the effect of the program on incidence of the disease, activity change, mortality, or morbidity. Depending on the nature of the marketing program, a different level of evaluation is required.

As has been indicated, the level of sophistication of evaluative research on marketing programs has not been very high. Most evaluation is performed at the process level. Nevertheless, marketing has a major role in health services management. Tucker says[12] (p. 37):

> Today, most hospital administrators would acknowledge that the well-being of their organization depends upon the attraction of resources to enable a hospital to meet the historical goals of patient care, teaching, and research. Attraction of the necessary resources and acceptance on the part of various publics of the hospital that the organization has attained its goals are vital to the long-term survival of the institution.

Marketing, with its explicit concern for resource allocation and public acceptance, can provide useful tools for hospital managers working for the survival of the voluntary hospital.

Marketing can be a powerful management tool. But a word of caution needs to be inserted. Gregg and Voyvodich provide it[13] (p. 144):

> . . . marketing in the hospital setting must continue to be viewed as a two-edged sword. It can be a valuable tool for identifying the unmet health services needs in a community, for helping to increase the rational development and deployment of hospital resources in a manner that maximizes efficiency, and for serving as a mechanism for increasing the satisfaction of all purchasers of hospital services. However, marketing clearly has the potential to excite appropriate demands for hospital services, cause hospital resources to be developed and deployed in an inefficient and irrational manner, and ultimately increase community health costs while lowering consumer satisfaction.

Thus there are ethical problems associated with hospital marketing efforts. These must be dealt with, as they arise, by the CEO. Failure on the part of the CEOs to pay due attention to ethical issues will doubtless result in a loss of not-for-profit tax status and in more regulation.

EPIDEMIOLOGY

Epidemiology is defined as "the study of the distribution and determinants of diseases and injuries in human populations."[14] Its purposes are stated in the following[15]:

1. To study the occurrence, distribution, and progression of disease problems and, more generally, to describe the health status of human populations so as to provide a basis for the planning, evaluation, and management of health promoting and restoring systems
2. To provide data that will contribute to the understanding of the etiology of health and disease
3. To promote the utilization of the epidemiological concept to the management of health services

As such it can serve as a basis for identifying needs in a marketing strategy.

Epidemiology is a recognized medical discipline and consequently provides a health service attitude and approach to strategic management and marketing. Although some physicians specialize in epidemiology today, most epidemiologists have master's or doctoral degrees without the medical degree. The Center for Disease Control (CDC) in Atlanta is the best known source of epidemiological studies—it is the center for determining the etiology of diseases such as Legionnaires and AIDS. State and local health departments have epidemiology sections and services. Some of the larger hospitals have epidemiologists for infection control. Increasingly, epidemiological methods are being used as the basis for clinical research to advance knowledge in the treatment, as well as prevention, of illness. We propose a broader role for epidemiology, that is, applying its approach to the health service marketing function.

Most health services focus on clinical medicine, that is, medical care to individuals. Physicians focus on care to their individual patients. Historically, the health services manager's primary role was to provide resources for physicians to meet the needs of their individual patients. Consequently, management focused on clinical medicine as well. Epidemiology, on the other hand, is population medicine where the community is the primary focus and concern. Managers must continue to focus on effectiveness of care to the individual patient and provide resources for physicians and other professional personnel to serve each patient. However, the community is becoming increasingly important to the ability of a health service to provide effective care to individuals, as well as to meeting needs of the community. Marketing focuses on the community; epidemiology provides a health service framework for a community focus.

Epidemiology is concerned with finding associations between states of health and disease and factors associated with them in a population. There are three types of epidemiological strategies—descriptive, analytic, and experimental. They are explained as follows:

1. Descriptive epidemiology describes the occurrence, distribution, size, and changes of health and disease in the population.
2. Analytic epidemiology uses three types of studies: retrospective, prospective, and cross-sectional. In a retrospective or case-control study, the epidemiologist collects data back in time (retrospectively) from two comparable groups of individuals: one with a specific disease or condition and one without. The objective of a retrospective study is to identify any history or exposure to one or more factors of interest (precursor condition). A prospective, cohort, or longitudinal study on the other hand starts with a group of people (cohort) characterized by some factor of interest (prescursor condition) and follows them forward (prospectively) in time (longitudinally) to determine the incidence (that is, observe the subsequent development) of some disease or condition. A cross-sectional or prevalence study collects data from a defined specific population at one time.
3. Experimental epidemiology also tests etiological factors, but it manipulates or controls the factors, as well as the controlled (usually random) assignment of individuals to the experimental and control groups. It consists of the evaluation of the effects of introducing, eliminating, or otherwise modifying the suspected factors on the occurrence or progression of some state of health or disease. Such experiments usually are referred to as "clinical" or "controlled" trials and are used mostly in the evaluation of new treatments, drugs, or services.

How Might a Hospital Take an Epidemiological Approach to Marketing?

Let us assume that one of the publics that a hospital wants to serve is the poor. In determining health needs of the poor in its community, the marketing department would want (1) to review studies done on this area by social welfare and other agencies, (2) to interview spokespersons for that population and the poor themselves who come into the hospital, and (3) to survey households if resources are available to do so. The planning and/or quality assurance department of the hospital, which maintains patient data, could be requested to do descriptive studies of the disease and demographic patterns of the hospitals Medicaid, general relief, and no-pay patients. Illness patterns and interventions vary widely among population groups; comparisons can also be made within and among communities and states.

What is the etiology of illness patterns among different population groups? What might be done to prevent problems to reduce the needs for such persons being hospitalized? How can the hospital work with other agencies to reduce the problems? Cross-sectional comparisons with the nonpoor population group might help identify unique factors among the poor that are amenable to intervention. Health department data and possibly cooperative studies with other organizations might be important to obtaining a study population sufficiently large for data analysis.

Satisfaction of needs would depend on the problem. For example, it might be found that the poor have a much higher rate of utilization of very costly neonatal intensive care services. Medicaid does not pay full costs of such services, or worse, the hospital may have to absorb the total cost if the patient is not eligible for Medicaid and has no other insurance. A high incidence of teenage pregnancies may be an underlying problem. Although effects of teenage pregnancies are substantial contributors to hospital losses, they can cause even more suffering to the people and populations involved. A social market-driven service should consider opportunities for helping to prevent such problems, as well as repairing the damage after it has been done.

According to Kotler,[4] "a social marketing orientation holds that the main task of the organization is to determine the needs, wants, and interests of the target markets and to adapt the organization to delivering satisfactions that preserve and enhance the consumer's and society's well-being" (p. 32). A hospital, for example, could work with other organizations using social marketing to attack such problems as teenage pregnancy, AIDS, and other social diseases that contribute to the crises in hospitals. People are most receptive to educational efforts when they are hospitalized and face the consequences of lack of knowledge. Neighborhood and community health center programs described earlier provide models for attacking health needs in the broadest sense. A hospital might join with other organizations for grant funds to help attack broader social problems that lead to costly hospitalizations. For example, the Kellogg Foundation, Robert Wood Johnson Foundation, and other private or government sources fund innovations for meeting social problems that result in very large medical expenditures and social tragedies.

Analytic and experimental epidemiology is relevant to evaluation in the marketing process. For example, a prospective, cohort, or longitudinal study might be done to evaluate the effects of the interventions on teenage pregnancy. It might be an opportunity for an experimental study with teenagers randomly assigned to the experimental or control groups.

Dever[15] suggests that managers will have to assume an important role in solving health and health care delivery problems, a role that will be facilitated by the adoption of epidemiology as the following:

- A tool to better equate resources and services with the population's health needs
- A framework for a more global (holistic, ecological) understanding of health and its determinants
- A guide to the development and provision of comprehensive services

- An objective basis for communication between management and health professionals
- A method for reconciling organizational interests with the population's health interests

Community Medicine

In the late 1960s and the 1970s community medicine was fashionable, but in the 1980s it was not a frequently used term as social programs were dismantled. Nevertheless, the community is a primary source of health problems among the disadvantaged. Some inner-city hospitals have been active sponsors of community health center programs, such as those discussed in Chapter 2.

In Great Britian, especially in Scotland, the community medicine model has been integrated into traditional health services since the early 1970s. Community physicians replaced the former public health officer positions and were attached to health service delivery systems. Community physicians are charged with being the linkage to identify community needs and to marshal health and other service resources to meeting such needs. Their functions relevant to American health services are to do the following[16]:

Identify the health care needs of the population
Measure the extent to which these needs are being met
Coordinate the development of health care objectives and plans to meet them
Coordinate the preventive health services and the promotion of health education
Develop working relationships between the (governing) board and medical (services)
Provide linkages between health and other community services

We propose that services truly interested in providing access for health to all persons, especially those most in need, should consider organizing the above functions into their strategic and marketing plan.

MANAGING ACCESS TO CARE: BALANCING COMMUNITY AND INSTITUTIONAL HEALTH NEEDS

Assuring adequate health care to those in need is the primary responsibility of policy makers, not institutional managers. Managers in for-profit health services can distance themselves from such responsibilities. They pay taxes, and it is the government's role to use those taxes to provide care for persons without means. It is quite possible that after this book is published, hospitals and other not-for-profit health services will have already lost their tax-free status. However, even if tax-exempt status is lost or even if there should be a universal health insurance or service system, demands for service to the disadvantaged will likely continue to exceed institutional resources to serve them. How can hospitals survive and still provide access to the poor? Many cannot—witness the number of inner-city and rural hospitals that have had to close.

We propose a number of steps to help cope with the dilemma of community versus institutional health needs. First, the issue should be addressed in any strategic and marketing plan. Is it a mission of the organization to serve community needs, and if so which needs? In addressing needs, we suggest that health be considered in its broadest sense, not just curative services. Preventing illness may be the best way in the long run to reduce some of the financial burdens placed on health services by the disadvantaged. Second, goals for community services must be communicated and made operational throughout the organization. Third, resources must be available to implement such goals.

What might a health service do to obtain resources for serving those who cannot pay the costs of their care? An obvious way is to strive for organizational efficiency to ensure that maximum benefit can be obtained from limited resources. Another way is to seek resources from others, such as through fund raising for care to the indigent, obtaining grants for innovative services to the disadvantaged, and the current Robin Hood practices of shifting costs to those who can pay. Political efforts to obtain more resources is a widely recognized but frequently poorly implemented approach. Perhaps a less obvious but effective way is to develop interorganizational resource sharing with social services for consolidated efforts to meeting the broad health needs of the disadvantaged.

Because of rapidly rising costs, images of rich doctors and elegant hospitals, and marketing and demarketing practices, there is less sympathy for many struggling health services. A refocus on meeting the broad health needs of the community may elicit more public support for health services providers.

Mercy Health Services, Farmington Hills, Michigan, provides one model of social-driven marketing that includes services to the poor. They are currently striving to implement the following steps[17] (p. 5):

1. **Reach out.** Be sure that we are doing all that we can do in each of our service areas. For example, be actively in touch with community and social agencies to see how the health needs of recipients can be approached. Work with Medicaid to see who is being denied approval, why, and how people who are denied approval get care. Conduct marketing research studies, and develop action plans on what might be done at each local level for the uninsured, unemployed, and underinsured. Discover who these people are, how they can be reached, and how to best meet their health needs.
2. **Work collaboratively with concerned physicians.** Issue an invitation to these physicians to join with our Mercy hospitals in volunteering medical care, needed prescription drugs, and appropriate hospital inpatient care to the hard core of unemployed, uninsured, or grossly underinsured who are in all of our service areas. Volunteerism is not dead. Appeal to the neighboring hospitals to do the same.
3. **Continue payer responsibility.** Continue to insist on a level of payment from private insurance and the emerging HMOs that enables us to continue the historical practice of cost shifting. This should be done until the time when alternative funding sources of the type suggested in the long-term solutions are in place. Employers and unions do not wish to walk away from the local indigent in their rush to reduce health expenditures, but currently they do not understand the problem, the options, or the consequences if the problem goes untended.
4. **Priority in public policy.** Focus our public policy priorities and initiatives that exist in Iowa, Indiana, Michigan, and on the federal level on trying to solve the financing and delivery problems along the long-term directions previously outlined.

5. **Improve philanthropic giving.** Organize our fund development and fund-raising programs around the overarching theme of reducing and eliminating medical indigence in our service areas. Our creative responses should appeal to givers. Coverage of deficits will not be appealing.

6. **Cross-subsidize within our organization.** Pool our financial gains and risks in such a way to enable subsidization of our own "disproportionate share" hospitals and physicians. Internal reallocation can help in the short run and is needed and appropriate.

7. **Continue education and consciousness-raising efforts.** Institute a program of education, awareness raising, reflection, and discernment of what it means, individually and corporately, to provide a preferential option for the poor. Attack where practical the specific health status problems of the poor, for example infant mortality, in some of our communities.

8. **Establish new connections and new dialogue directly with the poor.** These connections should be established directly with the poor, not with political advocates for the poor, in order to be influenced by the legitimate expectations of this population group.

9. **Develop and implement an ethical screen in decision making.** A new question must be added to all of our analyses and decisions, i.e., what impact, if any, will this decision, this policy, this initiative, or this expenditure have on service to the poor in this service area? This internal discipline, as part of an "ethical screen" in decision making, should be as important as the legal, financial, organizational, and market impact set of questions currently dominating our approach.

These nine steps for the short term, plus constructive work on long-term solutions, will enable us with honesty, integrity and realism to be able to say we did all that we could.

We conclude with a statement by John R. Evans,[18] which summarizes our beliefs about the role of managers in addressing access to care (p. 33):

> The contributions of health services managers to resolving the major problems confronting the system is limited by two main factors. First, managers have been putting (and have been trained to put) the emphasis on their institution and not on the health needs of the population. Second, they have concentrated their attention on the support or hotel functions of their facility and have been reluctant to intervene in the health service functions where large savings might be possible.

> This reluctance to intervene is not due to lack of recognition of the problems: it is due to the conflict between institutional and health interests and the uncertainty that the administrator's leadership will be sustained in the face of the opposition from those adversely affected, particularly the medical staff. There is increasing recognition from those in practice in the field that familiarity with epidemiological methods and a more critical approach to review of evidence are invaluable tools for rational decision making in administration and for objective communication with health professions.

REFERENCES

1. Rynne TJ: Line managers as marketers, Hosp Prog 67(7):23, 1986.
2. Hospitals, p 64, Nov 20, 1986.
3. Burns LA: Hospital initiatives in response to reductions in Medicaid funding for ambulatory care programs. Working paper, Chicago, 1981, American Hospital Association.

4. Kotler P and Clarke RN: Marketing for health care organizations, Englewood Cliffs, NJ, 1987, Prentice Hall.

5. Levitt T: Marketing myopia, Harvard Business Review, p 45, July-Aug, 1960.

6. Simon JK: Marketing the community hospital: a tool for the beleaguered administrator, Health Care Manage Rev 3(2):11, 1978.

7. Fink DJ: Marketing the hospital: MBA 12(9):50, Dec 1978/Jan 1979.

8. MacStravic RE: Health care marketing needs rational, ethical approach, Hosp Prog 61(5):60, 1980.

9. Healthy people: the Surgeon General's Report on health promotion and disease prevention, Washington, DC, 1979, U.S. Department of Health, Education and Welfare.

10. Longe M: What's going on in the community? Hospitals 53(18):171, 1979.

11. Green LW: How to evaluate health promotion, Hospitals 53(19):106, 1979.

12. Tucker SL: Introducing marketing as a planning and management tool, Hospital Health Serv Admin 22(1):37, 1977.

13. Gregg TE and Voyvodich ME: Marketing: fast becoming a necessary tool for hospital administrators, Hospital 57(7):141, 1979.

14. Mausner JS and Kramer S: Mausner and Bahn epidemiology: an introductory text, ed 2, Philadelphia, 1985, WB Saunders Co.

15. Dever A: Epidemiology in health services management, Rockville, MD, 1984, Aspen Publishers, Inc.

16. Brotherston J: The specialty of community medicine, Royal Society of Health Journal 93(4):203, 1973.

17. Connors EJ: Delivering health services to the poor, Farmington Hills, Mich, © 1986, Mercy Health Services.

18. Evans JR: Measurement and management in medicine and health services: training needs and opportunities, New York, 1981, The Rockefeller Foundation.

15

Management of Quality and Costs

Quality—*you know what it is, yet you don't know what it is. But that's self-contradictory. But some things are better than others; that is, they have more quality. But when you try to say what quality is, apart from the things that have it, it all goes **poof!** There's nothing to talk about. But if you can't say what quality is, how do you know what it is, or how do you know it even exists?*

PIRSIG RM: *ZEN AND THE ART OF MOTORCYCLE MAINTENANCE*

Fortunately there has been substantial progress in defining quality of health care services. However, any attempt to define quality will reflect the perspective of the person making the definition. Thus each definer will likely have a different definition. With this in mind, let us examine the quality of a health service. A patient might identify quality when treated with empathy, respect, and concern. A physician might define it as "delivering the most advanced knowledge and skills of medical science to serve the patient." A hospital trustee might say, "having the best people and facilities to deliver service." A hospital administrator would probably agree with the trustee, but also add that "the professionals who provide the service continually evaluate their efforts and provide education for continuing improvements." To those who fund hospital services, quality will also have a dimension of efficiency. We suggest that health services managers must look at quality not just from one perspective, but from the perspective of all who are concerned.

The Joint Commission on Accreditation of Healthcare Organizations (JCAHO) defines quality patient care as "the degree to which patient care services increase the probability of desired patient outcomes and reduce the probability of undesired outcomes, given the current state of knowledge."[1] In a 1969 publication Donabedian[2] proposed eight points of "good" medical care, which appear relevant today:

1. Good medical care is limited to the practice of rational medicine based on medical science.
2. Good medical care emphasizes prevention.

3. Good medical care requires intelligent cooperation between lay public and the practitioners of scientific medicine.
4. Good medical care treats the individual as a whole.
5. Good medical care maintains a close and continuing personal relation between the physician and the patient.
6. Good medical care is coordinated with social welfare work.
7. Good medical care coordinates all types of medical services.
8. Good medical care implies the application of all necessary services of modern scientific medicine to the needs of all the people.

In the past, quality control was the sole prerogative of the profession that had the knowledge and skills to evaluate quality, control licensure, and educate for improvement of quality, namely, the medical profession. Health care was not generally considered a right until very recently. Consumers usually obtain medical services on recommendations of friends who have limited technical knowledge and therefore base their recommendations on personal relationships with the physician and/or what they can afford. However, responsibility for quality service no longer rests only with the professions that have the knowledge and skills; it is now shared by the governors, managers, and payers of health services. The Darling case and other court interpretations confirm the "obligation of a hospital and its medical staff to oversee the quality of professional services rendered by individual medical staff members."[3] Social Security amendments (PL 92-603) confirmed the government's concern for quality as a major payer of health care through Professional Standards Review Organization (PSRO)—now Professional Review Organization (PRO)—requirements. Furthermore, consumer groups are concerned about the management of quality. For example, Ralph Nader's 1971 study group report on the medical profession's self-regulation concluded the following[4] (p. 153):

> Our study set out to discover what systems of quality control the profession has established to monitor each physician's service to his patients, to evaluate how well these systems perform, and to determine whether the profession merits the trust which society has placed itself into the hands, and relied on the hearts, of all its physicians. We have had to conclude that the medical profession has failed to meet that trust.
>
> . . . The study asked only whether or not a patient being treated by any physician in his office or hospital can be *reasonably sure:* that his physician is reasonably competent to treat that ailment (or that he will refer him to another whom the first believes to be reasonably competent); that his physician is reasonably up-to-date on diagnostic and treatment techniques, and on drug therapy information; that his physician will keep such records as to afford reasonable assurance that his work can later be effectively evaluated; that his physician's performance, no matter where given, will be monitored with reasonable frequency, objectivity and expertness by his peers.
>
> . . . We are forced to conclude that the patient cannot be reasonably sure.

There has been substantial progress since 1971. One would hope that there is a "reasonable" chance of competent treatment. However, there is still considerable evidence of malpractice in medicine. It is widely recognized that the problem of malpractice suits is malpractice. Our own experiences reviewing a number of court cases supports

such findings. For example, in one especially blatant case a fully accredited hospital with a reputation for high quality care did not appropriately scrutinize qualifications of at least one applicant for medical staff membership. They did not really check prior hospital privileges or training and gave full surgical privileges to a doctor who had falsified his surgical training and eligibility for board certification. What was worse, this doctor was not adequately supervised in accordance with medical staff bylaws in the 10 years he was on the staff, until a malpractice suit alerted them to a number of questionable practices.

The prestigious JCAHO, with all its efforts to assure high quality health care services, was recently charged as providing only minimal evidence that quality care can be assured in an accredited institution.[5] The JCAHO is a voluntary organization controlled by providers, not payers or patients. It has a 22-member governing board appointed by the American Medical Association, American Hospital Association, American College of Surgeons, American College of Physicians, and the American Dental Association. Its funding is derived from fees charged to organizations surveyed. It has a quasiregulatory role in that it qualifies services for Medicare reimbursement, and 42 states accept accreditation for licensing facilities.

The JCAHO reports that only 7% of hospitals they survey have inadequate quality assurance plans, and 29% of those showed no evidence of taking corrective action. On the other hand, the JCAHO reported 47% of hospice programs, 55% of mental health institutions, and 35% of nursing homes surveyed had inadequate quality assurance plans. Of these, 56%, 57%, and 50%, respectively, showed no evidence of corrective actions.[6]

There is convincing evidence of wide discrepancies in quality of care among various providers. Although quality assurance procedures are improving, the competitive environment pressures providers to relax quality standards. Hospitals trying to fill beds have incentives to attract more doctors and are less likely to impose sanctions for fear of losing doctors and thereby patients. By the same token, doctors in competitive environments are less likely to refer patients to other physicians who may have more skills related to a patient's specific needs. Shortell and Hughes[7] found relationships between intensity of hospital competition and mortality. (They also found state regulations helped to predict higher hospital mortality.) Another recent study by the Rand Corporation[8] found that doctor errors led to as many as one fourth of the deaths of patients treated for heart ailments, strokes, and pneumonia. Moreover, the evidence substantiating the effectiveness of many current and emerging medical practices is frequently questionable and in many instances entirely lacking.[9]

Certain factors are emerging as being related to higher technical quality of care. There is convincing evidence that volume of services is related to more favorable outcomes of care. That is, doctors and hospitals that have more experience treating specific illnesses provide higher technical quality of care.[10-12] Some studies found evidence of lower mortality in teaching facilities,[12] whereas others found no significant relationships between teaching status and patient outcomes.[13] There is some evidence that physician specialization and limiting treatment to patients whose disease is related to the specialization predicts better care.[13] The importance of board certification on the other hand has not been consistently related to performance.[11,12] In several studies a strong medical staff organization related to higher quality care,[14,15] but in another study the tightness of control measures for the surgical staff was associated with higher adjusted mortality.[16]

Most important to this book is the increasing evidence that management practices are related to quality of care.[14,17,18] Management cannot abrogate responsibility for technical quality of care to individual physicians. In the hospital the governing board has ultimate responsibility for quality of care in the institution. The CEO and management in general must execute board policy for high quality care. Managers have responsibility for promoting and assuring quality of care. In short, managers have an important role in life and death of the organization's clients, just as do physicians and other professionals.

FORCES FOR MORE ATTENTION TO QUALITY

One might think that with increasing emphasis on containing the costs of health care, pressures for quality control would recede. However, because of measures to contain costs, there is increasing concern that high quality care will be a casualty. Cost-containment practices of (1) prospective pricing systems and DRGs, (2) HMOs with gatekeeper and capitation reimbursement, and (3) larger deductibles and copayment disincentives to seeking care raise potential dangers of patients not receiving needed services. To guard against such problems, payers, such as Medicare, Medicaid, and private employers, demand more intensive surveillance of quality of care. In addition, malpractice litigation and court decisions that broaden corporate responsibility for quality of care force management to exercise more control over quality. The nursing shortage and nursing demands for quality care pressure management to address such issues. JCAHO accreditation standards are becoming tighter, and consumer groups, such as the American Association of Retired Persons (AARP), Business Groups on Health, and Ralph Nader's organization are exerting more pressures for quality of care. In 1989 the National Practitioner Data Bank was established to provide hospitals and other medical groups (but not the public) with information about misdiagnosis, mistreatment, and professional misconduct of individual practitioners. Increasing consumer awareness of quality through some of these groups, advances in methods for measuring quality, the publication of quality measures, and competitive marketing by providers also add pressures on management for higher quality health services performance.

APPROACHES TO EVALUATING QUALITY OF CARE

Who should be evaluated to control quality of care? Pellegrino[20] (p. 309) suggests three types of functional classification of the team concerned with care: the *health care team,* which consists of all who are engaged in providing or planning for some service to improve the general or community health, without neecessarily being in direct or indirect contact with the specific needs of a specific patient (this would include administrators and office personnel, in addition to physicians and nurses); the *medical care team,* which consists of those professionals, semiprofessionals, and nonprofessionals who provide some service for the patient without any direct or personal contact, for example, central supply personnel and laundry workers; and the *patient care team,* which comprises any group of professionals, semiprofessionals, and nonprofessionals who jointly provide services that bring them into direct personal and physical contact with the patient and that are part of a program of management for the patient. In this chapter we will focus on the more restrictive level of the patient care team, because that is where most of quality control efforts have been made; nevertheless, we believe the broader considerations deserve much more attention than they have received.

Three approaches to evaluation of quality have been identified by Donabedian[20] as: (1) structure, (2) process, and (3) outcome, or end results. These are currently the most frequently used classifications. He defines the three approaches as follows:

> *Appraisal of structure* involves the evaluation of the settings and instrumentalities available and used for the provision of care. While including the physical aspects of facilities and equipment, structural appraisal goes far beyond to encompass the characteristics of the administrative organization and qualifications of health professionals. The term *structure* as used here also signifies the properties and resources used to provide care and the manner in which they are organized.

> Two major assumptions are made when structure is taken as an indicator of quality: first, that better care is more likely to be provided when better qualified staff, improved physical facilities and sounder fiscal and administrative organization are employed. Second, that we know enough to identify what is "good" in terms of staff, physical structure and formal organization. That staff qualifications, physical structure and formal organization are not equaled with quality must be emphasized. It is only expected that there be a relationship between these structural elements and the quality of care, so that given good structural properties, good care is more likely (though not certain to occur). Devices like licensure, certification of facilities, and accreditation are based largely on these assumptions.

It appears that most informed consumers, hospital governing board members, and probably many administrators appraise quality of hospitals on a structural basis. Hospitals with teaching programs and medical school affiliations, the most modern facilities, the highest percentage of board-certified specialists, and a strong financial and organizational structure are assumed to have the highest quality services.

Donabedian goes on to define

> . . . *assessment of process* as the evaluation of activities of physicians and other health professionals in the management of patients. The criterion generally used is the degree to which management of patients conforms with the standards and expectations of the respective professions. . . . When evaluation of process is the basis for judgments concerning quality . . . there is the explicit or implicit assumption that particular elements and aspects of care are known to be specifically related to successful or unsuccessful outcomes or end results.

Assessment of process is the basis of quality review techniques used by hospital medical staffs through medical records committees and other medical audit or quality review committees that review the process of patient care by reviewing patient charts. Process techniques rely on generally accepted norms or defined criteria, on subjective judgments, and on the diligence of reviewers.

> *Assessment of outcomes* is the evaluation of end results in terms of health and satisfaction. That this evaluation in many ways provides the final evidence of whether care has been good, bad, or indifferent is so because of broad fundamental social and professional agreement on what results are brought about, at least to a significant degree, by good care.

Although outcome would seem to be the ideal appraisal of quality, it is also the most difficult to measure. Blood pressure, for example, is a single measure of outcome for hypertension, but for most illnesses there is no single sign. Mortality can of course be measured, but morbidity, that is, the state of being diseased, and survival time are difficult to measure. Moreover, even when outcome can be measured effectively, there are problems correlating it with diagnosis and treatment. Psychological and social factors also can confound the outcomes of appropriate care.

In a study of five methods of process and outcome evaluation, Brook and Appel[21] found the evaluation of care depended on the method used. For 296 patients reviewed in a major city hospital, from 1.4% to 63.2% of the patients were judged to have received adequate care, depending on the method used to evaluate the quality of patient care. Judgment of *process* using explicit criteria yielded the fewest acceptable cases (1.4%). Brook[22] (p. 37) states:

> The method currently in vogue, assessment of quality care based upon explicit process criteria is likely to produce the most stringent judgment of quality of care. The use and acceptance of this method is likely to double if not triple the number of personal health services provided without substantially improving the health of the American people. Thus, the result of the admirable intention of both physicians and general public to raise the quality of care by assessing the process of that care may have dire economic consequences and actually lower the health level of the population by directing money away from other social needs such as housing into medical care processes which are only thought to have an effect on health level.

The ultimate goal is a decrease in disease, death, disability, discomfort, and disaffection. Outcome measures are receiving more attention, and progress is being made toward the development of effective indicators by investigators at a number of universities.

METHODS FOR MANAGING QUALITY OF PHYSICIANS' SERVICES

Peer review, medical audit, quality assurance, and utilization review are terms commonly associated with the management of the quality of medical care. Peer review refers to physicians reviewing the quality of work done by other physicians. It can be done on a prospective, retrospective, and/or concurrent basis. Prospective review could be a consultation from another physician before a procedure is done. The medical audit or medical care evaluation is usually a retrospective review of patient medical records. In medical audit, quality is defined as degree of conformity with standards of accepted principles and practices. The medical audit was initially promoted by the

American College of Surgeons and has been continued through efforts of the JCAHO. Quality assurance suggests integration of quality-assessment activities into a practice or delivery system with the effect of raising standards. The concept implies that an evaluation system supplies reliable data to health care providers about their practices, induces behavioral changes that improve these practices, and provides reassessment to assure conformation to standards. Utilization review is a method for evaluating appropriateness of patient use of hospital services. It was mandated in Medicare legislation in 1965. The JCAHO defines utilization review in the context of appropriate allocation of hospital resources to provide high quality and efficient patient care. Peer review, medical audit, quality assurance, and utilization review, consequently, are terms that go hand in hand.

Peer review can be on an implicit or explicit basis.[22] Implicit review is based on overall physician judgment of the quality of care rendered by another physician. Explicit review refers to a specification of criteria and/or standards.

In 1981, the Joint Commission on Accreditation of Hospitals (JCAH), as it was known then, implemented more flexible but presumably more rigorous standards for quality assurance, calling for each hospital to develop its own plan. The standard follows[23] (pp. 152-153):

There shall be evidence of a well-defined, organized program designed to enhance patient care through the ongoing objective assessment of important aspects of patient care and the correction of identified problems. Included in the interpretation is that:

It is the governing body's responsibility to establish, maintain, and support, through the hospital's administration and medical staff, an ongoing quality assurance program that includes effective mechanisms for reviewing and evaluating patient care, as well as an appropriate response to findings.

. . . To obtain maximal benefit, any approach to quality assurance must focus on the resolution of known or suspected problems (that impact directly on patients) or, when indicated, on areas with potential for substantial improvements in patient care. It is incumbent on a hospital to document evidence of an effective quality assurance program.

The essential components of a sound quality-assurance program in the aggregate shall include:
- Identification of important or potential problems, or related concerns, in the care of patients
- Objective assessment of the cause and scope of problems or concerns, including the determination or priorities for both investigating and resolving problems. Ordinarily priorities shall be related to the degree of adverse impact on patient care that can be expected if the problem remains unresolved
- Implementation, by appropriate individuals or through designated mechanisms, of decisions or actions that are designed to eliminate, insofar as possible, identified problems
- Monitoring activities designed to assure that the desired result has been achieved and sustained
- Documentation that reasonably substantiates the effectiveness of the overall program to enhance patient care and to assure sound clinical performance

The medical record remains an important data source in the identification of problems. However, other potentially useful sources include morbidity/mortality review; monitoring activities of the medical and other professional staffs; findings of hospital committee activities (for example, safety, infection control); review of prescriptions; profile analysis, including PRO and other regional data; specific process-oriented/outcome-oriented studies; incident reports relating to both individual safety and clinical care; review of laboratory; financial data (for example, hospital charge data on services rendered, liability claims resolutions); utilization review findings; data obtained from staff interviews and observation of hospital activities; patient surveys or comments; and data originating from third-party payers and/or fiscal intermediaries.

Once an actual or potential problem is identified, it may be assessed prospectively, concurrently, or retrospectively. Whatever time frames for review and whatever quality assessment activities are used, representative care (that is adequate sampling) provided by all clinical departments or disciplines and individual practitioners must be evaluated. Whereas the evaluation of physician-directed care must be performed by physician members of medical staff, nonphysician health care professionals should assess those aspects of care that they provide. However, the participation of both physicians and other health care professionals in the same quality assessment activities when appropriate is strongly encouraged.

Structure, process, or outcome criteria; standards of practice of professional organizations; or criteria developed within the hospital or in cooperation with local hospitals may be utilized as appropriate. . . .

Appropriate action must be implemented to eliminate or reduce the identified problem. Such action may include but is not limited to educational-training programs, new or revised policies or procedures, staffing changes, equipment or facility change, or adjustments in clinical privileges.

Beginning in the early 1990s, the JCAHO will focus on outcomes and comparisons among similar hospitals instead of defining quality in terms of structure or process.[24] Quality will be measured by a hospital's degree of conformity to a performance standard. The JCAHO expects to use the clinical indicators, as well as other factors, to grade a hospital. The clinical indicators collect data on patient complications caused by poor quality of care, for example, anesthesia indicators, which are related to anesthesia and to aspiration of gastric contents. In addition to clinical indicators, there will be organizational indicators, which will include measures of management and organizational factors affecting quality. It will also include case-mix and severity adjustments, so that quality can be measured and compared across institutions. This will result in a national data base of clinical and organizational indicators, comparisons, and trends.

The JCAHO will not monitor quality itself, but feed back the data so that each hospital can compare its performance with other hospitals and with standards developed by the JCAHO. In other words, accreditation will focus on problem identification, and analysis, action, and follow-up procedures of the institution. Failure to comply will result in a limited probationary period and loss of accreditation if not corrected promptly.

A task force is attempting to develop organizational indicators for the new JCAHO agenda. Relevant to this book, organizational indicators are likely to include the organization's mission; culture; strategic, program, and resource plans; change and innovation; and leadership.[25]

Professional review organizations (PRO) are mandated by Health Care Financing Administration (HCFA). HCFA is the federal agency responsible for administering Medicare and Medicaid within the Department of Health and Human Services. PROs were described in Chapter 2, but pertinent to this chapter is that PROs too are moving from primary concerns about unnecessary utilization of services to quality, effectiveness, and outcomes. Under DRGs, there are financial incentives for early patient discharge. PROs are therefore examining timeliness of care to guard against premature discharge. PROs are also studying effectiveness of various interventions that result in protocols. In other words, if they find that certain procedures are no more efficacious than another less costly procedure, they will not pay for them. PROs will also mandate educational programs for physicians who are found negligent in doing certain procedures.

Until recently, quality review procedures focused almost exclusively on hospital inpatient care. Increasingly, however, quality reviews are being mandated in other health services. JCAHO has had an accreditation program for nursing homes, mental health services, and now HMOs. States have their own quality and licensing review programs for such services. More recently, ambulatory services have come under quality review surveillance by Medicaid agencies and other payers.

Clearly we are in an era of managed care. Autonomy of physicians has been substantially eroded. Although the United States presumably has a free-enterprise health care system, our experience in England and in the United States suggests that even though physicians in the United States have more *economic* autonomy, they have substantially less clinical autonomy than their counterparts in the so-called "socialized" systems, as in Great Britain. Doctors in England and most other countries are not subjected to utilization, quality, and cost reviews that are faced by physicians in the United States.

The United States is considered a model for high quality health care; certainly quality review procedures contribute to greater assurance of quality. Nevertheless, there are substantial variations in quality of medical care. Managers have an obligation to their patients to evaluate and continually improve the quality of care in their services.

MANAGEMENT OF QUALITY OR COST?

The assumption in the United States is that quality costs. That is, the higher the quality, the more it costs. "The Cadillac is better than the Hyundai, and it costs more." "Medical care is expensive; therefore the higher the quality, the more it costs." At certain levels the cost/quality relationship is valid, such as comparison of health services in a developing country (with expenditures of $2 per capita) with that of the United States (expending more than $2000 per capita). However, within a given range, it is a myth that higher quality necessarily relates to higher costs.

The Japanese invasion of the United States' auto industry demonstrated that higher quality can be achieved with lower costs. Indeed, W. Edwards Deming,[26] an American statistician who was instrumental in establishing the Japanese managerial revolution after World War II, proposes that poor quality increases "complexity," which in turn increases cost. Complexity is defined as (1) mistakes and defects, (2) breakdown and delays, (3) inefficiencies, and (4) variation. Conversely, he shows how improving quality reduces complexity, and higher productivity and lower cost follows. Crosby[27] suggests that 40% of operating costs are spent on nonconformance to quality. An example of the cost of nonconformance to quality in health services is rework, such as rehospitalization and complications from service, and other iatrogenic (disease induced by a physician or other professional) problems. Duplication of service is another example, as are the costs of inspection and regulating health services. Inefficiencies and the high cost of liability insurance are other examples of high costs of nonconformance to quality.

In health services there is some evidence that higher quality hospital care, for example, may be related to lower costs. Shortell et al.[15] in their study of 31 Massachusetts hospitals found that hospitals with higher cost per case had higher medical and surgical mortality after controlling for severity. Longest[28] examined direct costs and quality in 10 general hospitals in Atlanta, Georgia, and found evidence that hospitals that provide higher quality services tended to have lower direct costs and to take fewer person-hours to provide them. On the other hand, Scott et al.[16] report better outcomes of surgical care related to higher expense per patient day. These discrepancies are at least partially attributable to different units of measure, but together are consistent with findings of Schulz et al. of no relationship between cost and quality measures. That is, higher quality doesn't necessarily mean either lower or higher costs. In their study of psychiatric units, Schulz et al.[18] found that some units had both lower cost and higher quality, some had high quality but also higher costs, others had lower cost but also lower quality, and another group had unfavorable outcomes of both lower quality and higher costs. As stated by Donabedian[29]: (1) quality costs money, (2) money does not necessarily buy improvements in quality, and (3) some improvements in quality are not worth the added cost.

The above examined quality/cost relationships from an organizational viewpoint, but what about that of an individual patient? Fig. 15-1 portrays relationships between costs and patient outcomes. In a terminal illness, such as AIDS, increasing quantity of care and resulting increase cost of care may have little benefit to the patient's outcome. Highest cost per illness is for terminal cases. However, the ethical dilemma is at what point, if any, should intervention cease and services be limited to comfort and maintenance? No one should give up hope. Advances in medical science suggest that a breakthrough is possible with each passing day. On the other hand, the crisis in health care costs raises questions of how many thousands of dollars should be spent on high technology for patients who are likely to die anyway. Such questions are increasingly relevant when many people go without care because of a lack of funds.

For patients shown in Fig. 15-1 as having an illness amenable to medical intervention, the question arises as to when to stop adding more services. Until point A, the benefits minus the costs improve. After point A, benefits versus costs decline. At point B, increasing services are detrimental to patient outcomes, such as unnecessary

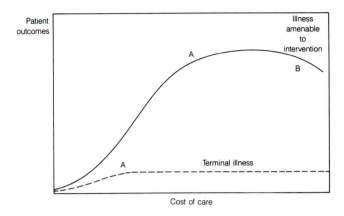

Fig. 15-1   Hypothetical relationships between costs and patient outcomes.

surgery that increases risk of death or complications. Payers, such as Medicare through PROs, are trying to find ways to learn when point A is reached for different diseases. They will then publish protocols for what will be reimbursed based on cost effectiveness of point A.

THE BOTTOM LINE AND THE RATIONAL MANAGER

The rational manager will attempt to buffer the organization from environmental forces to protect its technology.[30] The environment for health services is rapidly changing from very benevolent to rather hostile, at least in terms of funding. Survival of both the organization and the CEO is at stake. After all is said and done, if the organization's bottom line on annual income and expense statements is continually in the red, the CEO is not likely to survive. Nor will the organization survive if it continues. With many health services in a financial struggle, it is no wonder that health services executives and governing boards do indeed focus on the bottom line, sometimes seemingly to the exclusion of patient, staff, and community needs. What are alternatives for achieving a bottom line that is in the black?

Until the 1950s, patient revenues were limited, and, consequently, cost containment and fund raising signaled managerial effectiveness. Since then, patient income through increasing prices, expanded services, and marketing to attract more physicians and paying patients has predicted managerial success. A summary of some of the ways favorable bottom lines can be achieved follows.

Maximize Income to Meet Rising Expenses

Maximizing income to meet rising expenses can be expressed also as maximizing costs to increase income. In a cost-based, fee-for-service system, there are few restrictions to raising prices to meet increasing costs. Indeed there have been rewards to increasing costs. Increasing costs provided new technologies, larger and more elegant facilities, larger and better-trained staff, abilities to meet physician requests, higher wages and salaries, and more amenities to both staff and patients. All of these provided structural evidence of higher quality care.

Increasing prices has been the easiest way to increase income. Many rural hospitals missed opportunities to raise prices sufficiently to build strong institutions. Trustees were small businessmen and farmers who were unfamiliar with income maximization and who saw their role as one of containing rising hospital costs. Yet when such hospitals had to sell out to chains, the first action of the new owner was to raise prices substantially and add costly services that are structural indicators of high quality.

Increasing patient volume and number of services per patient is also a way to maximize income. Marketing to physicians who admit patients and to patients directly not only increases income, but justifies larger and improved facilities. Currently, with reimubursement discrepancies among Medicare, Medicaid, private insurers, and the uninsured and underinsured, marketing is even more important. The rational manager focusing on the bottom line will market to the private, fully insured and to Medicare patients in favorable DRGs (and try to have them discharged as soon as possible), but demarket to those who will be costly to the institution.

Other opportunities for increasing income are fund raising, lobbying for increased federal and state support for care to the elderly and medically indigent persons, procurement of grant funds for special programs, and favorable reimbursement practices from private payers.

Reduce Unit Costs

An adaptation of increasing income is to achieve economies of scale to reduce unit costs. In other words, as income increases, costs per unit of service should decline. The application of economies of scale to health services is unclear. Berki[31] suggests the following (p. 115):

> . . . whatever its exact shape and depending on methodologies and definitions used, economies of scale exist, may exist, or do not exist, but in any case according to theory, they ought to exist.

For example, hospital chains have been able to implement principles of bulk transactions by achieving discounts from suppliers because of large quantity purchases. Marketing for a vertically integrated system should be only slightly more costly than marketing for individual units. Economies of scale have also been shown in certain procedures where volume is related to quality.

Although consolidation of services should result in lower unit costs, evidence of this is elusive as noted in Chapter 3. Sharing costly capital expenditures, such as a lithotripter or MRI, between hospitals is a way to lower unit costs. Contract services for dietary or housekeeping or even management of the entire organization is another example of potential economies of scale.

Curtail Expenditures

Personnel costs consume the largest expenditures in health services. Personnel costs can be constrained in a number of ways, such as decreasing staffing ratios or substituting lower-cost personnel or machines for physicians, registered nurses, and other highly skilled personnel. Such opportunities are limited in health services however. Variable budgeting and patient classification systems, which relate staffing to patient volume and needs, have been shown to help contain staffing costs without sacrificing quality of care.

Increased surveillance of costs through management information systems helps to pinpoint high cost centers, deviations from expectations, and opportunities for savings.

Employee incentive systems have been used to increase motivation for cost containment. Ranges of employee incentive systems from which health services can develop their own plan include the following:

- Individual incentive plans related to standards based on work measurement techniques
- Team incentive systems based on productivity of the team
- Large group incentive systems based on the productivity of a department or whole hospital, such as the following:

    A profit-sharing plan, which is not applicable in a pure sense in not-for-profit services, but of which variations are possible

    Cost-savings sharing, which is more appropriate in not-for-profit services because it is based on cutting costs rather than increasing revenue and profits

    A labor-savings (Scanlon) plan, whereby payoff to the employee is based on a reduction of the percentage of total produce revenue involved in paying labor costs; usually employee management committees review suggestions for improvements.

    A value-added (Rucker) plan in which payoff is based on the ratio:

$$\frac{\text{Revenue Material Cost}}{\text{Labor Cost}}$$

where the numerator is an estimate of the value added by the health service to the service provided.

Although most of these systems appear to have limited application to nonprofit service industries, a few hospitals have reported significant results.[32] Some hospitals have given bonuses to medical directors where savings have been shown with utilization control systems. However, such incentive systems present at least appearances of ethical dilemmas.

Savings from Quality Improvements

Quality improvement as a methodology for containing costs is a relatively recent phenomenon in United States' industry. As noted, it is based on the theories of W. Edwards Deming, who helped to establish Japanese industry after World War II. It is now being reimported into the United States. One of the larger hospital for-profit chains has adopted quality as its primary management philosophy because it expects competition in health services to be based on quality more than price. It assumes that prices will be set, such as in prospective pricing systems using DRGs; consequently, quality will separate the successful from unsuccessful services. It is basing its quality improvement program on the Deming method described at the end of Chapter 7. A number of HMOs, hospitals, and other services have adopted "total quality management" principles based on the Deming philosophy, such as Harvard Community Health Plan, Hospital Corporation of America, NKC Hospitals, Rush-Presbyterian-St. Luke's Medical Center, and Meritor Health Center.

Fig. 1-2 presented the variables related to patient outcomes and management's role in improving such outcomes. Paraphrasing Paul Ellwood, Jr.: patients would be better served if management would focus on improving the quality of patient outcomes rather than the quality of hospital services.[33] Management philosophy and management strategy need to create a culture for total quality care. NKC Inc.,* which consists of three hospitals in Louisville, Kentucky, provides an example of "total quality management" (their phrase). Their ten steps to quality are designed to implement a strategy to improve patient outcomes[34]:

1. **Mission, values, quality policy, corporate goals.** NKC's mission statement asserts that it exists as an organizational framework to provide quality health care. Their values are: (1) respect for every individual, (2) delivery of quality of service, and (3) constant pursuit of excellence. "Quality is everything we do, and every decision we make is an attitude that we must create and nurture."

2. **Management's commitment to the quality process.** Action plans were developed for the CEO, the senior managers, the middle management, and the first level supervisors, and each manager rates the next level manager in terms of quality.

3. **Organizing for total quality management.** An internal quality management organization was structured to include a quality management council chaired by the CEO. Each member of the council chairs a group of hospital employees who design specific strategies for implementing parts of the quality action plan. A physician advisory group was also formed.

4. **Education and training.** Program strategies for education and training included management awareness briefings and special workshops in which the scope of service and the identity of the customers were defined for each department. The entire orientation program for new employees was revamped with a special emphasis on the quality process.

5. **Customers and their requirements.** A system to identify all NKC external customers and their requirements was implemented. Through such methods as written surveys and personal interviews, they ask their customers to define quality and judge whether the hospitals meet those requirements.

6. **Improvement opportunity identification.** A program to get employees to identify the barriers to error-free work was established. Employees who have their idea accepted are rewarded.

7. **Quality review.** The emphasis of quality review is on quality improvement, not

---

*Now Alliant Healthcare.

quality measurement. Designated as the primary management reporting system for the corporation, the components are the following:

competency—Are we capable?

appropriateness—Did it need to be done?

resource utilization—What is the cost of doing it well, and what is the cost of doing it incorrectly?

effectiveness—Was the desired outcome achieved? Were our requirements met?

risk management—Medical/legal and safety issues.

customer satisfaction—Were our perceived requirements met?

8. **Recognition and reward.** A number of programs to recognize and reward employees who identify areas that need improvement were developed. Quality has also become the predominant factor in the evaluation of all managers, and the performance appraisal system for all nonmanagement employees was also redesigned to make quality and its improvement the primary focus.

9. **Communication.** NKC formulated a comprehensive communication plan that uses multiple vehicles.

10. **Integrating total quality management with existing management programs.** A system has been developed to seek out policies, practices, and procedures that are barriers to the new corporate values, goals, and quality policy.

Some of Deming's theories conflict with other management theories, such as management by objectives. On the other hand, many points are consistent with management theory that has been proposed for years but is not adopted. Managers will declare their support of quality. In our experience with a large number of health services, however, we find they say it and believe it, but many do not manage for it. Managers do need to be wary of management fads. Many fade away in time, but the principles of those based on human and organization needs and outcome objectives are timeless, even though labels may be forgotten or come into disfavor.

REFERENCES

1. Modern Health Care, p 10, Dec 16, 1988.
2. Donabedian A: A guide to medical care administration, vol II, Medical care appraisal—quality and utilization, Washington, DC 1969, American Public Health Association.
3. Hedgepeth JH: Darling revisited, Hospitals 46(16):58, 1972.
4. McCleary R: One life—one physician: Ralph Nader's study group report on the medical profession's performance in self regulation, Washington, DC, 1971, Public Affairs Press.
5. Wall Street Journal, Oct 12, 1988.
6. Roberts JS: Reviewing quality of care: priorities for improvement, Health Care Finan Rev Ann Suppl 1987. Reported in The Medical-Economic Digest, p 7, Feb 15, 1988.
7. Shortell SM and Hughes EF: The effects of regulation, competition, and ownership on mortality rates among hospital inpatients, N Engl J Med 318(17):1100, 1988.
8. The Milwaukee Journal, p 5A, Oct 1, 1988, reporting on the Rand study published in that weeks Annals of Internal Medicine.
9. Eddy DM and Billings J: The quality of medical evidence: implications for quality of care, Health Aff 7(1):19, 1988.
10. Hughes RG, Hunt SS and Luft HS: Effects of surgeon volume and hospital volume on quality of care in hospitals, Med Care 15(6):489, 1987.
11. Payne BC, Lyons TF, and Neuhaus E: Relationships of physician characteristics to performance quality and improvement, Health Serv Res 19(3):307, 1984.
12. Kelly JV and Hellinger FJ: Heart disease and hospital deaths: an empirical study, Health Serv Res 22(3):369, 1987.

13. Flood AB and Scott WR: Hospital structure and performance, Baltimore, 1985, The Johns Hopkins University Press.

14. Roemer MI and Friedman JW: Doctors in hospitals: medical staff organization and hospital performance, Baltimore, 1971, The John Hopkins University Press.

15. Shortell SM, Becker S, and Neuhausen D: The effects of management practices on hospital efficiency and quality of care. In Shortell SM and Brown M, editors: Organizational research in hospitals, Chicago, 1976, Inquiry Book, Blue Cross Association.

16. Scott WR, Flood AB, and Ewy W: Organizational determinants of services, quality and cost of care in hospitals, Milbank Memorial Fund Quarterly: Health and Society 57:234, 1979.

17. Longest BB, Jr: The relationship between coordination, efficiency and quality of care in general hospitals, Hosp Admin 19:65, 1978.

18. Schulz R, Greenley J, and Peterson R: Management practices cost and quality in inpatient psychiatric services, Med Care 21(9):911, 1983.

19. Pellegrino E: The changing matrix of clinical decision making in the hospital. In Georgopoulos B, editor: Organization research on health institutions, Institute for Social Research, University of Michigan, Ann Arbor, 1972.

20. Donabedian A: The definition of quality and its approaches, Ann Arbor, Mich, 1980, Health Administration Press.

21. Brook RH and Appel FA: Quality-of-care assessment: choosing a method for peer review, N Engl J Med 288 (25): 1323, 1973.

22. Brook R: Quality of care assessment: what is the most appropriate method? In The hospital's role in assessing the quality of medical care, proceedings of the fifteenth annual symposium on hospital affairs, Center for Health Administration Studies, University of Chicago, May 1973.

23. Accreditation Manual for Hospitals, Joint Commission on Accreditation of Hospitals, Chicago, 1982.

24. Hospitals, pp 38-43, July 5, 1988.

25. Dowling W, Chairman, JCAHO Organization and Management Quality Indicators Task Force. Presentation to tenth annual fall conference of Health Services Administration Alumni Association, University of Wisconsin-Madison, Madison, Wis Oct 7, 1988.

26. Deming FE: Out of the crisis, Massachusetts Institute of Technology, Center for Advanced Engineering Study, Cambridge, Mass, 1982.

27. Crosby PB: Absolutes of quality management: transfer from industry to health care, Health Care Manage Q 9(1):3, 1987.

28. Longest B, Jr: An empirical analysis of quality/cost relationship, Hospital Health Serv Admin 23(20):1978.

29. Donabedian A: Five essential questions frame the management of quality in health care, Health Care Manage Q 1:6, 1987.

30. Thompson JD: Organizations in action, New York, 1967, McGraw-Hill, Inc.

31. Berki SE: Hospital economics, Lexington, Mass, 1972, Lexington Books.

32. Jehring JJ: The use of subsystem incentives in hospitals, Center for Study of Productivity Motivation, University of Wisconsin, Madison, 1967.

33. Modern Healthcare, p 26, July 15, 1988.

34. Powers MB: Quality takes steps forward, Healthcare Forum Journal, pp 29-34. Sept/Oct 1988.

16

The Management of Human Resources

The human resources responsibility of all health care services managers is to obtain qualified people and develop and use their capacities and abilities to best meet the objectives and expectations of the organization. This basic responsibility should be attained so that the needs of the individual employee are also met insofar as possible. The net result of this philosophy is optimum effectiveness of employees in delivering quality care, as well as a satisfied work force.

From a historical perspective, the need for obtaining qualified people and for developing and using their capabilities has been recognized for as long as men and women have worked together to achieve the objectives of an organization. In interpreting this aspect of the general philosophy, innumerable advances have been achieved in such functions as the recruitment, selection, placement, orientation, training, evaluation, and compensation of employees.

Of more recent development are study and interpretation directed toward human resources responsibilities so that a positive reaction (motivation) is attained by each employee of the organization. It is in this area that the behavioral scientists have made their greatest contributions.[1,2] However, much remains unknown about the numerous needs and expectations of people and their responses and adaptations to given situations. Despite the ramifications in this area, it is recognized that fair and equitable treatment of employees by managers significantly improves employee acceptance of policies and procedures because they experience adequate recognition and dignity.

In health care organizations there are additional factors that are significant. As organizations in the general service industry, there is no product involved, but a service. Berry[3] defines a service as "a deed, a performance, an effort. Although the performance of most services is supported by tangibles, the essence of what is brought is performance rendered by one party for another." There are few employees of health care organizations who do not have direct contact with the patients, residents, or clients of the organization. Not only is skill involved in rendering the service, but of significance is the approach, the attitude, and often the compassion of the employee in exercising his or her skill. In many situations the recipient of the service evaluates the organization

261

to a large extent on the interactions with employees. Therefore it behooves managers when exercising their human resources responsibilities to keep in mind the tremendous importance of employees in meeting the objectives of the organization.

Another aspect of health care organizations that is important to human resources management but also has broader significance is the role of the physician as the provider of information sought by the patient, resident, or client. It is difficult to attach a value to that information. In addition, the physician is the representative, or surrogate in many cases, for the patient in his or her relationship to the organization and its employees. Freidson[4] argues that the heart of the powerful role played by physicians is their claim of "medical emergency" on behalf of their patients (p 118):

> The physician is able to intervene in many places in the hospital and justify his intervention on the basis of a "medical emergency"—a situation in which the well-being of a patient is said to be in jeopardy and in which it is the physician alone who knows what is best done. We are all familiar with the dominant symbolic image: the interruption of orderly routine by a violent convulsion, heart failure, a hemorrhage. . . . while this no doubt happens on occasion, far more common in a hospital is the labeling of ambiguous events as emergencies by the doctor so as to gain the aid of resources he believes he needs.

Luke and Begun[5] argue that this claim to medical emergency has enabled physicians and some other medical professionals to create dual lines of authority for employees, that is, the employee's immediate superior, as well as the physician. This of course can be very confusing and disconcerting to employees because they are expected to serve two masters who may have conflicting ovjectives, such as cost savings versus advanced level of patient care. These same professionals have achieved great autonomy and influence over the health care industry in general.

A second factor Luke and Begun suggest as unique to health care organizations is equal access to health care. If treatment is not provided, the person could be impaired from functioning normally for life. Need is seen as an argument for equality of opportunity. This gives a special public dimension to health care. Employees, in turn, need to recognize the power of this external force, which indeed has resulted in such programs as Medicare and Medicaid, but also malpractice suits brought by patients against health care organizations and employees.

Thus the development of a human resources philosophy and its execution is not only necessary for health care managers, but also complex with changing ramifications because of the influence of internal, as well as external, forces. The balance of this chapter will summarize (1) the nature of the human resources management function and (2) managerial tools of value in exercising the human resources management process.[6]

THE NATURE OF THE HUMAN RESOURCES FUNCTION

There are five major components in what we will refer to as the nature of the human resources function. They are the following:

1. The job

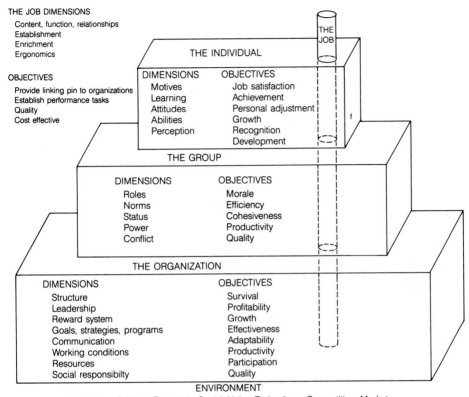

THE JOB DIMENSIONS
Content, function, relationships
Establishment
Enrichment
Ergonomics

OBJECTIVES
Provide linking pin to organizations
Establish performance tasks
Quality
Cost effective

THE INDIVIDUAL

DIMENSIONS	OBJECTIVES
Motives	Job satisfaction
Learning	Achievement
Attitudes	Personal adjustment
Abilities	Growth
Perception	Recognition
	Development

THE GROUP

DIMENSIONS	OBJECTIVES
Roles	Morale
Norms	Efficiency
Status	Cohesiveness
Power	Productivity
Conflict	Quality

THE ORGANIZATION

DIMENSIONS	OBJECTIVES
Structure	Survival
Leadership	Profitability
Reward system	Growth
Goals, strategies, programs	Effectiveness
Communication	Adaptability
Working conditions	Productivity
Resources	Participation
Social responsibilty	Quality

ENVIRONMENT
Regulatory--Political--Economic--Social--Union--Technology--Competition--Market

Fig. 16-1   The nature of human resources management.

2. The individual
3. The group
4. The organization
5. The environment

The first four items will be discussed in terms of objectives and dimensions. Our purpose is to present an integrated view of the function. To this end we include Fig. 16-1 as a representative model. The terms *function* and *model* will be used interchangeably.

The Job

The central idea of the model is the job as a connecting rod that holds together the various components of the model. If a person does not occupy a job or position in the health care organization, he or she has no direct connection with hospital, long-term care facility, clinic, or health service enterprise. Thus the major objective of the job is to provide a linking pin to the entire organization. A moment's reflection will establish the significance of this objective. The job represents the tie of the individual occupying the job to the organization. Obviously, if the job is ill-defined or deemed to be unimportant, the occupant is not likely to be an effective employee. Also, this concept of the job goes far to explain why change may be difficult to accomplish if it changes the content of the job and the purpose of the change is not obvious to the employee.

The job establishes (1) the performance tasks for the employee and (2) those tasks that will permit the organization to function. Any manager who notes that the organization is not performing well would be wise to look at the tasks that have been established for the jobs in troublesome departments. In addition, he or she would be wise to look at the interrelationship among jobs, especially when coordination among departments or units is required.

A major objective of the job is quality performance on the part of the incumbent. Tasks of the job must be clearly identified and delineated for quality performance to occur. The incumbent must also have the necessary skills, ability, and motivation to perform. An aspect of a job is also cost effectiveness. This assumes that the tasks are not superfluous and that the incumbent actually performs them. The importance of the job to overall organization cannot be underestimated.

To present some ideas of the scope—the width, length, and depth—of the job, we will make a few comments about what we will call the dimensions of the job. The first concept we have already mentioned entails the content, functions, and relationships. We have also discussed the significance of the establishment of the job. Another dimension is that of enrichment. Our concnern here is not basically with adding tasks to the job, but making the tasks more interesting to the incumbent and significant to the organization. A goal of management should be to make jobs more important and interesting but not necessarily to expect more production. If the employee becomes more proficient, there should be an increase in pay or other suitable recognition. When the incumbent's abilities and skills increase beyond the present job, he or she should be considered for promotion. Finally, there is the ergonomics aspect involving interactions between human beings and machines. As new equipment, such as the computer, has been introduced into health care organizations, the interactions between people and machines have increased and become more complex. Indeed, some pieces of equipment, such as x-ray and other complex body-scanning equipment, have caused employees to become increasingly concerned about their own well-being, as well as the well-being of the patient. Concern also must be held for hiring employees with the necessary skills and providing continued reinforcement of these skills so that the skills are not lost.

The Individual

Obviously, a position must be filled by a person who fulfills the job requirements. The employee has a number of objectives relative to the job and the organization. Although we will consider the interrelationship between the job and the person in the health care organization context, one should keep in mind that there are broader implications. For example, today increasing numbers of people view the job relative to the impact of that job on other family members and on their leisure time activities. Earlier, when people worked 60 to 70 hours per week and the man was considered to be the primary breadwinner, these factors were not as important. No manager can lose sight of the mores of the present and expect employees to behave as they would have a number of years ago.

A major concern of the individual is job satisfaction. Satisfaction can probably best be considered in terms of a job fulfilling a need. Almost all employees have a need for money. Does the job meet monetary expectations (assuming that the employee's requirements for money are consistent with the skill required in the job and prevailing rates for similar jobs in the community)? Other aspects of job satisfaction include challenging work, a low level of boredom, good working conditions, and satisfactory relations with other employees and supervisors. Given the broad nature of job satisfaction, one could question whether an employee can ever be completely satisfied. Although it is true that most jobs have their "down sides," most employees are realistic in their expectations or they probably never would have accepted the position or would already have looked for and relocated to a different job.

Most of us think that we have achieved some goal and are considered to be good workers. It really is a "sad day" when an employee leaves work with the feeling that he or she has achieved nothing. In fact, many believe that the need for achievement is the key to motivation. The idea is to match the job level with the achievement level of the employee. Some would argue that the achievement level should be slightly higher so that the employee has to "stretch" a bit. Others would argue that this situation would only lead to despair because the employee never accomplishes a goal. There is no perfect answer because people are different; they are not cast from the same mold. It behooves the manager to study and understand employees sufficiently so that the actual achievement can be matched with the expectation and abilities of the worker insofar as possible.

Every change in the job requires a personal adjustment by the employee. A similar situation exists for the remaining employees when a new person is hired. However, the group adjustment problems are slight compared with those of a new employee. Most people like to "settle in" and learn the routine of the job and the organization. Such settling in can lead to complacency and result in a serious problem when it becomes necessary to make changes in the treatment of a patient or in a procedure to follow in making or reporting a diagnostic test. However, most people adjust well and quickly to new situations. Indeed, most people have acquired the necessary skills to cope with adjustment from life experiences.

People grow on the job. In fact, if there is no room for growth on the job, the employee is probably over-qualified or, stated another way, underemployed. Either way, this kind of situation represents a real problem for the employee as to whether he or she should look for another place of employment. This situation also presents problems for the employer, because the employee, if over-qualified, is likely to become bored and dissatisfied, which will contribute to poor performance, both in quantity and quality.

The manager should also consider not only growth on the job, but also growth of employees in the organization. Because of the degree of specialization in most health

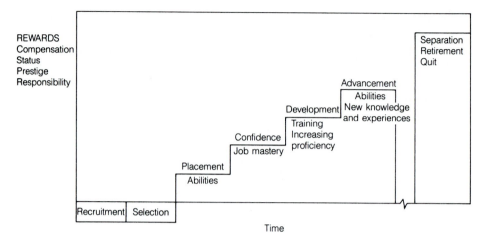

Fig. 16-2 Career development.

care organizations, this concept of growth may be difficult to achieve. However, if one considers the possibility of achieving a leadership position in a work team or a project, the objective of growth becomes more feasible.

All of us want to be recognized, especially when we know that we have accomplished a difficult task. All too often managers believe that employees will be satisfied as long as they are not being criticized. In fact, one of the authors was told by his superior that he could conclude that his work was satisfactory unless his superior "was on his back." But when the manager must be critical, it is too late for remedial action that could have prevented a problem from developing in the first place.

Many believe that unless recognition is tangible (money, a certificate, or a symbol, such as a watch), it is not very meaningful. We do not want to detract whatsoever from tangible rewards, but the manager must remember that a cheerful appearance, a friendly greeting, or a word of thanks as a statement of a job well done will go far with most employees. Most of us recognize that everyone has this need for recognition, but often managers just seem to be too busy or worried about themselves to take the time to recognize others. Of course the employee should be deserving of recognition. One should never praise an employee if the performance does not meet or exceed the standard expected.

Today most employees are interested in their own development and advancement. People are accustomed to development. Probably a source of this expectation is the school system, where students are promoted from grade level to grade level and to graduation. But graduation is considered a beginning of a new series of opportunities. Perhaps managers should recognize to a greater extent the kind of conditioning employees have received in today's society and consider how their organizations can best use these experiences in their development programs.

Fig. 16-2 represents a model for career development in a typical organization. The vertical axis represents rewards in the form of compensation, status, prestige, and/or responsibility. The horizontal axis is time, but note that the line is broken to indicate a longer time span than can be represented on one page.

The concept behind the model is that after a person is recruited and selected (hired) by the organization, he or she goes through a sequence or series of events in learning the present job, preparing for a new job, and eventually advancing to a higher level of compensation, status, prestige, and responsibility. The steps represented by the model are the following:

1. Placement according to one's abilities
2. Confidence arising from job mastery
3. Development or preparation for a higher level job through training and increasing proficiency
4. Advancement based on abilities acquired from new knowledge and experiences

The employee in an ideal organizational situation should expect to go through several series of these developmental phases. For some people in an organization, this process can be completed many times. For others who are not as capable or willing or who are unable to prepare themselves, the number of series could be few. This is not to imply, however, that all persons would be dissatisfed if they did not rise to the top levels of organizations. Whatever the situation relative to the individual, the process of development should continue until the employee retires, quits, or is separated for poor performance. One would expect that few employees would be dismissed unless the recruitment and selection processes are poorly executed. Note that recruitment and selection are placed below the horizontal axis. The rationale for this placement is that the prospective employee is not a member of the organization until he or she is hired and placed on a specific job. Also, many health care organizations are able to arrange employee schedules so that they can complete courses at a local educational institution. Some will pay tuition if the employee completes the course with a satisfactory grade.

Of more interest is the possibility of using present employees to train employees for new jobs in the organization. Some business organizations have found this practice to be significant from at least two perspectives. Present employees know more about the tasks to be performed than someone from outside the organization. Therefore the results are better. Second, there is a feeling of accomplishment on the part of the teacher, as well as the learner. Of course the teacher must have some training in teaching and be proficient in performance of the job he or she is teaching.

Among the dimensions relative to the individual are motives, learning, attitudes, abilities, and perception. Motives are discussed in Chapter 7 as part of roles of managers and employees. Motives become important in learning. In fact, the very basis of learning is motivation. If the employee does not have a positive motive toward learning, either the manager will have to develop motivation through inducements, such as a salary increase, or little learning will take place. Fortunately, most individuals do want to learn. The more complex problem is learning new job components as jobs and organizations change. This is an aspect of the implementation of strategy discussed in Chapter 6. Related to motives and learning is the dimension of attitude. Managers would like to see all employees have a positive attitude toward their job. Unfortunately, this is not always possible, and conflicts will develop. Chapter 17 explores the problem of conflict in more detail.

Not everyone has equal abilities relative to the job for which they are trained. However, probably the most difficult situation a manager can face in employee relations is when an employee wants to be promoted but doesn't have the abilities to perform the tasks of the higher level job. Sometimes training can resolve these kinds of problems, but in some cases the employee must be told that a promotion to the job in question is not possible. Sometimes the impact can be softened by suggesting an alternative or alternatives so the employee can choose.

No doubt the reader has already concluded that the dimension aspects are subjects with many ramifications and that it is impossible to do more than outline the basic dimensions. However, probably the most difficult of all the subjects is that of the perceptions the individual has about the job and the organization. For example, employees often have no standard or a very poor standard of comparison because they have had few experiences other than with the present job. In addition, they may have been given information by other employees that is not correct. The information may even come as a part of the "hazing" a new employee receives. Let it be said that the new employee is almost always highly motivated to succeed in the position. It is the responsibility of the organization and especially the employee's immediate superior to provide the necessary information and support so that the employee maintains a high degree of the original motivation and a positive perception of the job and the organization. It is the wise manager who devotes time and attention to the new employee and does not delegate the task to someone else.

The Group

In most work situations in health care organizations, employees do not work alone but perform their tasks relative to others in groups or teams. Most employees prefer to work with others although everyone would admit that working in a group environment becomes exasperating from time to time. Obviously the reason for group activity is synergy—the expectation that the group can accomplish more as a group than the individuals working alone. Thus the organization expects greater efficiency and productivity, together with an improvement in quality. It is generally believed that the cohesiveness of the group members in performing their tasks will meet and improve these organizational objectives. Hence the development of cohesiveness by the group leader or supervisor is expected. Cohesiveness is also believed to be important for the morale of the group and the job satisfaction of the individual member.

But most of us have had some sort of experience where these organizational ideals were not achieved. We recall the group setting its own standards, which were lower than management's expectations. Also, newcomers to the group were carefully coached regarding the group's norms or standards. We recall other situations where members of the group were at odds with each other and there was little cohesiveness. In some situations, cliques formed so that some members were ostracized. These and other related kinds of actions on the part of the group are frustrating to management and members alike. Because the supervision or leadership of a team or department is likely to be the first managerial responsibility of employees in health care organizations, we will devote more attention to this subject.

The first consideration is that of the dimensions of the group. Each individual member in the group has a role or specific series of tasks. We have examined the concept of role in Chapter 7 so we need only review some highlights here. First, the supervisor's superior is the key role sender, as well as is the organization itself in terms of its mission. The receipt of information often becomes confused because of the expectations of specialists, such as the physician, as well as other members of the group and the patient. The supervisor or even all members are all vulnerable to pressure of this type.

Despite the possible problem of employees taking advantage of the supervisor who believes in group participation, we still believe it is an excellent approach, especially in health care organizations. To this end we will discuss several aspects of the supervisor's managerial approach. Incidently, these comments are equally appropriate for higher level managerial positions.

There are three major components of the supervisor's job behavior: competency in (1) supervising subordinates, (2) meeting administrative responsibilities, and (3) relating with superiors and supervisors in other departments. Administrative details, such as planning activities of department members, adhering to organization policies, and exercising good judgment, can be learned, although judgment does require experience. If the relationships with subordinates are good, most likely superiors will be satisfied with the group's performance and hence the supervisor and peers will respect the group's performance and the supervisor's ability. Therefore it is appropriate to focus on the aspect of supervision of subordinates.

Supervisors should begin with giving close attention to employees and their needs. Skills needed are primarily social skills, which can best be improved through self-study of experiences and creative problem solving. Not all people are the same or motivated by the same factors. For some, money is important; others, challenging work; and still others desire the respect of their peers. Generally, the more approaches to satisfying needs of employees, the more successful the supervisor will be in creating a motivational climate. In health care organizations where there are many knowledgeable workers, one soon learns that they are difficult to control and one should avoid direct authoritarian methods insofar as possible. Peter Drucker, a well-known management author, suggests self-motivation and self-direction. This in turn suggests the development of coaching skills and counseling with employees. One must provide the environment whereby needs are satisfied and where self-motivation is most likely to develop.

The supervisor must build a team by developing a feeling of trust and concern for each other. Concern will be noted when employees begin helping one another. This is obvious when a sense of pride in the group is apparent, as well as a sense of belonging to the group. If employees are treated with dignity and respect, they will treat others the same way. This is significant relative to patient care. Helping employees stretch and reach for improvement will help the overall satisfaction of employees with the department. It should be noted, however, that there is no magic formula.

Some of the administrative responsibilities of the supervisor include the following:

1. Setting goals for the team and helping the team members set their own goals and reach them

2. Selecting and training new employees
3. Establishing the budget for the unit
4. Stopping problems through anticipation and prevention or quick solutions of them
5. Scheduling work, assigning work, establishing hours of work and vacations, and evaluating performance
6. Making work improvements
7. Giving workers say about their job, listening to their suggestions, and accepting those that are appropriate
8. Selecting employees for upgrading
9. Acting on grievances
10. Checking on adequacy of equipment and supplies
11. Communicating

The supervisor, as well as all managerial personnel, should keep in mind that management is more than the implementation of strategies and policies. Most important is the creation of a service mentality on the part of employees. Continued adherence to this philosophy will go far indeed in creating a favorable environment for members of the group and the attainment of a service orientation.

The Organization

Much has been said about the objectives of the organization. Chapter 4 defines strategic management and sets forth a model with both positive and negative aspects. The goal of health care organizations should be to continually serve the health needs of the community. Survival, profitability (for investor-owned organizations), growth, effectiveness, and adaptability, productivity, participation, and quality are all objectives setting the stage for this overall goal of service.

The dimensions of organization structure, leadership, reward systems, goals, strategies, and programs, communication, working conditions, resources, and social responsibility all relate to the internal environment of the health care organization. Each is discussed elsewhere in this book. The importance of repeating the organization aspect in this chapter is to point out that the total organization sets the stage for managing human resources. Unfortunately, some executives in organizations are of the apparent opinion that the personnel department can resolve all human resource problems. Certainly members of that department can provide advice and counsel on total organizational issues and problems, but they do not have the authority to effect changes in the total organization. On the other hand, chief executive staff members would be remiss if they did not seek the advice of functional managers in making organization decisions.

Note too that the model (Chapter 4) includes reference to the total environment, which is the subject of early chapters of this book. The impact of regulatory bodies, political factors, economic conditions, social changes, the union if there is one, changes in technology, competition, and changes in the market demand for health care services are all significant elements. In fact, these elements are the major factors in the development of the need for strategic management in health care organizations.

MANAGEMENT'S HUMAN RESOURCES TOOLS

Given the complexity and interrelationships involved in our model, one would expect that there are a large number of tools available to managers to change the effectiveness of people and the organization. In fact, they are relatively few, but all can be powerful with effective execution. The following are important:

1. Culture
2. Personnel planning
3. Selection
4. Job assignment
5. Training
6. Supervision
7. Personnel appraisal
8. Pay
9. Promotion

Some of these tools were discussed in early sections of this chapter. It is difficult to convey the real power of these tools unless one has been involved in their execution. With these two caveats in mind, let us look briefly at each of the tools. Taken together they represent an integrated approach to the management of human resources.

Culture

The significance of culture to the organization is discussed in Chapter 6, and we need not repeat this information at great length in this chapter. Although there are many definitions of culture, the simple statement by William B. Renner, vice chairman of the Aluminum Company of America, is best for our purposes: "Culture is the shared values and behavior that knit a community [health care organization] together." Culture involves people, and where large numbers of people are involved in providing personal services, their values are important factors. Kilmann[7] suggests that culture is "most controllable through norms, the unwritten rules of the game." He said (p. 212):

> A good way to assess a health services organization's culture is to ask members to write out what previously was unwritten. . . . members are willing and able to write out their norms under certain conditions: (a) that no member will be identified as having stated or suggested a particular norm (individual confidentiality), and (b) that no norm will be documented when one's superiors are present (candid openness). Furthermore, the members must have faith that the norm will not be used against them but will instead be used to benefit them as well as their organization.

When the guiding norms have been identified, the executives and personnel planners are asked to identify any new directions and then the norms associated with those new directions are determined. The difference between what is and what is desired is the culture gap. Even the identification of the gap together with the new norms often will cause change, provided of course that management is willing to change. Beyond this situation, agreements for change are usually required and new ways of behavior recognized and reinforced by managers and employees alike. Changing culture is a powerful tool but may require specialized consultants, at least initially.

Personnel Planning

It is only reasonable to expect that the personnel plan for human resources would be integrated with overall plans for the health care organization and with plans in other functional areas, such as finance and marketing. The personnel plan should be long range in nature and have some means for monitoring results.

More specifically, the development of the personnel plan has a number of components. First, it is necessary to determine current needs. Sources of information would be job surveys of the various departmental units in the health care organization, recording specific requests for replacements in vacant positions and for new positions to meet increasing demands. In addition, forecasts of short-term occupancy rates also need to be made. These sources will suggest short-term personnel needs. It is also necessary to determine the skills of the present work force in the health care organization.

As we indicated earlier in this section, there are long-term needs that must be considered. Usual data sources include anticipated turnover, absenteeism patterns, retirement, and growth expansion of various departments or the entire organization, such as the addition of a new treatment center in a hospital. Consideration also must be given to training of present employees to move into positions resulting from increases in usage or occupancy patterns. These data when analyzed result in a forecast of personnel needs. Consideration must also be given to the community growth or retrenchment patterns, as well as the availability of trained professionals. For example, many hospitals established schools of nursing to provide trained people for the hospital and the community when such educational facilities were lacking.

Although personnel planning can be a powerful tool, it is also complex in nature. Indeed, we reiterate that it requires the working together of personnel specialists, planners, and executive level representatives, as well as inputs from all departments, to achieve viable results. Also, the personnel plan should be recorded and made available to interested parties.

Selection

Selection is often referred to as staffing and includes the recruitment and the hiring decision (selection). The two general approaches to selection follow:

1. Program staffing: employment of personnel to carry out the objectives of a specific program, such as substance abuse education or a weight loss program
2. Career staffing: employment of a person with the organization on a permanent basis

Program staffing puts a person in a particular job for a specific or limited time. When the objectives of the program are met, the person will not continue as an employee or will be moved to another and usually longer-term program. A special emphasis is put on the employee's performance in reaching the objectives of the program and not necessarily on long-term commitment or pension benefits. Career selection, on the other hand, places a person in the organization with an organizational commitment whereby he or she is expected to remain with the organization for a long period.

In considering whether an organization is adequately staffed, it is first necessary to determine the criteria for such an evaluation. The most important criteria are the following:

1. Whether the goals/objectives of the organization are being met
2. The availability of resources—money, state of the labor market, hours of work, attractiveness of the organization
3. Quantity—actual number of people required by the organization
4. Quality—interpreted in its broadest sense: educational achievement, abilities, aptitudes, attitudes

All health care organizations need to be involved in recruitment activities. A good source is the organization's present employees, either through promotion or recommending a friend or acquaintance. A widely used source is the newspaper advertisement. Colleges and universities, associations, and professional recruiting companies are additional possible sources. The objective is to motivate a person to apply for a position.

Among the selection (determining which applicant to hire) tools are: the application form, interview, background/reference checks, tests, and physical examinations. The application form, interview, and physical examination are the most usual tools employed in health care organizations. The personnel specialists in the organization provide much technical assistance in the selection process.

Job Assignment

Once the decision is made to offer a job to the applicant and he or she accepts, the new employee's immediate supervisor begins the task of job assignment. Among the concerns of the supervisor are the following:

The qualifications of the new employee relative to the job
Where the person will work more effectively
Orientation of the new employee to the job, the work unit, and the organization
Determining and communicating how well the job is to be performed
The methods to be used to acknowledge accomplishments
Making the new employee feel welcome
Determining the employee's strengths and weaknesses
Ascertaining how to use the employee's strengths to overcome weaknesses
The kinds of experiences the new employee will need for improvement

It is wise for managers to remember that new employees also have questions and concerns. Some of these are the following:

What are the working conditions and work rules?
Will I get along with my supervisor and other employees?
When will I be paid? What are my benefits?
Can I really do the work that is expected of me?
How will I advance in the organization?
Will it be possible to transfer if I do not like this department?
Is there a training program? When and how can I participate?
How can I make this a place of permanent employment if I like my job and the organization?

Too often the employee's immediate supervisor forgets what it feels like to be a new employee and does not perform the orientation well, so that the new person is frustrated, dissatisfied, and decides that it is necessary to leave. It is not good for any manager to have higher-than-average unexplained turnover.

Training

Learning is a lifetime project. Managers and employees should continue to grow mentally and professionally. They need to keep up with the developments in their fields of expertise. As teachers, they must be able to impart to others the information and knowledge needed and to train others in new jobs and to help them succeed if they are promoted. An understanding of the nature of determining training needs is paramount.

Training needs may be determined by staff appraisals, informal program evaluation, surveys or inventories, job descriptions, or formal program evaluations. Attention must be directed to the individual employee. Consideration must be given to the following:

What the employee is doing now and how his or her work can be improved by a training program

Day-to-day observations of the behavioral patterns of the employee

Discussions necessary to determine the employee's needs, aspirations, motivation, and abilities

The philosophy and policies of the organization should be put in writing and made available to staff members. The immediate supervisor should clearly understand and implement the point of view of the overall organization. Such a statement creates better understanding and can provide a basis for the evaluation of training. The items receiving attention in a statement of intent include the following:

1. The overall philosophy toward training
2. A definite statement of the intent to train
3. Assignment of general responsibility for training
4. Types of training to be offered
5. Provisions for determining training needs
6. Evaluation of training programs
7. Incentives and recognition for those trained

Training should not be viewed as a fringe benefit of the organization. It should be a valuable program with measurable results. The quality of service should increase, and the benefits should be greater than the costs of training.

Supervision

Throughout this chapter references have been made to the importance of supervision. Therefore it is unnecessary to devote more attention at this point other than to reiterate that it is a critical aspect of managing human resources. Perhaps if we underscore the fact that the employee's immediate supervisor, in addition to the job, is a critical link between the employee and the organization, the significance of the position becomes more apparent. It is difficult to overvalue the impact of the supervisor in implementing human resources policies and procedures.

Personnel Appraisal

Personnel appraisal is the process of evaluating employees in an orderly and systematic manner so that both present and potential contributions of each individual are ascertained. The process involves judging people, which is a normal activity but is too often not objective.

Evaluation of employees should be made continually (an ongoing process), systematically, and orderly so that a fair assessment can be made. First impressions should not be the basis of appraisal, since they do not always represent an accurate picture of the employee. Objectives of personnel appraisal follow:

To measure the level of understanding and professional performance of all employees in the unit

To identify the relative strengths and weaknesses in both the understanding and the performance of the individual relative to the job and organization

To provide a basis for each individual to improve job performance

To assist in making decisions for professional advancement or to place the employee in a position for which he or she is better qualified

To provide a basis for pay increases

Guiding principles include the following:

1. Top executives must be sincerely interested in the personnel appraisal program.
2. Managers should thoroughly understand what the process calls for and how it operates.
3. The plan should be geared to the organization's own needs.
4. The plan should provide for effective and efficient administration.
5. In developing the plan, the judgment of all segments of the staff should be considered.
6. The plan should be thoroughly and skillfully designed, and factors that are going to be used should be valid and reliable.
7. Every appraisal program should be flexible to meet the professional employee's situation.
8. The person being evaluated should be known by the person making the evaluation.
9. Training of people making the evaluation is the best and most successful approach for improving appraisals.

Personnel appraisal began centuries ago. Emperors of the Wei Dynasty (221-265 AD) employed an "Imperial Rater," who evaluated the performance of administrators. Ignatius Loyola established a procedure for formally rating members of the Jesuit Society. Changes and adaptations have been made since these early periods. For example, Boissoneau and Edwards[8] suggest the use of multiple-rater appraisal system in hospitals. The important fact to remember is that managers then as now must make evaluations of their employees. The problem is how to make such judgments as fair and accurate as possible.

Pay

Pay is a major factor in the lives of employees. Their primary concerns are the amount of the wage or salary and the equity relations between jobs and people. The basic concerns relative to pay are the following:

Pay levels. This pertains to the relationship of the organization's pay to the community, legal minimum wages, and the pay schedules of other organizations so that pay is equitable with external criteria. Wage surveys are used by individual organizations or associations to determine how much organizations are paying. The orientation is external, and the aim is to determine a competitive pay situation.

Internal pay structure. This refers to the relationships between jobs within the organization. Basically, the jobs with higher skill, ability, and responsibility should receive higher pay. This is a generalization that can be circumvented by a community shortage of employees or by pay programs that emphasize length of service.

Method of payment. Most people in health care organizations are paid a wage per hour or a monthly (perhaps semimonthly) salary. However, there are a few incentive plans, such as for typists or word processors transcribing information to medical records. There appears to be some increasing interest in cost-savings plans in health care organizations. These plans are similar to profit-sharing plans in business except that employees share in the savings difference between budgeted costs and actual costs.

Fringe benefits. These range from pension plans to day care centers. On the average, the total expenditure for fringe benefits is about 30% (depending on what is counted in total wage costs). In most situations, the ramifications of the benefit package become so complex that specialists are employed to administer the various programs.

The objectives of compensation programs include:

1. Attracting and retaining qualified personnel
2. Equitable pay for work performed
3. Equal pay for equal work
4. Promoting a positive relationship between pay and organizational goals
5. Motivating workers to perform effectively

Health care organizations cannot function without effective employees. If the organization does not provide effective service, it will find it difficult to compete and survive. Wages, salaries, and fringe benefits are costs that must be controlled. Therefore compensation programs must be managed effectively by the organizations' chief executives and functional managers assigned to develop and administer the pay programs.

Promotion

The last tool to be discussed is that of promotion. As is true for all personnel tools, there are many ramifications to promotions. Promotions concern upward, lateral, downward, and outward movement of employees. We all like to think of promotion as upward—an increase in pay, prestige, and responsibility. Because of the specialized nature of many jobs in health, together with the licensing or certification requirements that are often based on educational attainment, mobility tends to be more limited, compared with business organizations, for example. However, there are two possibilities.

The first possibility is movement into a supervisory or managerial position. A second possibility is the development of promotion or pay levels within a given classification of employees, such as nurses. This system has worked well in organizations that employ a large number of professional people, such as engineers or researchers. The payment or prestige level is usually based on a combination of performance, in terms of innovative contributions, length of service, and leadership within the group or classification of employees.

Promotion outward or firing is usually a very difficult and traumatic experience for both the employee and manager. As a result of the increasing possibility of discrimination or unfair action charges brought against the manager and organization, it is necessary to maintain proper records regarding lack of performance, absenteeism, substance abuse or whatever. Of course the need for such documentation should also result in more unbiased performance evaluation of the employee.

Downward mobility, or demotion, does not happen often in health care organizations. However, it may occur as a result of mergers or perhaps an employee desires less responsibility or uses the lower-level position in preparation for retirement.

The management of human resources is complex. Executives should realize that it is not as much managing as providing an environment for employees to work and grow. Most organizations that are successful have something distinctive, such as gourmet meals, unique management styles, or high-tech employee centers. However, there are certain basic factors or themes that occur. Levering, Moskowitz, and Katz[9] in their studies of "100 Best Companies" conclude that going beyond good pay and strong benefits, the following themes contribute to an effective high quality organization (p. IX):

1. Make people feel that they are part of a team or, in some cases, a family.
2. Encourage open communication, informing its people of new developments and encouraging them to offer suggestions and complaints.
3. Promote from within; let people bid for jobs with outsiders.
4. Stress quality, enabling people to feel pride in their products or services they are providing.
5. Allow its employees to share in the profits [or cost savings] through profit-sharing or stock ownership [bonuses] or both.
6. Reduce the distinctions of rank between the top management and those in entry-level jobs; put everyone on a first-name basis; bar executive dining rooms and exclusive perks for high-level people.
7. Devote attention and resources to creating as pleasant a workplace environment as possible; hire good architects
8. Encourage its employees to be active in community service by giving money to organizations in which employees participate.
9. Help employees save by matching the funds they save.
10. Try not to lay off people without first making an effort to place them in other jobs either in the [organization] or elsewhere.

11. Care enough about the health of its employees to provide physical fitness centers and regular exercise and medical programs.
12. Expand the skills of its people through training programs and reimbursement of tuition for outside courses.

These authors also caution that such actions should not be looked at as "quick-fix" approaches or be considered to be manipulative. They caution that the sense of the approach should be "we are all it it together." This attitude certainly is prevalent in the best managed health care organizations we have observed.

SUMMARY

This chapter essentially has two sections. The first section centers on a discussion of a model explaining the nature of the human resource function in health care organizations. This section is primarily philosophical in nature and is designed to present an overall perspective and describe the interrelationships of the major contributing factors to managing human resources.

The nature of the job is stressed, pointing out its significance and integrating function. Performance of a job is the activity that binds a person to the organization. The role of the individual, group, and total organization in human resources management is discussed. Finally, it is stressed that organizations do not exist in a vacuum and the environment in terms of external forces impacts the human resources function of the organization.

The second part of the chapter is devoted to a discussion of the nature of the tools of personnel management. They are culture, personnel planning, selection, job assignment, training, supervision, personnel appraisal, pay, and promotion. Each of these is a complex subject. Therefore summary comments are made from the point of view of managers versus technical specialists.

The ability of all employees to perform depends to a large degree on their opportunities to learn and be trained for specific jobs. Each department or unit has its objectives and goals, as does the overall health care organization. Job-related objectives and goals must be explained to the employees so they can understand their relationship to the overall organization. Managers must give employees ample opportunity to question, to show individual interests, and to express their own ideas. Furthermore, the employee must be permitted to make mistakes, especially the new employee, and receive guidance and counseling so that the mistakes will not be repeated. Finally, chief executives must establish an overall environment conducive to enabling the employee to feel that the health care organization is indeed a good place to work.

REFERENCES

1. Schwab DP: Motivation in organizations. In Bittel LR and Ramsey JE, editors: Handbook for professional managers, New York, 1985, McGraw-Hill, Inc.
2. Schwab DP: Motivation in organizations. In Heneman HG III and Schwab DP: Perspectives in personnel/human resources management, ed 3, Homewood, Ill, 1986, Richard D. Irwin, Inc.
3. Berry L: Services marketing is different. In Lovelock C, editor: Service Marketing, Englewood Cliffs, NJ, 1984, Prentice Hall.

4. Freidson E: Profession of medicine: a study of the sociology of applied knowledge, New York, 1970, Dodd, Mead & Co, Inc.

5. Luke R and Begun JW: Industry distinctiveness: implications for strategic management in health care organizations, J Health Admin Educ 5(3):387, 1987.

6. Heneman HG III et al: Personnel/human resource management, ed 4, Homewood, Ill, 1989, Richard D. Irwin, Inc.

7. Kilmann RH: Management of corporate culture. In Fottler MD, Hernandez SR, and Joiner CL: Strategic management of human resources in health services organizations, New York, 1988, John Wiley & Sons, Inc.

8. Boissoneau RA and Edwards MR: Multiple rater performance appraisals: solutions for hospital personnel, Hospital Health Serv Admin 30(2):54, 1985.

9. Levering R, Moskowitz M, and Katz M: The 100 best companies to work for in America, Reading, Mass, 1984, Addison-Wesley Publishing Co, Inc.

17

Managing Conflict and Labor Management Relations

Much has been written about the roles of managers. In a recent article Ninomiya[1] relates his lifelong experiences in management and concludes that the following eight roles are used by managers:

Decision maker
Listener and communicator
Teacher
Peacemaker
Visionary
Self-critic
Team captain
Leader

Our concern in this chapter is the subject of conflict and the peacemaker role. This is what Ninomiya said (p. 88):

> Effective managers know how to minimize conflict. Some supervisors simply ignore its existence or become abusive and threaten to dismiss everyone involved. But managers who want their organizations to function productively face day-to-day problems directly. One way is to confront employees in order to determine the causes of the conflict. Another is to encourage work groups like quality circles; a third is to rotate jobs and reassign people. Every workplace has conflicts. Effective managers sense them early and deal with them head-on.

The first section of this chapter addresses the subject of conflict. Suggestions are made concerning the mitigation of conflict and managerial/organizational stress. The emphasis is on the individual. Conflict also exists relative to groups—the most significant group in organizations today is the union and resulting union/management conflict relationships. Relative to unions, the collective bargaining process is reviewed as are the managerial aspects of contract administration.

THE NATURE OF CONFLICT

A certain amount of conflict is beneficial to organizations. Conflict creates tension, which can lead to change and innovation. However, the potential for excessive conflict in health care organizations is readily apparent. It is doubtful that any other organization has such a wide range of specialized personnel gathered together in one work group. Managers are continually faced with eruptions of personal or departmental conflict. Periodically these conflict situations break into public view. Consumers of hospital services level charges of inefficiency and inattention to consumer expectations, and strikes by employees receive wide publicity. In addition, the unexpected and emergency nature of many of the treatments provides situations of stress that can lead to conflict. Conflict can affect the quality of patient care adversely. Although conflict may foster institutional innovation and progress, the welfare of the individual patient or resident is served more effectively by institutional stability and harmony. Moreover, conflict can adversely affect participants and the social system established in the organization and distort reality for many people. Thus we assume that controlling conflict is an important goal for health care organizations as we examine the sources and mitigators of conflict.

INDIVIDUAL CONFLICT

Conflict can be intrapersonal, that is, within individuals themselves. We sometimes hear of the employee whose standard of living exceeds the pay he or she receives from the job. If there is no change in this situation, he or she soon comes in conflict with self because needs are not met. One reaction is to strike out at supervisors and fellow employees as an escape from this dilemma. We sometimes note this type of reaction when other needs, such as security or self-esteem, are not met. An individual employee in a hospital may find the work situation frustrating because there are no promotional opportunities without more education. To complicate the situation even more, education is costly and means loss of income while it is pursued.

Individual values, capabilities, and administrative style can contribute to conflict. Influences of the formal health care organization environment, peer groups, and professional associates also affect the way a person perceives his or her role. Personality characteristics affect the degree of individual conflict and tension. Individuals who are relatively inflexible and those who are achievement-oriented are more susceptible to conflict pressures. This is usually referred to as a person/role conflict and involves a situation in which the individual feels incompatible with the role he or she occupies.

INTERPERSONAL CONFLICT

A second type of conflict relates to interpersonal factors. An individual's role in the hospital can have a major effect on the conflict to which he or she is subjected. His or her personal characteristics and experiences will determine how well a person can cope with role conflict. Role conflict involves a situation where an employee receives conflicting orders and it is difficult or impossible to comply with both directives. It is easy to imagine the role conflicts faced by physicians, nurses, and administrators. Physicians, for example, function as agents for the individual patient, their own specialty, their profession, their staff, their institution, and their community, as well as in the role of individual practitioners. The physicians' obligations to these individuals and groups and their obligations to themselves are periodically in conflict. The nurse is frequently caught between multiple lines of authority (intersender conflict). The manager often functions in a boundary role, between nurse and physician, two physicians, patient and employee, and so on.

Role ambiguity is related to role conflict. It can be defined as uncertainty about the way one's work is evaluated by superiors and about scope of responsibility, opportunities for advancement, and expectations of others for job performance. A variety of studies has demonstrated that there is frequently a wide disparity between what a superior expects of a subordinate and what the subordinate thinks is expected.[2]

Related to role ambiguity is role overload, in which the employee has too many tasks to perform. The result of this situation is likely to be "burnout," requiring a period of reduced effort for recovery, if indeed recovery is possible. In the hospital environment, role overload is certainly possible on those days when there are great demands for treatment and continuation of role overloads will result in decreased quality of care.

Thus interpersonal conflict is defined broadly to include both (1) interpersonal disagreements over substantive issues, such as policies and practices, and (2) interpersonal antagonisms, that is, the more personal and emotional differences that arise between independent human beings. Both forms are very common in the health care setting, although interpersonal antagonisms would seem to be more prevalent because by nature they deal with emotions.

Considerable basic conflict occurs if nursing status is a source of conflict. In years past, nursing was one of the few careers women could enter and attain some degree of professional prestige. Today, many more vocational opportunities are opening to women as sex discrimination continues to decline. Women can, or at least sometimes believe they can, gain greater recognition in fields such as business, government, medicine, and teaching.

Whereas in the past nurses were virtually the only professionals in the hospital besides physicians, they are now receiving increasing competition for status from a proliferation of allied health professionals, many of whom have higher standards of education, pay, and autonomy. Organizational forces present conflict for nurses. Nurses' career advancement has shifted from an individual to an organizational context in which a nurse must move through the management hierarchy to gain recognition. In this hierarchy, however, rewards are not given for professional patient care, but rather for administrative skills. The development of clinical nurse specialization is a reaction to person/role conflict.

GROUP CONFLICT

Certain internal characteristics inherent in the health care organization foster conflict. For example, interdependence, specialization, and heterogeneity of personnel, and levels of authority all appear to be related to conflict. In fact, few organizations require as many diverse skills as the hospital, which averages about three employees for each patient and uses a heterogeneous health team influenced by more than 300 different professional societies and associations.

In industry, top executives usually enjoy both formal and informal power and status. In the hospital organization, however, power and status do not appear to be centered in the same individuals. This characteristic, probably unique to hospital organization, is a basic source of administration/medical staff conflict.

Power has been defined as the maximum ability of a person or group to influence individuals or groups. Influence is understood as the degree of change that may be effected in individuals or groups. Observation tells us that a hospital administrator usually has (1) legitimacy from delegated authority for hospital affairs from the governing board; (2) effective control of funds, beds, and other resources; (3) increasing expertise, particularly as management information systems improve; (4) personal liking, and (5) the ability to coerce through the demands of outside agencies, such as the Joint Commission on the Accreditation of Healthcare Organizations. Deregulation may result in increased power for CEOs because of the objective of meeting competition. However, the unionization of hospitals, resulting in action that calls for managers to deal with employees as a group or groups rather than individually, tends to decrease the power of executives as far as unionized employees are concerned.

THE STATUS FACTOR

Changes in the status of minority groups and women have been major sources of conflict in society at large, both in the course of gaining change in status and after the changes are in place. Of course hospitals have not been insulated from the effects of those changes. In addition, nurses' status vis-à-vis physicians' adds another dimension. Physicians, too, perceive threats to their status: administrators have received the title of president, and in many hospitals the medical staff has been reorganized under the leadership of a medical director who reports to a nonphysician CEO.

CLIENT/ORGANIZATION CONFLICT

Health care organizations have not been immune from conflict with consumers; however, few empirical studies have examined this problem. Patients have very little voice in hospital matters nor, until recently, have they seemed to desire one. We suspect this is largely because of their faith in the professionals' ability to decide what is best for them. Consumer activists apparently do not see current constituencies or activities of health care organizations' governing boards as an effective voice for the client. Increasing numbers of malpractice suits against health professionals have increased concerns for patient rights, as well as insurance costs.

A lack of clearly defined community service goals may be an underlying factor in client/hospital conflict. Indeed, sometimes short-run goals become more important than the long-run mission of the organization. In some cases the means seem to justify the end. Certainly, health care organizations are susceptible to this inversion of ends and means. The hospital financial statement, for example, is one of the few easily understood measures available to trustees and managers, but it usually stresses institutional as opposed to patient goals.

Conflict or competition among hospitals is evident, especially in communities with a surplus of facilities. It can be assumed that the displacement of community service goals by institutional goals has important consequences, since what is best for a particular health care organization is not always best for the community it serves.

Regardless of the source, it is evident that a considerable degree of conflict exists in health care organizations. The problem, then, is to find ways and means to mitigate, or at least control, conflict. The next section suggests some possible approaches.

MITIGATION OF CONFLICT

In the first section of this chapter we suggested that many policies, practices, and procedures in organizations tend to reinforce conflict. In part this is a perceptual problem; however, in health care organizations, as in other organizations, there are certain traditional loyalties, and conflict may arise if these are challenged. If, for example, a situation is pushed to the point where employees must take a prounion or propatient position, this may result in person/role conflict. Such situations, and the work-flow patterns and pressures that result from emergency events, cannot be completely eliminated. However, the wise manager will try to eliminate situations that tend to reinforce conflict behavior and the resulting lack of effectiveness.

Historically, one of the earliest approaches to mitigating conflict was to eliminate the opposition. In the animal world we see many examples of the stronger eliminating the weaker in the battle. The weaker member is not necessarily killed, but is certainly excluded from the battlefield. The history of warfare gives us sufficient examples of people's use of this approach.

We do not expect to see warfare situations in health care organizations. However, the tactics of dominating or eliminating the opposition is certainly used. Opposing people are transferred or fired, departments are reorganized or eliminated, salary increases are withheld, or boycotts are conducted. Finally, we are all familiar with the "put-down" practiced by many individuals. In general, however, although the domineering approach may force conflict "underground," it is hardly a viable approach in this day and age. The recent "downsizing" practices of health care organizations, mergers, and buy outs could be considered by some as "warfare" activities whereby "we win—you lose." It is hoped that this attitude will not become rampant.

A second general approach is the development of bureaucratic rationality with its resulting policies, rules, and procedures. In this situation, the concept of authority is contained either in documents or in formal procedures. Deviations are examined in the light of policy, and a basis for eliminating the conflict-inducing practice is provided. This type of approach may seem very efficient but is probably not effective, especially as far as employees or patients are concerned. We have all been refused a request for an explanation with the comment: "It's policy!" Again, conflict is probably not mitigated.

The third general approach involves bargaining. We devote a later section of this chapter to collective bargaining. Suffice it to say at this point that it often results in a win/lose situation: "I gain what you give up." Probably if bargaining were thought of as a problem-solving process rather than in terms of balance of power, it would be more useful in settling conflict. In fact, it can be argued that bargaining cannot exist unless there is conflict.

Another approach—one in which third-party arbitration or the use of bribes or under-the-table payments is frequently seen—often results in a lose/lose situation. As the name implies, in lose/lose situations, neither party gains, or each gains only a small portion of its original goal.

WIN/WIN STRATEGIES

Basically the win/win strategies of conflict mitigation focus on the problem or issue rather than the parties involved, be they individuals, groups, or institutions. Parties focus on the problem rather than on themselves, look for facts, avoid behavior that is self-oriented, and do not trade, vote, or use averages in mitigating conflict.

Veninga[3] suggests that administrators need to develop three competencies to facilitate conflict mitigation. The first is to develop a style of conflict mitigation that is compatible with the manager and the situation. He suggests that the confrontation or win/win style is most effective. A second competency involves the need to clarify messages—the ability to understand and clarify the meaning behind words. The third competency is the utilization of the problem-solving approach. The problem-solving process involves an initial investigation, problem identification, consideration of various solutions, and implementation of evaluation.

ACTION PROGRAM FOR MITIGATION OF CONFLICT

This section discusses some approaches that can be useful in the mitigation of conflict.

Comprehensive Institutional Goal Setting

Comprehensive institutional goal setting is a formalized program to define goals and objectives explicitly. Too often goals are defined implicitly, for example, "high-quality care at low cost." Explicit goals list measures that will affect quality and costs. Often goals can be stated in terms of specially attainable objectives, an important aspect of strategic management.

As suggested in previous chapters, goal definition should begin with a study of the needs of the community the institution intends to serve to obviate displacement of goals. Medical staff members and employees, in addition to managers and trustees, should participate. Sociologists, political scientists, and economists, as well as planners and citizens of the publics served, could provide appropriate resource personnel. Explicit institutional goals aid community understanding, assist internal and external evaluation of outputs by reducing overemphasis on inputs, such as costs and facilities, help sublimate personal differences by focusing efforts on end results, and help to marshal required resources for attaining goals.

Organizational Changes, Public Relations Programs

Communications can be improved by broadening the official lines of communication with the citizens served by the institution. Policies for governing board membership might be revised to represent more appropriately the constituencies served. Or, an advisory board might be established to review expressed needs of constituencies and hospital programs to meet needs. A public relations program based on appropriate client attitude surveys might be beneficial.

Community Goal Setting

Although many communities are beginning to prepare plans for community health services, some have not effectively articulated the explicit goals and objectives that the plans are meant to serve. Appropriate comprehensive health planning by the community should stimulate institutions to focus on community needs and objectives rather than just on institutional needs and objectives. It would also be wise to discuss health needs with employers in the community.

Management by Objectives and Role Definition

Management by objectives (MBO) is the participation between the subordinate and his or her superior in setting the subordinate's goal. Through interaction and discussion, a subordinate can determine precisely what is expected, thus reducing the anxiety that results from ambiguity. MBO is designed to improve work independence in task performance while increasing accountability. However, employee development for advancement purposes is generally not a part of most MBO programs.

Role definition through job descriptions and administrative manuals can also help reduce role conflict and ambiguity. These tools are familiar to most administrators.

Creative Problem Solving

Creative problem solving uses techniques that sublimate antagonistic conflict and foster creativity (for example, stressing "choice behavior," which is an examination and a selection from the alternatives, and "problem-solving," which is a searching or idea-getting process). When choice situations are turned into problem-solving situations, participants are apt to focus on end results rather than on who is presenting or standing for what. This approach maximizes creativity and sublimates hostility, self-pity, and rigidity. Creative problem solving promotes end results in which everyone wins, rather than choice situations in which there is a winner and loser or compromises in which everyone loses.

Transactional analysis, the "I'm OK, you're OK" adult-to-adult communications approach, is another approach based on the philosophy of trying to avoid interpersonal conflict.

Constructive Confrontation

Issues of conflict tend to proliferate when there are interpersonal antagonisms between individuals. A manager can take certain steps to avoid issues that may result in open interpersonal conflict. However, the indirect effects of interpersonal antagonism will frequently persist and in the long run may be more damaging than open confrontation. Walton[4] suggests using constructive confrontation with third-party intervention, particularly by consultants from outside the institution. The components of confrontation include (1) clarifying the issues with parties, (2) expressing feelings descriptively, (3) expressing facts and fantasies, and (4) reaching resolution and agreement. It would appear, however, that third-party intervention should be used sparingly.

PARTICIPATIVE MANAGEMENT

Participative management is a philosophy of management in which hospital employees and physicians participate in a meaningful way in the administration of the hospital. It is a philosophy espoused by our type D administrator's role, by Likert,[5] and by McGregor,[6] who writes of "Theory X and Theory Y." Broad participation in authority systems minimizes major incidents of conflict, although minor incidents may be more frequent.

Management by objectives and comprehensive institutional goal setting are examples of participative management. Managers do not abdicate their responsibility; they share it. By sharing planning, coordination, control, and management information, administrators can actually gain more control over their responsibilities.

Health workers are expected to function as a team, yet they are seldom trained to do so. Because health care managers spend more time with physicians and nurses than with any other group, it would be beneficial if they had meaningful dialogues in their informative educational period. This could be arranged through seminars or research projects on subjects such as ethics, legal problems, group dynamics, or contemporary problems in health. Opportunities could be presented for informal and formal associations. Interdisciplinary study could also be arranged through the work environment.

MANAGERIAL/ORGANIZATIONAL STRESS

Managerial/organizational stress is a special aspect of conflict. Every person constantly strives to reach and maintain a level of equilibrium. As this equilibrium level is distorted by environmental and internal strains, the likelihood of physical and psychological disease increases. Each individual has his or her own level of stress tolerance. When this level is exceeded, the person "breaks down." We see the effects of breakdown in terms of increased irritability, stomach disorders including ulcers, hypertension, increased cholesterol level, and heart attacks. Although these are most likely to occur after repeated exposure to stress, stressful situations are likely to affect employees' productive ability. One of the major situations producing anxiety, fear, and stress is change. Because of the increasing numbers of changes in the health care system, stress is an increasingly important aspect of the system. In addition, many episodes involving patient care are stress producing, such as major surgeries and the intensive care unit. Another aspect of stress is upward mobility. Appelbaum[7] states (p. 10):

> All managers, as they move up the corporate ladder, are caught in a bind leading to stress: they want to lead and they want to be liked. But a leader usually has to deal with the anger and frustration of subordinates and cannot create a personality contest climate. Trying to accomplish both creates the need to suppress conflicts within subordinates and managers.

Because of the nature of the health care system, stress and burnout are unfortunate consequences. Therefore health care managers must not be unaware of the particular environmental forces, but need to take appropriate managerial actions to mitigate stress and intervene when appropriate to prevent escalation.

Stress is considered to be the basis of about 11% of employee's claims for occupational disorders and disabilities as reported by the Cincinnati-based National Institute for Occupational Safety and Health. Dr. Wilder, Professor of Psychiatry at Albert Einstein College of Medicine, New York, reports the following stress signposts[8]:

> *Absenteeism and tardiness.* When their work is not rewarding, people develop a lot of stress and they don't want to come to work.
> *Negative attitudes toward patients.* The patients are seen as "pests," and the health care worker's job becomes a burden.
> *Bickering.* Rivalries that have little to do with work issues will multiply when people are dissatisfied with their jobs.
> *Psychosomatic illness, depression and substance abuse.* These costly problems for employers can be particularly dangerous for health care workers who have access to drugs.

From a manager's point of view, Wilder sees the following as contributing to the stress experiences of health care employees: hospital bureaucracy, the growing complexity of most jobs, and more demanding but less appreciative patients.

White and Wisdom[9] report from a survey of administrators of short-term hospitals the following stressors indicated by the respondents (p. 115):

■ Time is usually an important factor in decision making.
■ More time is needed to deliberate my decisions.
■ I am caught between two or more groups with conflicting interests.
■ I have to cross functional boundaries frequently.
■ It is necessary to communicate with persons outside the hospital on matters of business.
■ Highly technical information is needed to carry out administrative duties.

The authors suggest the following implications for managers: (1) managing time and workload, (2) developing interpersonal and organizational relationships, and (3) managing technology. Along a similar vein, Quick et al.[10] suggest the following approaches to preventive stress management: goal setting and planning, time management, and social support ("By establishing a norm of information exchange and active dialogue, coordination among the hospital departments will improve, and conflict will either be reduced or worked through") (p. 109).

Let us end this discussion on conflict and stress with two quotations from *The Royal Bank Letter* of the Royal Bank of Canada[11] (p. 3):

> I have never known a man who died from overwork, but many who have died from doubt," wrote Dr. Charles Mayo of the famous Mayo Clinic. For the word "doubt" we might substitute "self-doubt." One of Sigmund Freud's most important discoveries was that fear of oneself and fear of the outside world were often related, and that they often interact. As the psychologist Abraham Maslow has pointed out, we are naturally afraid of our own impulses, memories, capacities, potentialities and destinies. We tend to transfer such apprehension to real or anticipated external events that might test our inner strength.

And on a positive action note (p. 4):

> After a lifetime of studying the medical aspects of stress, Dr. Selye concluded that the key to countering distress is to develop a philosophy of living which follows with nature's unbreakable pattern. He labelled his philosophical prescription, detailed in his 1974 book *Stress Without Distress,* "altruistic egoism." It takes account of the natural law that selfishness is central to all existence—that organisms will always look after their own interests first.

> Altruistic egoism, he wrote, is "the selfish hoarding of the good-will, respect, esteem, support and love of our neighbor [which] is the most efficient way to give vent to our pent-up energy and to create enjoyable, useful, and beautiful things." This is done by working to "earn thy neighbour's love." Anyone practicing Selye's philosophy will have little time to center on the strictly self-centered problems that cause distress.

And we might add that the person following Dr. Selye's prescription will not be the source of the conflict but will be a person involved in conflict mitigation and a peacemaker.

COLLECTIVE BARGAINING

Up to this point in the chapter, our primary attention has focused on individual conflict situations. We turn now to the group conflict environment, which is most clearly demonstrated in relationships with a union. A union need not be present for group pressures to occur. In union situations, however, there are federal laws governing the conduct of the union/management relationship.

CHANGING PHILOSOPHIES REGARDING UNIONS

A union is a group of employees who have joined together to seek common goals or objectives. The two "bread-and-butter" issues are wages and security. Other significant objectives are hours of work, working conditions, and work rules. In addition, unions are concerned about altering the arbitrary power of managers in decisions affecting layoffs, firing, changes in work assignments, and similar factors affecting the work environment.

Although the term *collective bargaining* was coined in approximately 1900 by Beatrice and Sidney Webb, the union itself is one of our early institutions. Unions of the early 1800s were local in membership and usually fraternal organizations. These unions had social aspects, but more important, they were formed to give some measure of security to the out-of-work person or to the family of a disabled or diseased worker. Until the organization of the large industrial unions (those accepting all members regardless of job or occupation affiliation) in the 1930s, most associations were craft associations.

The major reasons for the inability of unions to organize industrial workers was that such workers were highly replaceable. They did not require a long educational or training period, and our immigration laws permitted a constant supply of labor. In the 1930s, the simple principle of controlling the plant gate (employee entrance) was hit upon by employees as an effective power measure. After all, if the replacements could not enter the plant, the company could not operate. We see the same principle followed today in the form of the picket line, which makes employees and others feel self-conscious about entering even if they are not actually prevented from doing so. An understanding of the significance of the picket line is important to the hospital administration because most union members, whether employees, patients, or visitors, are reluctant to cross a picket line. Thus a small union representing a very small proportion of employees in a hospital may have a significant effect on hospital operations.

It is likely that a union in a hospital or a related health services facility will be craft in nature. That is, it will be for employees with a given skill or from a given professional group, for example, electricians, plumbers, medical technologists, or nurses.

The 1930s also saw a shift in the legal framework surrounding the rights of employees to join unions. The National Labor Relations (Wagner) Act of 1935 established the first national labor policy of protecting the rights of workers to organize and to elect their representatives for collective bargaining. The heart of the Act is contained in Section 7, which embodies the following enumeration of Findings and Policies contained in the introductory section of the Act:

> It is hereby declared to be the policy of the United States to eliminate the causes of certain substantial obstructions to the free flow of commerce and to mitigate and eliminate these obstructions when they have occurred by encouraging the practice and procedure of collective bargaining and by protecting the exercise by workers of full freedom of association, self-organization, and designation of representatives of their own choosing, for the purpose of negotiating the terms of their employment of other mutual aid or protection.

Section 7 states:

> Employees shall have the right to self-organization, to form, join, or assist labor organizations, to bargain collectively through representatives of their own choosing, and to engage in concerted activities, for the purpose of collective bargaining or other mutual aid or protection.

The Wagner Act apparently provided for hospitals to be unionized. In 1947 the Wagner Act was amended by the Labor Management Relations (Taft-Hartley) Act.

Two of the more controversial additions were: (1) the inclusion of employee or union unfair labor practices, and (2) allowing the states to prohibit union security provisions (the right-to-work concept). Of more significance to our discussion is the fact that the Taft-Hartley Act removed hospitals from coverage under the law. However, in 1974, after years of lobbying by groups such as the ANA, PL 93-360, the Nonprofit Hospital Amendments to the Labor Management Relations Act, was enacted. Some of the unique features of the amendments are as follows:

1. A 90-day notification to the other party is required to renegotiate a contract (it is 60 days for other covered organizations).
2. Unions must give a 10-day notification before a strike, to help hospitals make arrangements for patients who might be affected by the strike.
3. In the event of a threatened strike or lockout, the Director of the Federal Mediation and Conciliation Service can appoint an impartial board of inquiry.
4. Employees who hold religious conscientious objections to joining or financially supporting labor organizations may donate an amount equivalent to union dues to a charitable organization approved by the hospital and the union.

In general, these modifications are designed to protect patients from undue hardship and to meet the unique requirements of hospitals.

EMPLOYEES, MANAGERS, AND UNIONS

Barbash[12] has developed a model of industrial relations that involves managers, employees, unions, and the state or federal government. The key process in industrial relations, according to Barbash, is management efficiency or cost discipline. Management efficiency as it pertains to labor means economizing on the use of scarce labor resources. The application of efficiency techniques to labor stirs workers to organize into a protective work society (union) to pursue security. The goal of the workers is to bring about a security response to management efficiency. Barbash[12] suggests that the "acronym PEEP—standing for price, effort, equity, and power— identifies the specific interests which the work society seeks to protect and advance in pursuit of security" (p. 3). Price refers to the cost of labor; effort is mental and physical exertion; equity involves the comparison of employees with others in similar situations; and power is having a voice in developing the terms of employment.

Collective bargaining is the means by which management pursues efficiency and by which the employees (the union) maintain and attempt to advance security. In the private sector, the product market governs the parameter of the bargaining process. The union will not price its members' jobs out of the market and management will not pursue demands so that more harm comes to the company than to the union. The state or federal government, representing the general interest, participates in maintaining a balance between the parties through (1) labor market actions—full employment, education, and training; (2) labor standards—minimum wages, occupational health, and safety; (3) labor relations—laws such as the National Labor Relations Act; (4) wage-price stabilization; (5) social welfare—social security; (6) equal opportunity—Civil Rights Act of 1964; and (7) information—consumer price index.

The hospital does not fit well into the industrial mold. However, with the increased emphasis on managerial efficiency, the hospital is becoming more "industrialized." Nurses, for example, are in the transitional period between viewing their work as a calling and viewing it as a job. Many nurses groups are now unionized, a clear association with industrialization. Barbash[12] suggests that the conversion of a work group to unionism is subject to several conditions (pp. 13-14):

> The first condition is that the work group must experience a feeling of injustice which erupts into open conflict. The second condition turns on whether the management response aggravates or resolves the feeling of injustice. The third condition is whether the group commands sufficient cohesiveness and awareness to act collectively. The fourth condition is whether the union, if one comes in, can command resources and techniques to transform inchoate and informal protest into an organization. The final condition of union proneness is whether government aids or hinders unionization. Most unions lack the strength to gain recognition on their own. The state is, therefore, indispensable to unionization because managements do not recognize unions unless they are legally forced into it.

The adversary interactions between management and the union have worked well in the industrial setting. However, this adversary interaction does not work as smoothly in the health care system and hospitals. There are three primary reasons for this:

1. There is no real product market.
2. Management efficiency is limited with respect to professionals, such as physicians.
3. The greatest costs are likely to bear on those outside the immediate environment of the bargaining process—the patients.

Barbash[12] suggests that in light of this situation some sort of collaboration, problem-solving, and integrated bargaining is needed. Labor-management cooperation then could include creative leadership on the part of one group or the other (management or the union) and the utilization of third-party consultants to resolve differences. The cementing motivation in this exchange could well be the recognition of the need for high-quality of care in an otherwise "industrial" or business-like climate. Obviously such an approach to adversary interaction requires considerably more experience than we have at the present.

Why Do Employees Join Unions

A key factor in the decision to join unions is the desire for better economic and working conditions. Most people want to increase their income. Seldom do you hear of a person refusing a wage or salary increase, particularly if the wage or salary was low to begin with. Even more compelling is the *belief* that unions do help in getting increases in compensation and improved working conditions. Moreover, when the differential between lower- and upper-skill-level wages decreases, the higher-skill-level employees become more easily convinced that unionism is the answer, especially if there is a union present.

At the core of the compensation factor is the issue of perceived equity or inequity as the case may be. Unfortunately, in many situations, what might appear equitable to management is far from equitable in the eyes of the wage earner. A little wisdom and understanding and better communication on the part of the manager can go far to alleviate situations in which the inequity is perceived rather than real. However, all too often no one cares or takes the effort to make comparative studies or even to determine employee attitudes until after the union points out such problems.

Employees today are also asking for increased control over their destinies. Generally, we do not like to depend on others, nor do we want an adult/child relationship with our superiors. Immediate supervisors often appear (and often are) dictatorial, do not listen or try to understand, and enjoy their position of power. The union can bring group pressure on the recalcitrant supervisors, particularly by means of the grievance procedure.

Employees often believe that if only they could talk directly to the chief administrator, many problems could be redressed. However, it is very difficult for a lower-level employee to talk with the CEO in a bureaucratic organization. Very few people have the necessary perserverance even if such a procedure were feasible. A union changes all this. Representatives from the union bargain directly with top management. The employee believes that when management "gets the word," working conditions will improve.

Related to this is the opinion of many that no one listens or cares about what goes on in the lower levels. As long as no major problems arise, it is assumed that all goes well. In this connection, one should point out that the CEO can and does become isolated from actual operating situations. Managers reporting to the CEO may want to look good, and they are careful not to report problems that will reflect badly either on them or on the chief. Thus the communication network that on paper looks good may, in fact, be ineffective.

COLLECTIVE BARGAINING PROCESS

As unions employ more highly trained and professional organizers, as labor laws are extended, and as changes in public opinion relative to unions and collective bargaining occur, we are likely to see more unions among health care employees. Because of this, it is necessary that managers have an understanding and appreciation of the collective bargaining process. This is the objective of this section.

The first phase of the collective bargaining process involves negotiation. As Mintzberg[13] points out in his study of executives, negotiation is one of the key roles of managers. *The American Heritage Dictionary,* Second College Edition (1982) offers two definitions of "negotiate" that are useful to our discussion. To negotiate is "to confer with another in order to come to terms or reach an agreement" and "to arrange or settle by conferring or discussing: *negotiate a union contract." Note that these definitions suggest a give and take* to reach a meeting of the minds, an agreement, or a decision. Also, there is nothing to preclude an individual or one-to-one negotiation as when a CEO "negotiates" his or her salary with the governing board.

Mintzberg,[13] in a further examination of the role of the manager, suggests that the manager's work can be viewed as a programmed system. One of the programs he suggests is that of negotiation; that is, managers have several models or programs that they use in negotiating agreements either on an individual or a collective basis. For example, groups of employees do discuss through their representatives (department heads) requests (demands sometimes) for changes, such as in hours of work, working conditions, salaries, and procedures. Indeed, the entire hospital may discuss (negotiate) with the board of directors an across-the-board, cost-of-living salary increase. Managers may find themselves negotiating with the medical staff over such matters as arrangements with hospital-based specialists, emergency room service, house staff remuneration, or ethical issues. The medical staff boycotted hospitals in some instances when negotiations over issues of importance to both parties broke down. In the future this kind of action may well increase, as medical staff–hospital interdependencies become more critical.

The role of negotiation is a common one for the manager. What is new for the administrator is bargaining with a union that represents employees and has the power of work stoppage or arbitration to back up its demands. This bargaining process necessitates a programmed system that is different from the one that the manager employed before unionization.

The health care manager may be disturbed to discover that the union assumes a conflict of interest between it and management. This may indeed be an unhappy and unpleasant situation for managers who firmly believe in a team approach. Needless to say, most team concepts or Theory Y propositions accommodate unions. Despite this, if there are a number of unions involved in a hospital, there is bound to be some degree of rivalry between them. This will make the task of the manager more difficult from time to time.

What may be even more disagreeable to the manager is to find that the union wants to bypass him or her and negotiate directly with the board. Whether this procedure is ever followed, the very possibility of it may make many managers dubious about unionization.

The key issue involved, however, is recognition and certification of the union as the exclusive bargaining representative of a group of employees. With hospitals now under the National Labor Management Relations Act, the actual election and certification is administered by the National Labor Relations Board. This is done through the General Council, which is appointed by the President of the United States. Reporting to the General Council are 31 regional directors for the 31 regions of the United States. Petitions for elections are filed in the regional office, which also processes complaints and holds initial hearings on unfair labor practices as outlined by law.

Regardless of the legal climate now or in the future, negotiation from a collective bargaining point of view must begin with the recognition of a union.

The first step in the recognition procedure is a petition filed by the prospective union or group of employees within a bargaining unit. This "show of interest" petition is filed with the National Labor Relations Board and must include 30% of the employees in the bargaining unit. If the governmental agency finds the petition in order, a copy is sent to the employer. At this time, if the hospital administrator has heard nothing about unionization in his or her hospital and/or has no expert on staff, he or she would be well advised to call on a labor lawyer. The employer is also asked if he or she will submit to the election without a hearing. If a hearing is possible, an employer would be again advised to hold it so that details, such as the nature of the bargaining unit (the employees to be covered), can be determined. When everything is in order, an election is held, supervised by the governmental agency. If a majority of the employees votes in favor of the union, the union is certified as the bargaining agent for all the employees in the bargaining unit.

A second possibility in union recognition may be voluntary recognition. Here the employer agrees to recognize the union as the bargaining unit without going through the election process. This may be a proper procedure in the interest of peaceful negotiations; however, management cannot expect preferential treatment or even more favorable treatment on the part of the union. Concern should be expressed that management not be threatened or coerced into union recognition, since either possibility may not be in the best interest of patients. However, voluntary recognition does take place and is usually viewed by the union as a real accomplishment.

When the union has been recognized by the National Labor Relations Board as the bargaining agent, the collective bargaining process begins in earnest. Usually the union makes its demands through a small number of members chosen to represent it. Management representatives may make a counteroffer to the demands. At this time, the two groups of representatives sit down at the bargaining table and begin the give-and-take process of negotiation. There is no obligation by either party to agree to the demands or counteroffers made by the other. Eventually, agreement will result in a contract that will govern employee relations during the length of the contract period, usually 1 to 3 years. Both parties must "bargain in good faith." Bargaining in good faith is difficult to determine but may be described as bargaining willingly and conscientiously.

The union seeks to convince management that its demands are reasonable and realistic. Management is expected to remain cognizant of the many relationships and costs involved beyond the bargaining unit itself. When agreement is reached, the terms are reduced to writing in the form of the contract. Union members must then accept (ratify) the contract terms in its entirety by a majority vote. When the union has accepted, management signs the contract and it is officially in force. If no agreement is reached, a strike may result. Bargaining under strike conditions is a similar process but with added stress. Compulsory arbitration is an alternative in some states, as are contracts that have a no-strike clause. A strike does not really solve any problems. The stress evolved both during and after the strike requires a long period to resolve, if it is ever resolved.

It must be stressed that the first contract is usually the most difficult. There are no precedents, and everything is new including the bargaining teams themselves. Needless to say, this often leads to some hard-to-live-with clauses that must be altered during the next negotiating session.

CONTRACT ADMINISTRATION

The fact that a contract has been signed by both parties does not mean that all relationships are terminated until the next bargaining session. To the contrary, the administration phase means the day-to-day living experiences under the contract, the phase in which both parties try to make it work. It is through these experiences that the soundness of the contract is determined. Naturally, there will be some problems. For example, parts of the contract may not be clear. Also, the sincerity of the parties is tested in this period. There is no logic to spending a great deal of time negotiating a contract only to have it sabotaged by one or both parties.

Generally, management assumes the responsibility for the administration of the contract. The union observes this operation and is quick to point out significant (in the opinion of the union) deviations from the agreement.

Some parts of the contract require little administration, for example, posting seniority lists or posting of job openings. Others tend to be very difficult and require great care in administration. Items such as seniority lists, layoffs, discipline, promotions, and wage rate changes can be very controversial. Great care should be taken in the establishment of procedures, since they will set precedents for the future. Should there be items not specifically covered or not clear, it is good practice for management to sit down with the union and iron out these difficulties. Otherwise, management is usually courting a grievance.

Because department heads are likely to be most directly affected, particularly by a new contract and to a lesser extent by renegotiated contracts, it is highly recommended that these people receive training designed to acquaint them with the union and the contract. All too often department supervisors feel left out, especially if they do not understand union philosophy or the contract provisions. After all, a completely new relationship must be established in which the union is a wedge between former management/employee relationships. Needless to say, department heads are often quite unhappy with the situation.

The greater the understanding by the department head, the easier the contract administration will be. A training session can clear up many potential problems. Otherwise the informal grapevine will bring information, often faulty, to the department head. Management should be assured that the shop steward (the counterpart of the department head, who is elected by the employees to represent them at the department level) has received an in-depth briefing on the contract and on union procedures.

An important part of administration revolves around the grievance procedure. A grievance is usually considered to be any dissatisfaction or feeling of injustice regarding the work situation expressed by the employee. Some define a grievance more narrowly to refer only to those items stated in the contract. In this case, any dissatisfaction not related to the contract is not a formal grievance. This is usually likely to result in more dissatisfactions and poor employee/management relations, as well as items to be bargained for at the next negotiating session. Whatever definition management employs, it must find ways to get to the root of the problem and to acquire all salient facts and must reach a decision with respect to its (management's) position.

The grievance procedure provides a system whereby the union and management can solve their problems jointly. All too often it is viewed as a win/lose situation as opposed to some sort of win/win mutual agreement. In a grievance situation, an employee believes he has a problem. He works out a potential solution and offers it to the department head. If the department head cannot accept the employee's position or the employee is dissatisfied, the employee contacts the steward or committeeperson. If the steward thinks the employee has a "case" or feels it is politically wise for the union to support the demand even if it is weak, a written grievance is filed with the employee's supervisor and usually the personnel department.

When a satisfactory solution to the problem is reached by the department head, employee, and steward with the assistance of the personnel department, the problem or grievance is ended. If there is a clear-cut case of contract violation or if management clearly acted unfairly, the grievance is settled at this first level. When there is no settlement the grievance is passed on to the next level, which will involve administrators and the union president and perhaps a representative from the national union office. The same clinical approaches are used to see if a settlement is possible. Where there is no agreement, a third party is called in. This final step is referred to as arbitration. However, there are some alternatives, for example, calling in a fact-finder to investigate and make recommendations; these may or may not be acceptable to management and the union. Arbitration tends to be final, and both parties must abide by the decision, although it is possible in some cases, for example, discrimination, to extend the controversy through the court system. The grievance system is often a key demand of employees in the contract negotiation and is always protected by the union as a most significant right.

The role of the department head in the grievance procedure is a critical one. He must be aware of conditions in his department and understand the policies and procedures of administration. The more familiar he is with them, the more smoothly the grievance will be handled.

Grievances must be adjusted promptly and the grievance machinery (paper work and contacts) must be well understood and simple in process. Appeals from the first level (department decisions) must be readily available. Care must be taken in the selection of the arbitrator so that he understands the unique features of hospitals. Again, when administrators have questions about contract administration, especially grievances, they are well advised to seek expert advice.

An important addendum to contract administration is the interpretation of the contract in terms of changing laws. In addition, the period between the contract signing and the next negotiating session is one in which problems are brought to light, which may result in new demands by the union. Wise administrators will warn their managerial staffs to be on the lookout for problems so that these demands can be anticipated and evaluated before the stress period of actual negotiations.

The 1980s have seen a decrease in union activities in the United States. There have been a number of reasons advanced for this decline, and it has been a continuing point of study for industrial scholars. Speaking at the Fortieth Annual Meeting of the Industrial Relations Research Association in December, 1988, Arnold Weber,[14] president of Northwestern University, spoke to these changes. Among his comments are the following:

- There has been a breakdown of formal arrangements for multiemployer bargaining and stable pattern relationships including wage practices, concessionary bargaining, and downsizing practices.
- The National Labor Relations Board and the Reagan Administration have become more neutral, some would say antiunion.
- Employers have developed new tactics including the use of bankruptcy laws to undermine union agreements, contracting out work, and the sale of assets.

One of the key factors in these changes has been the role played by management. Instead of a passive actor who has little interest in the condition of the worker, management has changed its approach to industrial relations. Weber[14] suggests the following changes:

■ Labor relations within the firm has been upgraded from a passing *tactical* concern of top management to a high priority *strategic* issue" (p. 4).

■ Personnel administration, in its contemporary incarnation as Organization Behavior, has come of age as a legitimate management function. . . . it [Organizational Behavior] offers an alternative framework for a human resources strategy and sophisticated tools for the reorganization of jobs, new approaches to compensation, and elaborate systems of employee communications and participation (p. 15).

■ Management's approach to technology has been sharply different from the standard perspective of industrial relations analysts. . . . the impact of the technological change on employment and unemployment [has been refocused by management to] employee displacement and the development of programs to mitigate the consequences of this displacement (p. 15).

Lawler and Mohrman[15] call this approach the "New Management," a change in management style including the introduction of participation systems, structures, and practices, and new technologies requiring a highly skilled responsible workforce. They then comment (p. 299):

If these changes are developed and put into place without the involvement of unions it may be nearly impossible for unions to find a role. Unless their leaders take an active participative role, unions are headed for continuing decline. If this occurs, the New Management that will arise will lack workforce representation; employees will have only spotty input into the organizational changes that will determine the form and vigor of American business. In our opinion, this is not a desirable set of events.

However, Philbrick and Hass[16] question whether the "New Management" is legal according to labor relations legislation. Section 2 (5) of the National Labor Relations Act prohibits unlawful domination by management of a labor organization, which is defined as follows:

Any organization of any kind, or any agency or employee representation committee or plan, in which employees participate and which exists for the purpose, in whole or in part, of dealing with employers concerning grievances, labor disputes, wages, rates of pay, hours of employment, or conditions of work.

Although committees (quality circles as part of Quality of Work Life programs for example) and participative management are necessary and desirable, will they be found to be contrary of law where unions are involved? Probably not. However, it would be expected that as such managerial actions are challenged, such laws as pertain will be amended or rewritten if managerial actions actually result in better working conditions for employees. It should be noted that we are *not* in any way suggesting that management's real concern for employees should not be paramount in management's exercise of personnel policies and action. Our purpose is to suggest that in some cases there may be historical and even legal explanations for conflict. In the final analysis we believe that the team concept (the "New Management") is well worth the effort for employees and the organization.

It behooves health care managers to keep abreast of developments in the labor/management relations field. As an example of change, the National Labor Relations Board established rules identifying eight collective bargaining units in acute health care hospitals. The eight proposed bargaining units include those for registered nurses, physicians, all other health care professionals, technical employees, skilled employees, clerical employees, all other nonprofessional employees, and security personnel. The rules were to become effective May 22, 1989. However, on May 19, 1989, the American Hospital Association (AHA) was granted a preliminary injunction blocking implementation of the rules. According to AHA officials[17] the expected growth of bargaining units under the new rules "would affect labor costs, hospitals' largest expense comprising more than half of their budgets, by raising administrative expenditures at a time when hospitals are treating older and sicker patients who require more expensive care" (p. 1). The final outcome of these legal decisions remains to be seen at this writing. However, regardless of the final decision, this situation illustrates the need for health executives to keep informed about union and legal developments.

Will unions and collective bargaining continue to grow in the health care industry? Fennel[18] of the Service Employees International Union answers, "The question is not whether health care unionization will grow but, rather, how militant will it be" (p. 80). Fottler[19] suggests that "employee voice in the terms and conditions of employment will be the major junction of health care collective bargaining in the next decade" (p. 50). In fact, the future of unionization in the health care industry rests on the actions and resolution of conflict issues between management, employees, and the reimbursement policies, and practice stemming from public policy.

SUMMARY

Conflict in health care organizations is a complex issue. Although it deserves considerably more research, much can be done to apply available knowledge of the sources of conflict and of mitigating activities. In general, increased demands for service and attempts to diagnose and lessen conflicts will result in new policies and procedures. Among these will be research studies to identify the impact of various conflict situations. In addition, one can expect to see changes in goal setting, planning, organizational relationships, and training programs.

As a special form of conflict, we reviewed developments in collective bargaining and unionization of employees in hospitals and related health institutions.

Many labor relations experts are of the opinion that we will see more unionized employees in hospitals and probably more strife. The reasons cited for unionization include changing attitudes toward unions, which are now seen as serving white-collar as well as blue-collar workers, greater professionalism on the part of union organizers, poor personnel and business practices in some hospitals, racial complications, the increasing conviction on the part of workers that it is no longer possible to "go it alone," and the changing legal environment including the 1974 change in the National Labor Relations Act that removed the exemption of not-for-profit hospitals and eliminated the hodge-podge status of hospital labor laws. Others predict less union activity.

Whether a health care organization is actually organized, the manager is constantly engaged in negotiations. Earlier, this process was more likely to be on a one-to-one basis. To an increasing extent administrators and other management personnel now find themselves negotiating with groups of employees. This is a natural development as hospitals grow larger and more complex. It is a form of power and must be expected.

In health care organizations that are to be organized, the first bargaining session is crucial, since it sets the stage for all others. A key factor is the recognition of the union. This may be done through an election or by management agreement. Key issues to be negotiated are generally wages, hours of working, working conditions, and procedures important to the union, such as the place of seniority in promotions or layoffs. The bargaining session itself is sometimes a lesson in frustration, but eventually a contract is developed and submitted to the union membership for ratification. It is then signed by management and becomes the guide to union/management relations during the contract period.

Contract administration is of equal importance to union/management relationships. It is generally carried out by management with the union playing a watchdog role. When the contract is violated or management acts unfairly, a grievance is filed. The grievance procedure is an important right in the eyes of the union and must be recognized as such. Of vital importance is the training of department heads so that they understand union procedure and the contract provision.

There can be no question that unions in health care organizations will affect employer/employee relationships. Some hospitals with contracts will say that there has been a deterioration in the relationship; others will insist that there has been an improvement. Whatever their attitudes, thousands of managers have learned to live with unions, and many prefer the relationship to one in which employees have no outlet for their expectations, attitudes, and demands.

REFERENCES

1. Ninomiya JS: Wagon masters and lesser managers, Harvard Business Review 66(2):84, 1988.
2. Barnard C: The functions of the executive, Cambridge, Mass., 1938, Harvard University Press.
3. Veninga R: The management of disruptive conflicts, Hospital Health Serv Admin 24(2), Spring, 1979.
4. Walton RE: Interpersonal peacemaking: confrontations and third-party consultation, Reading, Mass, 1969, Addison-Wesley Publishing Co, Inc.
5. Likert R: New patterns of management, New York, 1961, McGraw-Hill, Inc.
6. McGregor D: The human side of enterprise, New York, 1960, McGraw-Hill, Inc.
7. Applebaum SH: Managerial/organizational stress: identification of factors and symptoms, Health Care Manage Rev 5(1), Winter, 1980.
8. Eaton K: Employee stress: it's a problem executives need to tackle, AHA News, American Hospital Administration 25(2):6, 1989.
9. White DB and Wisdom BL: Stress and the hospital administrator: sources and solutions, Hospital Health Serv Admin 30(5):112, 1985.
10. Quick JC et al: Health administration can be stressful . . . but not necessarily distressful, Hospital Health Serv Admin 30(5):101, 1985.
11. Stress in perspective, The Royal Bank Letter, The Royal Bank of Canada 70(1):1, 1989.
12. Barbash J: Toward an understanding of the labor problem in hospitals, Center for Advanced Study in Health Care Fiscal Management, Organization and Control, University of Wisconsin-Madison, Madison, Wis, 1979.
13. Mintzberg H: The nature of managerial work, New York, 1973, Harper and Row Publishers, Inc.

14. Weber AR: Understanding change in industrial relations: a second look, Proceedings of the fortieth annual meeting, Industrial Relations Research Association, 1988.
15. Lawler EE III and Mohrman SA: Unions and the new management, Acad Manage Exec 1(4):293, 1988.
16. Philbrick JH and Hass ME: The new management: is it legal? Acad Manage Exec 2(4):325, 1988.
17. Injunction puts bargaining-unit rules on hold, AHA News, American Hospital Association 25(22):1, 1989.
18. Fennel KS: The unionization of the health care industry: general trends and emerging issues, J Health Human Resources Admin 10(1):66, 1988.
19. Fottler MD: Health care collective bargaining: future dynamics and their impact, J Health Human Resources Admin 10(1):33, 1988.

V

FUTURE CHALLENGES, STRATEGIES, AND ETHICS

18

Managerial Performance and Ethics for Hospitals and Health Services into the Twenty-first Century

There is only one thing that we can say for certain about the hospital and health services environment into the twenty-first century and that is that it will be very different from what we are experiencing today. Not only are many changes occurring, but they appear to be accelerating. This book is symptomatic of the acceleration of change. Our first edition was published in 1976. By 1983 a revision was necessary because of many changes in the field of health services administration. However, much of the 1976 material was still relevant in 1983. Changes between 1983 and this 1990 edition have been much greater, so that an essentially new book had to be written. On the other hand, although there have been dramatic changes in the health services environment, needs for health service, objectives of the system, and recommended management practices have not changed all that much.

We predict that the environment in which health services operate will continue to change in the future at least as dramatically as it has in the past. There is no reason to expect that pressures for cost containment will abate. Indeed, they could become greater as sources of funding find rising health care costs increasingly burdensome. Concern for the underserved is not likely to diminish either; consequently, we might expect increasing pressures to facilitate access to care. Furthermore, technological advances are also likely to accelerate. Unlike manufacturing industries where technological advances increase productivity, in health services productivity usually declines with technological advances, because sicker patients are treated and more knowledgeable professional skills are needed. The clash of these forces focuses on rationing care and along with rationing, the ethical dilemmas of what might be rationed to whom. While policy makers struggle with ethical considerations, the implementation of these policies falls onto health services managers.

Standards, attitudes, and ideologies change as well. What might be unthinkable today may become quite acceptable and common in the decades ahead. One needs only to look at changes, shortening cycles of changes, and attitudes toward sex, civil rights, music, and art to predict that there will be changes in the future. Dilemmas related to bioethics will likely be another major force on health services in the future. Such issues as genetic engineering, transplantations, costs, and definitions of quality of life and life itself are current and emerging controversies.

The structure of health services can also change dramatically in response to cost, access, quality, and equity issues. As recently as the 1960s and 1970s few would have predicted the changes that occurred, or did not occur, in the 1980s. Although a universal health insurance scheme is again on the horizon at the time of this writing, it has failed to materialize a number of times in recent history. On the other hand, although it seems highly improbable today, given certain major environmental disruptions, a national health service is not impossible. More likely at the time of this writing is a privatized and "for-profitized" health system as the tax-free status of not-for-profit services is threatened by hospital management actions and governmental reactions. While health services managers struggle with current changes, it appears that the public is looking for a major overhaul of the entire system in the United States. A recent survey found that 89% said that the American health system requires significant change.[1] Given a description of the Canadian universal health insurance system, 61% of the respondents said they would prefer that system.

How might health services managers cope with accelerating changes and increasing pressures? More important, how might managers take advantage of changes to achieve higher performance and greater intrinsic rewards?

ORGANIZATION AND MANAGEMENT STRATEGIES FOR MEETING FUTURE CHALLENGES TO MANAGEMENT

Miles et al.[2] have developed a general model of the adaptive process, which they refer to as the "adaptive cycle." They indicate that there are three broad "problems of organizational adaptation": the "entrepreneurial problem," the "engineering problem," and the "administrative problem." The entrepreneurial problem relates to the identification of the organizational domain—the specific good or service and the market target or segment. The engineering problem operationalizes the management's solution to the entrepreneurial problem. This involves the proper transformation process—inputs to outputs. The administrative problem is the reduction of uncertainty within the system and rationalizing and stabilizing activities that solve problems faced by the organization in the entrepreneurial and engineering stages of strategy development and implementation.

Miles and Snow[3] suggest that organizations adapt to their environments in four different ways: as *defenders, prospectors, analyzers* and *reactors* (p. 29):

1. *Defenders* are organizations that have narrow product-market domains. Top managers in this type of organization are highly expert in their organization's limited area of operation but do not tend to search outside of their domains for new

opportunities. As a result of this narrow focus, these organizations seldom need to make major adjustments in their technology, structure, or methods of operation. Instead, they devote primary attention to improving the efficiency of their existing operations.

2. *Prospectors* are organizations which almost continually search for market opportunities, and they regularly experiment with potential responses to emerging environmental trends. Thus, these organizations often are the creators of change and uncertainty to which their competitors must respond. However, because of their strong concern for product and market innovation, these organizations usually are not completely efficient.

3. *Analyzers* are organizations which operate in two types of product-market domains, one relatively stable, the other changing. In their stable areas, these organizations operate routinely and efficiently through use of formalized structures and processes. In their more turbulent areas, top managers watch their competitors closely for new ideas, and then they rapidly adopt those which appear to be the most promising.

4. *Reactors* are organizations in which top managers frequently perceive change and uncertainty occurring in their organizational environments but are unable to respond effectively. Because this type of organization lacks a consistent strategy-structure relationship, it seldom makes adjustment of any sort until forced to do so by environmental pressures.

They applied this model to a study of 19 voluntary community hospitals in addition to other industries. The hospital industry was selected because they found it to be one of the more rapidly changing and turbulent industries in our society, thereby permitting them to study adaptations to change over a shorter time.

They found that hospital organizations adapted differently to environmental changes, as proposed in their model. *Prospector* and *analyzer* administrators engaged in more substantial organizational adjustment, they were more aware of environmental contingencies and they permitted more influence in decision making by other organizational members. They also conformed more to a "human resources" theory of management.

By the same token, Miles and Snow found that defender and reactor hospitals had implemented fewer and less substantial adjustments; they viewed organizational decision making as less contingent on the task environment; and they indicated that other organizational groups in the hospital exercised less influence on decision making. Defender and reactor managerial theories appeared to be more consistent with the "human relations" model (that is, more supportive or showing more concern for people and less concern for production).

The reader must be cautioned to recognize that a prospector or analyzer managerial adaptation is not necessarily appropriate for either the hospital or the hospital in its community at a given point in time. The CEO for example may have a "prospector" orientation, whereas the elite in the hospital who may have more influence over organizational destiny, such as the medical staff and trustees, may have a reactor orientation, leading to predictable conflicts between the two.

The health services environment is turbulent, but there are also opportunities for even greater service to health needs of individuals and communities through advancing knowledge and technology. Prospector and analyzer organization skills will be increasingly important, and managers should prospect ways to improve patient outcomes and community health. In this text we have proposed strategies for managing both the external and internal environment to achieve improved organizational outcomes.

If you were to ask most health services managers if their objectives were to efficiently improve patient outcomes and community health and to provide access to high quality care for those in need, they are likely to respond, "Of course!" Indeed, some do. However, there is substantial evidence of diversion from these objectives.

DISEASES OF HEALTH SERVICES MANAGEMENT

There are many potential diseases leading to mismanagement, such as lack of knowledge or skills, lack of attention, and ethical pitfalls. Two problems related to organizational outcomes are (1) inverting ends and means of the organization and (2) managing symbolically rather than to achieve outcomes. Diversion from objectives for improving health is evident from managers who focus almost exclusively on bottom line survival or growth of the institution. Granted survival is an issue for hard pressed services, but as proposed in Chapters 14 and 15, ensuring that the organization meets community needs is a way to gain support for organizational success, that is ultra-stability.

Inversion of ends and means is apparent in organizations where management itself becomes a primary goal. An example is when the manager's career goals become primary. For example, the young hospital administrator might spend a great deal of time in professional executive networks external to his or her unit of responsibility. This might further his or her own goals, but it can also neglect needs of the organization for which the administrator is responsible. Luthans et al.[4] in their exhaustive survey of 44 managers in a variety of industries found that the most **successful** managers did indeed spend more time in external networks; however the most **effective** managers spent more time on regular organizational management tasks. Another example of inversion of ends and means was evident in a remark made to one of us by a president of one of the larger not-for-profit hospital chains. He stated that "my philosophy is like that of one of my board members who heads a large auto battery manufacturing company. My board member says that his company is no longer in the battery business, it is in the transportation business. Similarly, we are not just in the hospital business; we are in the management business." We ask, "What happened to health?"

Symbolic management is another disease of managers. Some managers will implement the symbols of management, but for no particular purpose.[5] That is, they will do what managers are supposed to do, such as gather data on operations, hold meetings, and form committees, but as ends in themselves, not to help achieve particular goals. Schulz, Greenley, and Peterson[6] found that some of the poor-performance organizations with higher costs and lower quality had the trappings of management, such as many reports and meetings similar to the high-performance organization that had the higher quality and lower costs. However, reports and meetings in the poor performers focused on day-to-day problems rather than evaluation of progress for achieving longer-range goals for higher performance. On the other hand, the high-performing organizations focused their information systems, evaluation, and problem solving on organization service outcomes.

In Fig. 1-2 we proposed that through its influence on professional characteristics, organizational culture, and organizational performance, management can contribute in a major way to improving patient outcomes and community health. We also suggest that focus on such outcomes facilitates reaching ultrastability. However, there are times when a combination of hostile environmental forces can overwhelm even the best efforts.

MANAGEMENT OF ORGANIZATIONAL DECLINE

Although management strives for organizational ultrastability and management can influence internal and external environments to help achieve ultrastability, other forces move against it. For some health services, the environment will become too hostile and organizational resources inadequate to prevent organizational decline. Management needs to be realistic and take appropriate action, no matter how unpleasant. Rather than falling into organizational decline with rigidity, inflexibility, confusion, and disorganization, management needs to examine options for meeting challenges. If decline appears inevitable, nongrowth strategies of acquisition by others, divestiture or retrenchment in markets or services that drain the organization, or liquidation must be considered. Many hospitals and other health services have closed, and more are expected to close. Hoffman[7] argues that once a decision for "institutional euthanasia" is made, management must act decisively and compassionately. Prolonging uncertainty results in loss of many of the best people, feelings of abandonment among those left, and loss of managerial credibility, and it compromises quality of service. Strong, assertive management and visibility of managers become paramount in such periods.

Behn[8] argues that strategic management is at least as important in organization decline as in periods of organization growth. In a difficult period of organization decline, an explicit corporate strategy can provide a sense that the organization is at least partially controlling its own destiny. Retrenchment requires sacrifice. And, writes Levinson,[9] "Only a sense of purpose makes a sacrifice worthwhile." Goals are subsidiary to purposes: "When there are no purposes, people can't be for anything." Those in management need to be able to explain what it is that they and the organization's members are working for while they are retrenching.

Weiss and Filley,[10] in a management strategy for retrenchment, recommend a reexamination of the organization's mission to determine whether and how a new point of organizational resource equilibrium can be established. If survival is possible and the organization can still effectively meet its mission, a new structure must be designed that makes appropriate use of available resources. Then present members must be realigned within the new structure in a manner that minimizes helplessness and encourages commitment to a changed system. They suggest that consultants can be particularly useful to find a new point of mission equilibrium cutting through some of the organization's stakeholders' resistance to change. The goal should be, "Do more with less," not, "less with less."

Weiss and Filley note that the typical process for reorganization includes the following steps:

1. Identification of a planning group that includes experts in the work content and, very important, people whose acceptance of the new design is critical

2. Specification of criteria to be achieved in the reorganization
3. Specification of alternative structures that meet the criteria
4. Analysis of costs and benefits in feasible structures
5. Synthesis of findings into a final design

They suggest that the above process takes place most effectively if it does not deal with matters of staffing at the same time. They caution against making across-the-board cuts or resolving restaffing by means of seniority and perhaps attrition. They also concur with others that, "no news is far more dysfunctional than bad news." People with favorable or unfavorable information about the future were found to be coping, but those who had no information experienced symptoms of helplessness, low motivation, learning disabilities, and severe stress.

All organizations, just as all people, undergo periods of severe stress. The test of successful persons and organizations is how well they handle such periods. There are many prescriptions for coping; however, none that we are aware of include neglect of the people and organizations who must place trust in management.

AN ETHICAL FRAMEWORK FOR HEALTH SERVICES MANAGEMENT

What position would you take and what would you do if you were a hospital CEO and the following occurred:

- You receive a phone call at home at 10:30 PM from the head nurse in the emergency room who says, "I hate to trouble you at home with this, but I'm concerned about Dr. Delamater, who has been here the past 2 hours treating a motor accident case. Although he seemed to handle the case well, I smelled alcohol on his breath. This is the third time that he has been on call that I have smelled alcohol. I mentioned this to Alice (director of nursing) after the last time, but she said not to worry, if he doesn't show any manifestations of being intoxicated. I'm sorry to trouble you, but it just doesn't seem right." (Dr. Delamater is the president of the medical staff and is not only a very close friend, but one of the biggest producers for the hospital, and he has been the best staff president you have worked with.)
- The parents of a 12-year-old comatose girl come to you asking that life support systems be withdrawn. They have no insurance and their doctor says survival is probably hopeless, but he would not participate in ending life support because miracles do happen.
- The mayor and several leaders from a rural community approach you to set up a clinic in their town because their doctor left, they just can't recruit another one, and other towns are too far away to serve them. It is a poor town that has lost its main employer, and the patients you do get from there usually have no insurance or have Medicare or Medicaid, on which you lose money. You are already hard pressed financially from such patients.
- You have been invited to be a paid director of an HMO that negotiates contracts with your hospital for inpatient and certain ancilliary services.
- You read an article that suggests MRIs (magnetic resonant imaging) are frequently overused and that there are cheaper alternatives, such as ultrasound, for

many cases. Your hospital installed a state-of-the-art MRI a year ago, and its use has grown rapidly, assuring that it will be profitable for the hospital. Moreover, it has been a major part of this year's hospital advertising. No one has questioned its overuse. Should you?

These are just a few of the biomedical and managerial ethical issues regularly facing health services managers. Although managers have organizational support for addressing many ethical issues, "the manager is the organization's conscience." In this final section we examine some of the structural ways to approach ethical issues. We then examine them from a process viewpoint and finally from a managerial philosophy perspective. Much of this book has dealt with philosophy, as well as strategy, of management. We conclude by examining managerial philosophy for approaching ethical and managerial responsibilities.

Structural Approaches to Addressing Ethical Issues

An organization can provide a structure to help expose and solve ethical dilemmas. One way is to have a statement of organizational philosophy—an organizational credo so to speak. An organization philosophy provides a context for its mission statement and as such should preceed the mission statement. A philosophy or credo identifies moral values and principles reflecting right and wrong for the organization, or what is acceptable and unacceptable. It is a statement of the organization culture. Thomas Watson, former president of IBM, said that "the basic philosophy of an organization has far more to do with its achievements than do technological or economic resources, organizational structure, innovation and timing." Darr[11] suggests that few health services have credos or statements of philosophy.

A statement of philosophy might include how it relates to patients, staff, the community, and other health services. Statements can be very broad so as to be meaningless. For example, a philosophy to treat patients in a Christian manner is not much of a guide unless there is an elaboration of how it might be implemented. Being explicit, such as stating that the organization will be an advocate for the patient and community, has important operational implications. For example, implementing a belief of community advocacy implies that less costly alternatives to the MRI should be explored, even though it may sacrifice hospital earnings. A patient's advocate should investigate Dr. Delamater even though it could have serious repercussions for friendships and hospital earnings.

A committee structure can also facilitate solving ethical dilemmas. Most hospitals today have institutional ethics committees (IEC). They may have separate biomedical and administrative IECs or combine both functions into one. Table 18-1 presents purposes of biomedical IECs as presented in the report of the President's Commission for the Study of Ethical Problems in Medicine and Biomedical and Behavioral Research. Biomedical IECs have been euphemistically called "God squads" because they literally determine when life support is to be withdrawn. However, the role of a biomedical IEC is usually much broader, as shown in the table. Memberships on such committees are mostly interdisciplinary with physicians and clergy being most common. However, they also include nurses, attorneys, administrators, social workers,

Table 18-1 Purposes of biomedical institutional ethics committees

Purpose	Percent classifying this as a stated purpose	Percent classifying this as an actual function
Provide counsel and support to physicians	59% (10)	69% (11)
Make ethical/social policy for care of critically ill	47% (8)	38% (6)
Review ethical issues in patient care decisions	53% (9)	56% (9)
Provide counsel and support to other professionals	35% (6)	31% (5)
Determine medical prognosis	29% (5)	25% (4)
Provide counsel and support to patients and families	29% (5)	31% (5)
Make final decisions about life support	13% (3)	31% (5)
Determine continuing education needs	18% (3)	19% (3)
Other	12% (2)	12% (2)

From President's Commission for the Study of Ethical Problems in Medicine and Biomedical and Behavioral Research: Deciding to forego life-sustaining treatment: ethical, medical, and legal issues in treatment decisions, Washington, DC, 1983, US Government Printing Office.
Note: Numbers in parentheses refer to frequency of response.

and laypersons. Tertiary care hospitals with neonatal intensive care units will have a special infant care review committee for disabled infants with life-threatening problems. Administrative IECs focus on managerial ethics, such as potential conflict-of-interest issues of board members and others, allocation of resources with ethical considerations, such as service to the poor rural town noted previously, and patients' rights.

Codes of ethics, such as the Hippocratic oath and the American Medical Association, American Hospital Association (AHA), and American College of Health Care Executives (ACHE) statements, provide further guides to solving ethical problems for which there are no easy answers. Because of their relevance to management, we have replicated the ACHE and AHA statements in the boxes on pp. 313-315 and pp. 316-318.

Principles and a Process Approach for Ethical Issues

Using moral philosophies that have influenced western European culture, such as those of Immanuel Kant, John Stuart Mill, Thomas Aquinas, and John Rawls, Darr[11] suggests principles for delivery of health services.

They are *autonomy, beneficence, nonmaleficence,* and *justice. Autonomy* requires that one act toward persons in such a way that they are self-governing—able to choose and pursue a course of action. He assumes truthfulness is a part of autonomy. In other

STATEMENT ON ETHICAL CONDUCT FOR HEALTH CARE INSTITUTIONS

Introduction

Health care institutions, by virtue of their roles as health care providers, employers, and community health resources, have special responsibilities for ethical conduct and practices. The broad range of patient care, education, public health, social service, and business functions they undertake are essential to the health and well-being of their communities. In general, there is a public expectation that they will conduct themselves in an ethical manner that emphasizes a basic community service orientation.

These guidelines are intended to assist members of the American Hospital Association to better define the ethical aspects and implications of institutional policies and practices. They are offered with the understanding that individual decisions seldom reflect an absolute ethical right or wrong, and that each institution's leadership in making policy and decisions must take into account the needs and values of the institution, its medical community, and employees and those of individual patients, their families, and the community as a whole. The governing board of the institution is responsible for establishing and periodically evaluating the ethical standards that guide institutional practices. The chief executive officer is responsible for assuring that hospital medical staff, employees, and volunteers and auxilians understand and adhere to these standards and for promoting an environment sensitive to differing values and conducive to ethical behavior.

These guidelines examine the hospital's ethical responsibilities to its community and patients as well as those deriving from its organizational roles as employer and a business entity. Although some responsibilities also may be included in legal and accreditation requirements, it should be remembered that legal, accreditation and ethical obligations often overlap and that ethical obligations often extend beyond legal and accreditation requirements.

Community role

- Health care institutions should be concerned with the overall health status of their communities while continuing to provide direct patient services. This principle requires them to communicate and work with other health care and social agencies to improve the availability and provision of health promotion and education and services as well as patient care and to take a leadership role in enhancing public health and continuity of care in the community.
- Health care institutions are responsible for fair and effective use of available health care delivery resources to promote access to comprehensive and affordable health care services of high quality. This responsibility extends beyond the resources of the given institution to include efforts to coordinate with other health care providers and to share in community solutions for providing care for the medically indigent and others.

These guidelines were developed by the AHA Advisory Committee on Biomedical Ethics and approved by the Board of Trustees in November 1987. They are considerably broader than the document that they replaced, *Guidelines on Ethical Conduct and Relationships for Health Care Institutions,* which was last revised in 1981.

© 1987 by the American Hospital Association, 840 North Lake Shore Drive, Chicago, Illinois 60611. Printed in the U.S.A. All rights reserved. Catalog no. 058749. 12M-12/87-1638.

This guideline document is intended to provide general advice to the membership of the American Hospital Association. Reprinted with the permission of the American Hospital Association, Copyright 1987.

Continued.

STATEMENT ON ETHICAL CONDUCT FOR HEALTH CARE INSTITUTIONS—cont'd

Community role—cont'd

- All health care institutions have community service responsibilities which may include care for the poor and the uninsured, provision of needed services and educational programs, and various programs designed to meet the specific needs of their communities. Not-for-profit institutions, in consideration of their community service origins, Hill-Burton obligations, and tax status, should be particularly sensitive to the importance of providing and designing services for their communities.
- Health care institutions, being dependent upon community confidence and support, are accountable to the public, and therefore their communications and disclosure of information and data related to the institution should be clear, accurate, and sufficiently complete to assure that it is not misleading. Such disclosure should be aimed primarily at better public understanding of health issues, the services available to prevent and treat illness, and patients' rights and responsibilities relating to health care decisions.
- As health care institutions operate in an increasingly competitive environment, they should consider the overall welfare of their communities and their own missions in determining their activities, service mixes, and business ventures and conduct their business activities in an ethical manner.

Patient care

- Health care institutions are responsible for assuring that the care provided to each patient is appropriate and of the highest quality they are able to provide. Health care institutions should establish and follow procedures to verify the credentials of physicians and other health professionals, assess and improve quality of care, and review appropriateness of utilization.
- Health care institutions should have policies and practices that support the process of informed consent for diagnostic and therapeutic procedures and that respect and promote the patient's responsibility for decision making.
- Health care institutions are responsible for assuring confidentiality of patient-specific information. They are responsible for providing safeguards to prevent unauthorized release of information and establishing procedures for authorizing release of data.
- Health care institutions should assure that the psychological, social, spiritual, and physical needs and cultural beliefs and practices of patients and families are recognized and should promote employee and medical staff sensitivity to the full range of such needs and practices.
- Health care institutions should assure respect for and reasonable accommodation of individual religious and social beliefs and customs of patients whenever possible.
- Health care institutions should have specific mechanisms or procedures to resolve conflicting values and ethical dilemmas among patients, their families, medical staff, employees, the institution, and the community.

Organizational conduct

- The policies and practices of health care institutions should respect the professional ethical codes and responsibilities of their employees and medical staff members and be sensitive to institutional decisions that employees

---

STATEMENT ON ETHICAL CONDUCT FOR HEALTH CARE INSTITUTIONS—cont'd

Organizational conduct—cont'd

might interpret as compromising their ability to provide high-quality health care.

- Health care institutions should have policies and practices that provide for equitably administered employee policies and practices.
- To the extent possible and consistent with the ethical commitments of the institution, health care institutions should accommodate the desires of employees and medical staff to embody religious and moral values in their professional activities.
- Health care institutions should have written policies on conflict of interest that apply to officers, governing board members, physicians, and others who make or influence decisions for or on behalf of the institution. These policies should recognize that individuals in decision-making or administrative positions often have duality of interests that may not ordinarily present conflicts. However, they should provide mechanisms for identifying and addressing conflicts when they do exist.
- Health care institutions should communicate their mission, values, and priorities to their employees and volunteers, whose patient care and service activities are the most visible embodiment of the institution's ethical commitments and values.

---

words, patients should not be coerced. *Beneficence* is defined as acting with charity and kindness. *Nonmaleficence* means in effect do no harm. *Justice* is fairness.

A commission on ethical issues in health management sponsored by the Association of University Programs in Health Administration[13] proposed criteria for deriving value statements similar to Darr's, but added *confidentiality* and *utility* to the list. *Confidentiality* is guarding against the dissemination of private personal information. *Utility* is balancing the criteria in a manner that promises the best overall outcome in each situation.

Darr also proposes that a problem-solving process be used in analyzing ethical problems. This includes the following (pp 21, 22):

Analyzing separating the overall structure of a problem in a particular case into its major components

Weighing assessing strengths and weaknesses of various alternatives, which could be used in solving the problem by balancing them against one another

Justifying providing a compelling and sufficient moral reason that appeals to an established moral principle, such as "Always tell the truth." (Any such principle must be compatible with the organization's statement and the manager's personal ethic.)

Choosing selecting one or more of the available alternatives, preferably on the basis of a position that can be and has been shown to be justified

Evaluating reexamining the choices and their justifications, identifying unanswered questions, and relating decisions about one particular case to similar cases

AMERICAN COLLEGE OF HEALTHCARE EXECUTIVES CODE OF ETHICS

Preface

The Code of Ethics is administered by the Committee on Ethics, which is appointed by the Board of Governors upon nomination by the Chairman. It is composed of nine Fellows of the College, each of whom serves a three-year term on a staggered basis, with three members retiring each year.

Preamble

The purpose of the Code of Ethics of the American College of Healthcare Executives is to serve as a guide to conduct for affiliates. It contains standards of ethical behavior for healthcare executives in their professional relationships. These relationships include members of the healthcare executive's organization and other organizations. Also included are patients, clients or others served, colleagues, the community and society as a whole. The Code of Ethics also incorporates standards of ethical behavior governing personal behavior, particularly when that conduct directly relates to the role and identity of the healthcare executive.

The fundamental objectives of the healthcare management profession are to enhance overall quality of life, dignity and well-being of every individual needing healthcare services; and to create a more equitable, accessible, effective and efficient healthcare system.

Healthcare executives have an obligation to act in ways that will merit the trust, confidence and respect of healthcare professionals and the general public. To do so, healthcare executives must lead lives that embody an exemplary system of values and ethics.

In fulfilling their commitments and obligations to patients, clients or others they serve, healthcare executives function as moral agents. Since every management decision affects the health and well-being of both individuals and communities, healthcare executives must evaluate the possible outcomes of their decisions and accept full responsibility for the consequences. In organizations that deliver healthcare services, they must safeguard and foster the rights, interests and prerogatives of patients, clients or others served. The role of moral agent requires that healthcare executives speak out and take actions necessary to promote such rights, interests and prerogatives if they are threatened.

I. **The healthcare executives responsibilities to the profession of healthcare management**

The healthcare executive shall:

A. Uphold the values, ethics and mission of the healthcare management profession;

B. Conduct all personal and professional activities with honesty, integrity, respect, fairness and good faith in a manner that will reflect well upon the profession;

C. Comply with all laws in the jurisdictions in which the healthcare executive is located, or conducts professional or personal activities;

AMERICAN COLLEGE OF HEALTHCARE EXECUTIVES
CODE OF ETHICS—cont'd

I. **The healthcare executives responsibilities to the profession of healthcare management—cont'd**

D. Maintain competence and proficiency in healthcare management by implementing a personal program of assessment and continuing professional education;

E. Avoid the exploitation of professional relationships for personal gain;

F. Use this code to further the interests of the profession and not for selfish reasons;

G. Respect professional confidences;

H. Enhance the dignity and image of the healthcare management profession through positive public information programs;

I. Refrain from participating in any endorsement or publicity that demeans the credibility and dignity of the healthcare management profession; and

J. Refrain from using the College's credential or affiliation with the College to promote or endorse external commercial products or services.

II. **The healthcare executive's obligations to the organization and to patients, clients or others served**

A. *Commitments to the organization*

The healthcare executive shall:

1. Provide healthcare services consistent with available resources and assure the existence of a resource allocation process that considers ethical ramifications;

2. Conduct both competitive and cooperative activities in ways that improve community healthcare services;

3. Lead the organization in the use and improvement of standards of management and sound business practices;

4. Respect the customs and practices of patients, clients or others served, consistent with the organization's philosophy; and

5. Be truthful in all forms of professional and organizational communication and avoid information that is false, misleading, and deceptive or information that would create unreasonable expectations.

B. *Commitments to patients, clients or others served*

The healthcare executive shall:

1. Assure the existence of a process to evaluate the quality of care or service rendered;

2. Avoid exploitation of relationships for personal advantage;

3. Avoid practicing or facilitating discrimination and institute safeguards to prevent discriminatory organizational practices;

4. Assure the existence of a process that will advise patients, clients or others served of the rights, opportunities, responsibilities and risks regarding available healthcare services;

5. Provide a process which assures the autonomy and self-determination of patients, clients or others served; and

6. Assure the existence of procedures that will safeguard the confidentiality and privacy of patients, clients and others served.

Continued.

AMERICAN COLLEGE OF HEALTHCARE EXECUTIVES
CODE OF ETHICS—cont'd

II. **The healthcare executive's obligations to the organization and to patients, clients or others served—cont'd**

C. *Conflicts of interest*

A conflict of interest may be only a matter of degree, but exists when the healthcare executive:

- is in a position to benefit directly or indirectly by using authority or inside information, or allows a friend, relative or associate to benefit from such authority or information.
- uses authority or information to make a decision to intentionally affect the organization in an adverse manner.

The healthcare executive shall:

1. Conduct all personal and professional relationships in such a way that all those affected are assured that management decisions are made in the best interests of the organization and the individuals served by it;
2. Disclose to the appropriate authority any direct or indirect financial or personal interests that might pose potential conflicts of interest;
3. Accept no gifts or benefits offered with the expectation of influencing a management decision; and
4. Inform the appropriate authority and other involved parties of potential conflicts of interest related to appointments or elections to boards or committees inside or outside the healthcare executive's organization.

III. **The healthcare executive's responsibilities to community and society**

The healthcare executive shall:

A. Work to identify and meet the healthcare needs of the community;
B. Work to assure that all people have reasonable access to healthcare services;
C. Participate in public dialogue on healthcare policy issues and advocate solutions that will improve health status and promote quality healthcare;
D. Consider the short-term and long-term impact of management decisions on both the community and on society; and
E. Provide prospective consumers with adequate and accurate information, enabling them to make enlightened judgments and decisions regarding services.

IV. **The healthcare executive's duty to report violations of the code.**

An affiliate of the College who has reasonable grounds to believe that another affiliate has violated this Code has a duty to communicate such facts to the Committee on Ethics.

Although solving ethical dilemmas can be wrenching experiences, an even larger problem is identifying what might be ethical problems. We venture to guess that most breeches in ethics are the result of ignorance rather than conspiracies. It is easy to overlook conflicts of interest. For example, a person seldom recognizes a position that may be more favorable to self-emoluments than to organizational needs. We may not recognize that friendships and favors influenced decisions over what might have been more objective criteria. Moreover, one might rationalize actions, such as double-billing, by saying it makes up for my not being fully reimbursed for other expenses. An example of rationalizing practices is a large group practice on the West Coast to which one of us consulted. The purpose of the consultation was to help them improve their productivity. However, after getting into the organization, it became clear that they were earning twice as much as colleagues in other practices because of practice priorities for personal earnings. Although these were respected and otherwise honorable physicians, they gave credit to each physician for every test and procedure that physician ordered. The executive committee reviewed each physician's ordering practices. They called in physicians who did not order as much as their departmental colleagues, suggesting that those who ordered less were missing pathology and not giving "good care" to their patients. They totally ignored unnecessary utilization, greater risks to patients, and high costs to patients, yet the clinic's goal statements were clearly patient centered. No doubt the physicians believed they were practicing patient-centered medicine, even though it was obvious to us as outsiders that patients were being exploited. Needless to say, physicians were shocked when confronted with the discrepancies between their goals and practices. Rationalizing unethical and even illegal behavior is a terrible trap that one can slide into.

Fears for organizational survival is another ethical trap. For example, recent publicity concerning hospital kickbacks to physicians for each patient hospitalized not only reveals a questionable practice but is damaging to the reputation of the medical care system.[14] On the other hand, fiscal success that leads to greed, such as the example just described, or recent headlines reporting "Doctor-owned Labs Earn Lavish Profits in a Captive Market"[15] blemish the entire field and especially health services trying to implement a service mission.

PERSONAL APPROACHES TO MANAGEMENT

In the past 2 or more decades, management theory has been dominated by contigency models; that is, appropriate management practice depends on the situation. Although we do not reject contingency theories, it is important that in practice they be supported with an overriding and consistent personal values-driven leadership. Badaracco and Ellsworth[16] suggest three distinct philosophies of leadership: political leadership, directive leadership, and values-driven leadership. We do not see them as being mutually exclusive. Political economy issues are inherent in the health service system. Leaders must also be directive at times to achieve organizational goals. However, we agree with Badaracco and Ellsworth that consistency in the application of values provides a necessary integrity to management.

Considerable attention has been given in this book to roles of managers as different facets of management were presented. In conclusion, we propose that health services managers consider adopting a role of that of a "servant-leader" as described by Greenleaf.[17] The role of the health service is to serve the health needs of the people. As such, the manager is a servant to those needs. Management is not an end in itself, but a means to ensure the achievement of organizational goals. The manager is not a servant in the sense of a household servant. On the contrary, he or she must be a leader as well. That is, the manager must lead the organization to serve health needs.

Managers have to operate within conflicting public policy expectations that "implore [management] to act more and more like for-profit businesses, while chiding them for not acting enough like charitable institutions"[18] (p 3). These are not necessarily inconsistent expectations. In serving society, organizations must be efficient in meeting their needs. It is also contingent on management to ensure that society supports them to do just that. The combination of a values-driven servant and leader seems to us to be an appropriate role for health services management into the twenty-first century.

In conclusion, we state that although health services and their management are experiencing severe challenges at this time, we are optimistic about the opportunities for the future. Current challenges emphasize the importance of health services management and its responsibilities for improving care. Even though managers are crucial to effectiveness of service, they seldom receive direct gratification from grateful patients as do doctors, nurses, and other direct care personnel. Unfortunately, they are usually on the receiving end of problems and complaints. Managers have to rely on intrinsic rewards, knowing that, given all the pressures, their organization is doing better than it would have without them. In spite of increasing challenges, health services are doing better for those they serve and are doing it with better organizations. We see increasing opportunities for such intrinsic, if not extrinsic, rewards.

REFERENCES

1. AHA News, p 3, Feb 20, 1989.
2. Miles RE et al: Organization strategy, structure, and process, Acad Manage Rev 3(3):456, 1978.
3. Miles RE and Snow C: Organizational strategy, structure, and process, New York, 1978, McGraw-Hill, Inc.
4. Luthans F, Hodgetts RM, and Rosenkrantz SA: Real Managers, Cambridge, Mass, 1988, Ballinger Publishing Co.
5. Feldman MS and March JG: Information in organizations as a signal and symbol, Admin Sci Q 26:171, 1981.
6. Schulz R, Greenley J, and Peterson R: Management, cost, and quality of acute inpatient psychiatric services, Med Care 21(9):911, 1983.
7. Hoffman PB: Institutional euthanasia: little chance of turning back, AHA News, p 4, Feb 20, 1989.
8. Behn RD: Leadership for cut-back management: the use of corporate strategy, Public Admin Rev 40(6):1980.
9. Levinson H: The great jackass fallacy, Cambridge, Mass, 1973, Harvard University Press.
10. Weiss JW and Filley AC: Facilitating retrenchment in the public sector: issues and recommendations, Consultation: An International Journal 5(2):102, 1986.
11. Darr K: Ethics in health services management, New York, 1987, Praeger Publishers.
12. Watson T Jr: A business and its beliefs, McKinsey Foundation Lecture, New York, 1963, McGraw-Hill, Inc.
13. Hiller MD: Ethics and health administration ethical decision making, Association of University Programs in Health Administration, Arlington, Va, 1986.
14. Wall Street Journal, Feb 22, 1989.

15. Wall Street Journal, Mar 1, 1989.
16. Badaracco JL and Ellsworth RB: Leadership and the quest for integrity, Boston, 1989, Harvard Business School Press.
17. Greenleaf RK: Servant leadership: a journey into the nature of legitimate power and greatness, New York, 1977, Paulist Press.
18. Seay JD and Sigmond R: Community benefit standards for hospitals: perceptions and performance, Frontiers Health Services Manage 5(3):1989.

Index

Page numbers in *italics* indicate boxed material and illustrations; *t* indicates tables.

322